Introducing
Global Health

Introducing Global Health

Practice, Policy, and Solutions

Peter Muennig

Celina Su

JB JOSSEY-BASS™

A Wiley Brand

Cover design by: Michael Rutkowski
Cover images: © Kamran Khan

Jossey-Bass books and products are available through most bookstores. To contact Jossey-Bass directly call our Customer Care Department within the U.S. at 800-956-7739, outside the U.S. at 317-572-3986, or fax 317-572-4002.

Wiley publishes in a variety of print and electronic formats and by print-on-demand. Some material included with standard print versions of this book may not be included in e-books or in print-on-demand. If this book refers to media such as a CD or DVD that is not included in the version you purchased, you may download this material at http://booksupport.wiley.com. For more information about Wiley products, visit www.wiley.com.

Library of Congress Cataloging-in-Publication Data

Muennig, Peter, author.
  Introducing global health : practice, policy, and solutions / Peter Muennig, Celina Su.
–First edition.
       p. ; cm.
  Includes bibliographical references and index.
  ISBN 978-0-470-53328-4 (pbk.); ISBN 978-1-118-22041-2 (ebk.); ISBN 978-1-118-23399-3 (ebk.)
  I. Su, Celina, author.   II. Title.
  [DNLM: 1. World Health.   2. Health Policy. WA 530.1]
  RA418
  362.1–dc23

                                                         2013012274

Printed in the United States of America
FIRST EDITION
PB Printing   10 9 8 7 6 5 4 3 2 1

Contents

Figures and Tables

FIGURES

TABLES

The Authors

Peter Muennig is an associate professor at Columbia University's Mailman School of Public Health, where he teaches global health policy, comparative health systems, and health disparities to graduate students in public health. He has consulted for numerous foreign governments and has run a nongovernmental organization, the Burmese Refugee Project (which he cofounded while still a student), for twelve years. He has published more than sixty peer-reviewed articles, two books, and many chapters and government reports. He or his work has appeared in many media outlets, including the *New York Times*, the *Washington Post*, *Slate*, the *Wall Street Journal*, NPR, and CNN.

Celina Su is an associate professor of political science at the City University of New York. Her research concerns civil society, political participation, and social policy, especially health and education. Her publications include *Streetwise for Book Smarts: Grassroots Organizing and Education Reform in the Bronx* (Cornell University Press, 2009) and *Our Schools Suck: Young People Talk Back to a Segregated Nation on the Failures of Urban Education* (coauthored, New York University Press, 2009). Her honors include the Berlin Prize and the Whiting Award for Excellence in Teaching. Su was cofounding executive director of the Burmese Refugee Project from 2001 to 2013. She earned her PhD from the Massachusetts Institute of Technology.

Introduction: An Overview of Global Health

Before we can begin to think about global health, we must understand how institutions work. One example of an institution is a bank. Most of us deposit our money in banks because we are confident that we can retrieve our money whenever we want—that is, that the money will still be there and accessible to us, plus interest and minus fees. Banking is an *institution,* just as banks themselves are institutions. One way of thinking about an institution is that it constitutes the habits, cooperation, and behavior of large numbers of people. It is something that we as humans, within a given culture, collectively believe in. It is real and trustworthy because everyone believes it to be. When customers lose confidence in an institution, it collapses. This is because institutions must exist in our minds for them to exist in the real world. Just think of all the banks that went under worldwide during the Great Depression. When the banks' ability to securely hold deposits became precarious, thousands of average citizens participated in bank runs and attempted to withdraw their funds from banks and place their cash under their mattresses instead.

This, in turn, exacerbated the banks' already fragile accounting books and reserves. Many of the banking laws the United States has today stemmed from lessons learned from institutional failures in the Great Depression. The government stepped in to reinforce our collective belief in US banks and other financial institutions, or—at a bare minimum—in the existence of the currency we deposit there. If we deposit US$10,000 and the bank goes out of business, the government promises to pay that money back to us. It will do so even though this money is held only as zeros and ones on some accounting database somewhere and not in any tangible form, such as gold or even paper currency. The trust that we have in the institution, therefore, extends to a trust that we have in our nation's government.

As long as (almost) everyone in your society has agreed that a US$1 bill is worth $1 and a $100 bill is worth $100, the money has value even though each bill is nothing more than a piece of paper and ink with an actual worth of just pennies. Under this system, you can contribute a portion of your life to performing a task in a factory or office and be confident that the money you receive in return for your labors will always buy you a known quantity of avocados.

During times of financial stress, investors go to the currency that most people believe in most firmly. This way, despite the fact of the Great Recession that began in the United States in 2007, global investors bought US dollars. This sent the value of the dollar soaring relative to that of other currencies. Investors bought dollars precisely because the US dollar is widely recognized as the most reliable of the global currencies—at the time that we went to press, at least.

Institutions vary by geographical and historical context. Slavery was an accepted social institution in ancient Greece and Egypt. It was the rare leader who thought that people should not be owned by others. Now, slave-holding is rare. (The absolute number of slaves held is larger than at any point in history, but as a proportion of all inhabitants on earth, it is quite small [Bales, 2004].) Arranged marriage is a social institution in some places but not in others. Thus, institutions can be social or cultural in nature. They do not have to be inscribed into law or have official governmental agencies or buildings representing them.

Institutions—even ones that, at first glance, have little to do with an individual's health, such as banking or marriage—are important in global health in several key ways. First, much of what shapes population health around the world lies outside of the official medical and health care systems. As one example, traffic accidents are a leading cause of death globally, and whether we obey traffic light signals or drive into oncoming traffic is determined by institutions within each country. Another example might be whether we wash our hands after using the bathroom or a surgeon washes her hands before a surgery. Second, many areas around the world currently do not have rules and regulations that explicitly promote healthy institutions (such as ensuring affordable access to safe drinking water) and prohibit unhealthy ones (such as tobacco advertisements aimed at children). This is partly because some institutions that are considered "normal" in some settings—such as access to family planning, including condoms and safe early-term abortions—are quite contentious in others. Third, even if governments attempt to develop helpful public policies and programs, they may not be successful because corruption is often endemic in governmental agencies.

This last point is important for global health. Many institutions in many low-income countries—banks, currencies, or even rules of conduct, such as everyone driving in the same direction on an agreed-on side of the road—are weak. In fact, it might be argued that such nations have a low income and low life expectancy *precisely because these institutions are weak*. When the trust in institutions breaks down, it becomes difficult to build social infrastructure, such as roads and schools. That is, the banks can be too weak to lend money for such projects. If the money is acquired, institutionalized corruption may make it impossible to successfully pay for such programs. At every step of development, what we believe to be acceptable behaviors matters.

In extreme cases, when trust disappears, it becomes difficult to perform basic, everyday activities, such as buying basic goods by any means other than bartering or using some other nation's currency. At the time of this writing, the cost of a medical examination in most clinics in Zimbabwe was listed in terms of units of grain or livestock. This is because people had lost all faith in the value of their currency.

These institutions sometimes break down when individual self-interest overrides collective interest—this is sometimes known as the "tragedy of the commons." Those who take bribes in exchange for a road project break down the notion of trust that we hold in the overall institution.

In nations with weak institutions, it becomes not only almost impossible to run government programs but also to deliver aid. Thus, the real challenge of global health is to figure out how to make institutions work to get global agencies and individual countries functioning to improve health.

This is partly challenging because the needs of one region are so very different from those of another. In some areas, the average person can expect to live only thirty to forty years because there is no clean water to drink, and the soil is contaminated with feces because there are no toilets. This, in turn, leads to high rates of mortality, especially among children, because of diarrhea. At this level of health development, small sums of money can go a long way because the leading health problems—lack of clean water and sanitation—are so basic and cheap to fix. But this is precisely also the context in which institutions are often weakest. In fact, these problems still exist precisely because it is so difficult to get anything done.

In a wealthy country such as the United States, however, problems such as poor access to medical care, reliance on the automobile for transit, poverty, and weak pollution controls form the major institutional challenges. Nations solve these problems in different ways. For instance, the United Kingdom has a centralized, socialized medical system. Switzerland, however, relies on highly regulated private health insurance to get the job done. In both cases, these nations are successful because their institutions work well—there is logic to how their systems run, in a way that seems to reflect many of their respective peoples' overall wishes and reasoning.

This textbook focuses on institutions and the policies that might help government to develop them if they do not exist and to reform them if they are not running well. It covers most of the pressing global health problems from this angle. This way, the student not only will learn about the leading health concerns but also will get a sense of some of the ways that these problems might be fixed at the international, national, and local levels. As such we emphasize policies that either shape or bypass existing institutions. At a minimum, we point out the difficulties in doing so (as in our discussion of international aid in chapter 3).

At a very local level, if we wish to build latrines in a poor village, for example, we attempt to get buy-in, that is, we attempt to get the people in the village to believe in the idea of latrines. At a global level, the challenge is to build institutions that a much wider range of people (or at least their political representatives) view as legitimate and worthy of respect. Neither the World Health Organization (WHO) nor its parent, the United Nations (UN), has always instilled a great amount of trust among those who are aware of their existence.

Building stronger institutions at the global level, though, is not a straight-forward process. This is difficult when the UN has few regulatory powers to punish nation-states and agencies that flout its rules and recommendations. Then, for every recommendation that the UN or the WHO writes but is sub-sequently ignored, the institution becomes weaker, provoking a vicious cycle. The institutions fail because people believe they are ineffective, and people believe they are ineffective when they fail. Organizations work best when local branches are built around a central list of priorities and each arm is staffed with an outstanding manager who is accountable for his or her department's performance and who can operate with relative independence and agency.

Of course, getting everyone to collectively believe in a solution—to insti-tutionalize a solution—is very challenging. Moreover, "solutions" can backfire. These unintended consequences of our policies frequently arise when we fail to fully consider the systems that gave rise to the problem in the first place. Our world is a world of paradoxes. Building a healthier world requires at best an understanding that these paradoxes are possible and concurrently and sys-tematically thinking about public health at the individual, social, local, regional, national, and global levels.

WHY A PUBLIC HEALTH PERSPECTIVE?

The place you live is the single most important determinant of how healthy you will be and how long you will live. Imagine that you are a fetus nestled comfortably in your mother's womb. If you are borne in rural eastern parts of the Democratic People's Republic of the Congo (DPRC), the chances of you or your mother dying during your birth or shortly thereafter can be as high as 50 percent (WHO, 2012). Bleeding, infection, or other labor complications are easily managed by a health worker with just a few months of training, but chances are that your mother was never able to get these services (Kruk, Galea, Prescott, & Freedman, 2007). If you make it out of the womb, your chances of seeing your fifth birthday are also low, with about a 20 percent chance of death in many areas (WHO, 2012). The lack of basic sanitation or clean water means that you are almost certainly likely to be exposed to bacteria and parasites that cause diarrhea and intestinal bleeding. Poor mosquito control means that you are also likely to contract malaria. You mother probably does not make much in a day, and lacking access to basics such as fertilizers and seeds, local farmers are unlikely to produce food at a cost that your mother can afford. Weak from poor nutrition, you immune system probably cannot fight off all these infectious diseases.

Now imagine that you were born in Malmo, Sweden. Your mother not only has free access to high-quality medical care at birth, but she also started receiving care as soon as she discovered that she was pregnant, including free essential vitamins, such as folate. After a carefully monitored birth in a cutting-edge hospital, you are discharged into a comfortable home. Even if your mother is single and unemployed, the government ensures that she has access to high-quality housing, health care, and nutrition. There are no infectious agents in the water, no mosquitoes infected with malaria, and no West Nile virus. Your chances of making it to your seventieth birthday are greater than your chances of making it to age five in the DPRC (CIA, 2012; Oeppen & Vaupel, 2002; WHO, 2012).

You might see this Congo-born you as having low chances of survival because there is lousy medical care and bad economic circumstances. That is true. But where do the bad economy and lousy health system come from? Health systems cannot be repaired unless political institutions are repaired as well.

THE GLOBAL HEALTH LANDSCAPE

Water, water, everywhere,
Nor any drop to drink.

—Samuel Taylor Coleridge, "The Rime of the Ancient Mariner"

With global climate change and the human destruction of natural protective barriers, such as mangrove forests, many of the world's coastal regions are now exposed to cyclical flooding. This, in turn, leads to destruction of homes and livelihoods. Many of these areas will one day be permanently under water because global warming exacerbates the destruction already done by human habitation (Bush et al., 2011).

The Polynesian island nation of Tuvalu, for example, is only 4.5 meters above sea level, and it will be uninhabitable by 2050 (Connell, 2003). It is one of twenty-two Pacific island nations. Together, these nations contain seven million inhabitants that, altogether, contribute 0.06 percent of global greenhouse gas emissions. But these nations will suffer a disproportionate blow from the climate changes caused by their wealthy, industrialized neighbors, particularly China and the United States. On Tuvalu, the government is arranging to move the remaining ten thousand residents off the island. The residents will try to establish themselves and earn their living in countries such as New Zealand and Australia. They will disperse, and linguists expect the Tuvalu language to disappear within two or three generations (Farbotko, 2005; Hammond, 2009).

Even without forced migration and displacement, flooding greatly increases human exposure to infectious agents. Sanitation systems become useless as sewer water mixes with rising ocean waters. On a planet with an expanding population, *there is too much water.*

Perhaps an even bigger problem arises from the damming of rivers and water pollution from industry and human settlement, choking off vital international waterways. With irrigation and damming, many major rivers fail to reach the sea at all. Those that do are often contaminated with salt, lead, mercury, pesticides, trash, and sometimes with thick black toxic sludge that no one dares to test. Some inland seas and lakes, such as the Aral Sea, have become either too dry or too polluted to sustain life, let alone use as a source of drinking water (figure I.1.). This water shortage problem is only getting worse with climate change. *There is too little water* to sustain the rising human population.

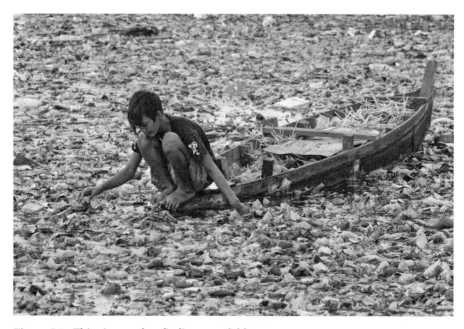

Figure I.1. This river makes finding recyclables easy.
Source: Copyright © Jurnasyanto Sukarno/epa/Corbis.

Thus, the global water supply presents major public health challenges not only because there is massive flooding resulting from human activities, but also drought resulting from human activities. There is simultaneously too much water in some places and too little water in others.

Low-income nations are growing at a blinding pace, even as they are having trouble supporting the people that are already there with their already weak institutions. Rising populations lead to poverty, pollution, human waste, and overcrowded schools. Sub-Saharan Africa and India are growing at such a rapid pace that it seems that many regions cannot overcome the **poverty trap.** A poverty trap occurs when the conditions underlying poverty prevent poor people (or their children) from escaping poverty. In this case, they cannot eat, and without adequate nutrition they cannot fight off infectious diseases or learn in school. This combination of disease and undereducation makes it almost impossible for future generations of children to escape poverty, thus perpetuating the trap from one generation to the next. *There are too many people.*

At the same time, rich nations are in stark population decline. Japan's birthrate is so low that, by 2050, the country is projected to be half the size it was in 2004 and its social services will be straining under the load of one million people over the age of one hundred. If trends continue, most European nations, along with Chile, Singapore, South Korea, and China, will soon follow in Japan's footsteps. *There are too few people.*

Thus, there are no simple trends in public health. We do not simply have too much water or too little, too many people or too few. The fundamental questions in public health are complex and sometimes paradoxical. Most common health problems are local. Nevertheless, there is emphasis on the *global,* the buzzword of the early twenty-first century. This suggests that our policies are best directed transnationally.

Economic and public health projects fail time and again because global institutions tend to take one policy and apply it to all localities as one giant bandage. Many of the misadventures of global health agencies can be attributed to thinking globally rather than locally. For instance, the International Monetary Fund (IMF) and World Bank got together in the 1980s and contributed to the **"Washington Consensus,"** or the idea that rising debt in low-income countries can be addressed only by tough love. (This is a simplification of a very complicated and controversial topic. We will keep it at this simple level for now and expand later.) The Washington Consensus probably worked in some places, but in others it probably set the development agenda back a few decades.

The **structural adjustment programs** recommended by the IMF and World Bank (described in more detail in chapter 1) essentially led to the wholesale destruction of the middle class in sub-Saharan Africa. These "programs" required cuts to nations' social programs, such as health, education, and transportation, along with other economic changes. As a result, sub-Saharan Africa has never really recovered. The WHO's recommended tuberculosis treatment program did not take into account local patterns of drug resistance (Khan, Muennig, Behta, & Zivin, 2002). People living in areas where the drugs simply did not work were treated so many times they sometimes died from the treatment rather than the disease (Farmer, 2004).

Although there is no such thing as a one-size-fits-all solution to economic, health, or education policies, global public health *does* exist. Pollution, infectious disease, people, and products all cross borders. These problems exist because countries with weak pollution controls and cheap labor tend to be more attractive for business investors. Global environmental regulations would go a long way toward solving problems like these.

A more nuanced vision of health is needed to solve "global" problems. Poverty might be viewed as a global phenomenon, but if so, it is certainly very different in Germany than it is in Sierra Leone. Despite a proliferation of doctors, journalists, and even clowns "without borders," borders most definitely exist, with very real consequences to the lives of those who live within them. Habits, laws, social networks, means of grievance, economic stability, and stratification and mobility by class, race, space, caste, and language— institutions—vary profoundly from one place to the next. So, why would a one-sized formula for development or public health fit all?

If *global* is such a misused word, why is it in the title of this book? Ultimately, policy responses to most local public health problems are shaped by and require global governance. And this brings us to the focus of this book. We ask, "How can we better understand global health problems and strengthen the institutions that fix these problems?" We do our best to teach students the status quo and then try to tear it apart. We ask whether the current set of buzzwords and policies are really going to address the problems that they set out to fix. By dissecting these problems as critically as possible, we hope that the student can come to a better understanding of the issues altering the world's health and well-being.

ABOUT THE BOOK

The remainder of the book is organized as follows. Part 1, which consists of chapters 1 and 2, focuses on the foundational basics of global health. In chapter 1, we give a brief history of major historical forces, such as industrialization and urbanization, that helped to shape the major epidemiologic trends and public health challenges we face today. Because population health outcomes are integrally tied to economic and human development overall, and because they increasingly cross national borders, we emphasize the ways in which intergovernmental institutions and international actors have struggled to implement policies that are coordinated and appropriately contextualized.

In chapter 2, we introduce China, Chile, and a state in India called Kerala as case studies. We use these case studies to explore how different types or sets of social and economic investments influence health and why. We chose these case studies because they represent different types of governance (democratic and nondemocratic) and different types of social investments (social investments versus free market). Kerala has generally been democratic in governance but has elected communists to power for long stints punctuated by more market-leaning officials. Chile has experienced periods of heavy social investment and periods of heavy social divestment. We revisit these three political economies again in chapter 7.

For instance, some nations that make effective investments in basic education might gain more in longevity than nations that invest in universal medical care. Although medical care treats disease after it has already struck, basic education provides a survival toolkit. In Darwinian terms, education can be used to optimize one's environmental niche for survival over the course of an entire life. This way, in some cases, education can prevent disease before it has a chance to strike.

Part 2, "Global Health and the Art of Policy Making," will help students to identify the major policies shaping global health and will critically investigate how these policies might be improved or better implemented. Chapter 3 presents the predominating diseases in different development contexts. Chapter 4 looks at the aid that is delivered to address this burden of disease. Chapter 5 explores health delivery systems that are charged with using this aid to reduce the burden of disease, and chapters 6 and 8 investigate how effective global governance is at helping low-income nations stem disease and to prevent it from spreading between nations (first examining social policies and then the global governance institutions that implement these policies).

Finally, part 3 takes a look at some of the issues and cutting-edge solutions in global health today. Chapter 9 discusses poverty as the central node in a complex web of public health challenges, the ways in which poverty manifests differently in low- versus high-income countries, and what antipoverty programs should look like. Chapter 10 reviews some of the ways in which poor physical environments—especially lack of sanitation, air pollution, and outer-ring development and urbanization—lead to poor population health. Chapter 11 takes a look at how our social environments, especially social forces such as race and gender, shape patterns in health outcomes. Chapter 12 examines challenges in trade liberalization, especially nations' attempts to avoid the so-called resource curse, whereby countries with great natural resources surprisingly do worse in terms of economic, social, and human development. Chapter 13 focuses on cutting-edge solutions to addressing these problems.

These include changes in how we think about the cities we live in, innovative ways of incentivizing people to be healthier, and radical reshaping of our drug and immigration policies. As these chapters suggest, students studying global health need to analyze problems and potential solutions on many levels—individual, local, national, and international—at once. Chapter 13, our conclusion, attempts to articulate emerging trends and next steps in global health by presenting several prominent case studies of social policy interventions.

As a final word, we should note that instead of listing key concepts in sequential order, we try to revisit and discuss certain complex themes throughout the book. So, for example, we do not have a chapter on **epidemiology** (the study of health problems in populations). Such a chapter would be full of information on how to calculate disease rates and how to conduct public health studies. Instead, we mention the major bits of epidemiology that you will need to understand how to study global health as they arise in real-life situations or in the news. For example, when we discuss the politics of making policies, we talk about how to understand how policies are tested and improved. It is here that the relevant concept in epidemiology is briefly discussed, and always within the context of a real-world example. In social environments and health in chapter 13, for instance, we discuss how, from the standpoint of maximizing health, girls tend to benefit more from education than boys. This is because girls respond to education by having fewer children when they become women (partly because it may allow them to make better-informed decisions and to participate in the workforce). Many researchers believe that educated women also tend to pass their knowledge on to their children and thereby help increase their children's survival to a much greater extent than educated men. But in some nations, such as India, boys tend to be favored over girls. This is true not only when it comes to deciding which children go to school but also which children get fed when food is scarce. Because food is needed for education, girls lose out twice over. In fact, in India, China, and parts of the Middle East, there are many fewer girls than boys because some families abort female fetuses and some starve or otherwise neglect female children in order to better provide for males. This has led to massive gender imbalances, a phenomenon known as *missing women.* Although this has been a long-standing problem, it may have been made worse by the advent of low-cost ultrasound machines that allow for the quick determination of fetal sex and sex-selective abortions. This section builds on discussions on the root causes of health, governance structures, and disparities in outcomes from previous chapters.

Because of the pedagogical approach we use, readers who read this book front to back will benefit most. It also helps to read it completely through because, after introducing a concept, we try to revisit it, building on it in a fresh way. This allows the mind to naturally learn and absorb the material without the need for notes. Although readers who skip around may occasionally encounter unfamiliar concepts, the good thing about our approach is that we redefine and reintroduce more-complex ideas as they arise and let less-complex ideas relax comfortably where they first appear.

One consideration that readers should keep in mind is that all works in the social sciences—be they works of journalism or academic articles—are influenced by the opinions of their authors. Researchers tend to focus on topics and concerns that they believe in or feel emotionally compelled by and—often unwittingly—interject their beliefs in a search for truth in numbers. Negative findings often go unpublished in the academic literature because editors do not see them as likely to promote their journals. Few fields are as rife for editorials presented as fact than global health. Authors of textbooks are no different. We attempt to bring you informed opinion that covers multiple sides of the issues we present.

ACKNOWLEDGMENTS

Elly Schofield, who worked hard to smooth and unify the text, and Jana Smith, who wrote most of the class exercises, were graduate students at Columbia University at the time of writing. Muhiuddin Haider, Marilyn Massey-Stokes, and Joyce Pulcini provided thoughtful and constructive comments on the complete draft manuscript. Javeria Hashmi and Amira Ahmed, then students at Brooklyn College, provided invaluable research assistance.

KEY TERMS

epidemiology	*structural adjustment*	*Washington Consensus*
poverty trap	*programs*	

REFERENCES

Bales, K. (2004). *Disposable people: New slavery in the global economy.* Berkeley: University of California Press.

Bush, K. F., Luber, G., Kotha, S. R., Dhaliwal, R. S., Kapil, V., Pascual, M., et al. (2011). Impacts of climate change on public health in India: Future research directions. *Environmental Health Perspective, 119*(6), 765–770. doi: 10.1289/ehp.1003000.

CIA. (2009). *Life expectancy at birth.* Available online at www.cia.gov/library/publications/the-world-factbook/rankorder/2102rank.html

Connell, J. (2003). Losing ground? Tuvalu, the greenhouse effect and the garbage can. *Asia Pacific Viewpoint, 44*(2), 89–107.

Farbotko, C. (2005). Tuvalu and climate change: Constructions of environmental displacement in the *Sydney Morning Herald*. *Geografiska Annaler: Series B, Human Geography*, *87*(4), 279–293.

Farmer, P. (2004). *Pathologies of power: Health, human rights, and the new war on the poor*. Berkeley: University of California Press.

Hammond, R. (2009). *Tuvalu: Islands on the frontline of climate change*. London: Panos Pictures.

Khan, K., Muennig, P., Behta, M., & Zivin, J. G. (2002). Global drug-resistance patterns and the management of latent tuberculosis infection in immigrants to the United States. *New England Journal of Medicine*, *347*(23), 1850–1859.

Kruk, M. E., Galea, S., Prescott, M., & Freedman, L. P. (2007). Health care financing and utilization of maternal health services in developing countries. *Health Policy Plan*, *22*(5), 303–310. doi: 10.1093/heapol/czm027.

Oeppen, J., & Vaupel, J. W. (2002). Broken limits to life expectancy. *Science*, *296*(5570), 1029.

WHO. (2012). *World Health Organization health statistics: Mortality*. Available online at www.who.int/healthinfo/statistics/mortality/en/index.html

Introducing
Global Health

PART ONE

The Basics of Global Health

CHAPTER 1

A Very Brief History of Global Health Policy

KEY IDEAS

- Although people often think of health as a question of genetics and biology, the field of global health is now largely focused on how policies and social environments affect mortality and morbidity.

- The past century, marked by the second Industrial Revolution and economic development around the world, has brought improvements in standards of living. But industrialization in low-income countries poses new threats to human health, primarily through environmental degradation and occupational hazards.

- Better nutrition and basic infrastructure such as sanitation systems have helped many societies to experience an epidemiologic transition, when infectious diseases drops and life expectancy greatly increases.

- Global health policies are now partly shaped by intergovernmental institutions, such as the United Nations (UN), formed after World War II. These institutions are chiefly concerned with economic development, human development, and preventing war.

- Although fiscal austerity, trade liberalization, and the so-called Washington Consensus dominated many intergovernmental policies in the 1980s and 1990s, more recent policies have begun to acknowledge that multiple models for development are needed.

HEALTH AND PUBLIC POLICY THROUGH THE TWENTIETH CENTURY

People tend to think of health as a question of genetics and biology but our environment, more than our genetic code, probably explains why our feet would pop out of the bottom of the Renaissance-era beds you see in current museums. Over time, the environments around us have tended to improve our health prospects. New medical technologies, access to better nutrition, and fewer life-threatening hazards in our everyday work lives have helped increase global life expectancy. In the healthiest nations, life expectancy has increased from fifty years in 1900 to sixty-five years in 1950 to eighty years in 2000. In a much more extreme trajectory, Cuba's life expectancy moved from nineteen in 1900 to fifty-seven in 1950 to seventy-seven in 2000 (figure 1.1).

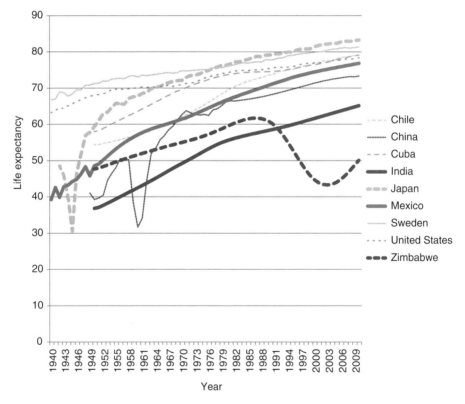

Figure 1.1. Changes in life expectancy from 1940 to 2009 in some of the nations that we discuss extensively in this book.

Source: World Health Organization. Rendered by Gapminder.org.

In this chapter, we give a very brief history of some of the key trends that have shaped population health worldwide in the past few hundred years. Along the way, we will introduce some of the key public health issues that we will dive into more deeply later in the book.

Communities and Health

In the days when humans lived as hunters and gatherers, the best hunters and the best gatherers were almost certainly more likely to get the hottest partner around. But for most people, eating and being eaten were probably bigger concerns than one's position in the social pecking order (Diamond, 1998). These two problems—finding food and fending off attacks—were greatly mitigated by agrarian lifestyles, introduced around ten to twelve thousand years ago (Denham et al., 2003). By keeping livestock, farming, and gathering in communities large enough to scare off predators, humans greatly increased their chances of survival.

When food could be had with less physically demanding work, a sedentary lifestyle and more rapid population growth occurred. But the agrarian life also introduced new problems. For one, there was a need for division of labor and governance. Thus, formal **social hierarchies** were introduced. Those at the top were more or less ensured access to food, a mate, and superior protection from threats than those at the bottom.

Europe and Asia had some native plants and animals that really benefited the people there, including barley, two types of nutritious wheat, and easily domesticated goats and sheep for wool, leather, and meat. The grains could be stored for a long time without getting spoiled, unlike fruits and vegetables. European and Asian people were also lucky because their lands were contiguous on an east-west axis so they could reach one another and trade products by land. Donkeys and horses from the Middle East also helped these people trade and flourish. With luck, work, and trade, the people of Europe, the Middle East, and Asia cultivated a wide range of nutritious crops and domesticated animals. Folks in Africa, however, mostly dealt with untamable animals, such as lions and leopards; they continued to hunt and gather (Diamond, 1998).

Of course, up until relatively recently in human history, few people died of diabetes and hypertension. It is true that the automobile, television, and high-caloric food all play big roles in the predominance of heart disease as a major cause of death (Lowry, Wechsler, Galuska, Fulton, & Kann, 2002). But few people died of these conditions mostly because more often people died of infectious disease before they had a chance to get their first heart attack. Over time, the people outside of the Americas developed immunity to common pathogens. There is even evidence that they evolved by natural selection to become resistant to some diseases, such as the plague (Galvani & Slatkin, 2003). When Europeans encountered Native Americans during the colonial period, they brought diseases, such as smallpox, that cut down half or more of some tribal populations. Likewise, endemic malaria in Africa and yellow fever in parts of Asia killed many Europeans during the colonial era (Diamond, 1998).

Thus, by transitioning from hunter and gatherer lifestyles to an agrarian and feudal life, old threats to survival were conquered but new ones were introduced. These newer problems tended to require higher-scale cooperation and collective problem solving so that health policies began to evolve not just in small villages or clans but also in nation-states and civilizations.

These problems included, among many others, the need to dispose of all the feces produced by large collections of people living together and to ensure clean water to drink. Some human civilizations were able to tackle these problems quite early on. Many ancient civilizations show evidence of complex water delivery and basic sewage disposal systems. Other nations to this day cannot effectively provide these basic provisions, even though it has never been cheaper or easier to provide them. Thus, we see that a given community or nation can unambiguously benefit from new ideas and technologies only if it can govern well enough to counteract the unintended consequences of collective living and make full use of technology so that it does more benefit than harm. (See figure 1.2.)

National Policies and Health

In the late 1700s and 1800s, manufacturing technologies and processes gave rise to the first **Industrial Revolution.** This opened the door to the development of new medicines and life-saving goods. In the first Industrial Revolution, the development of refined coal and the steam engine helped create a new manufacturing sector, one in which machines helped with agriculture and transport. New tools and machine parts were also made. This, in turn, led to new machines that greatly facilitated the production of textiles (with cotton spinning machines), paper, and glass. Water was easier to pump out of mines. The advent of the coal-powered steam engine transformed trade and migration along new rail routes, and the rediscovery of concrete (which had been lost for thirteen hundred years) reinvigorated building construction techniques.

The second half of the nineteenth century brought the second Industrial Revolution, with assembly-line production of goods, the internal combustion engine, and electricity power generation. This era is renowned for the development of steel, chemical industries, petroleum refinement, the car industry, and hydroelectric power.

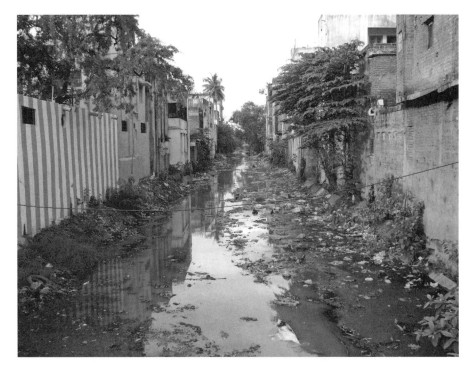

Figure 1.2. Residents live near a waterway containing raw sewage and trash in Chennai, India, 2013.

Source: Flickr/McKaySavage.

But just as agrarian living created some problems and solved others, industry posed new health threats. In England, for example, the population had remained steady at six million from 1700 to 1740. After the first Industrial Revolution, the population increased from eight million in 1800 to seventeen million in 1850 and then to almost thirty-one million in 1900 (Ashton, 1997). Yet, despite this population increase, childhood survival rates remained abysmally low. Children were not afforded the chance to receive an education, and they were expected to work. The Industrial Revolution made the hazardous conditions of child labor a lot more visible than they were before and was documented by writers such as Charles Dickens. Children died in explosions in mines; they were burned and blinded making glass. "Matchstick girls" developed phossy jaw, or phosphorous necrosis of the jaw, and then organ failure while making matches (Myers & McGlothlin, 1996). The new, dense

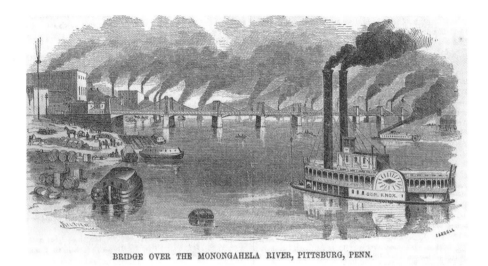

BRIDGE OVER THE MONONGAHELA RIVER, PITTSBURG, PENN.

Figure 1.3. During the Industrial Revolution, the advent of coal and steam use as energy sources became widespread.

slums brought open sewers, polluted water and air, and persistent dampness, leading to widespread cholera, tuberculosis, lung diseases, and typhoid (Ashton, 1997). (See figure 1.3.)

Technological advances such as steel provided bold new opportunities to bring consumer goods to market that have greatly improved our quality of life, but they came at an enormous cost in terms of pollution, depreciation, and global climate change. Cancers, heart disease, neurological diseases, kidney disease, and liver disease slowly began to take center stage as infectious diseases were conquered and lifelong exposure to toxic hazards increased in industrializing nations (Parkin, Bray, Ferlay, & Pisani, 2005; Trichopoulos, Li, & Hunter, 1996). Mass cultivation of food products allowed society to feed its rapidly growing population, but it also allowed the tobacco industry to greatly expand production and market its product to a broader portion of the population.

In the United States, environmental degradation culminated in a number of river fires that took large crews of firefighters to extinguish. Factories along the Cuyahoga River in northeastern Ohio had been dumping flammable solvents into the water, which were probably ignited by a passing train. When this river caught fire in 1969, the last of many fires, it called national attention to waterway pollution in the United States.

WAS THE INDUSTRIAL REVOLUTION A PUBLIC HEALTH DISASTER OR BOON?

The Industrial Revolution is widely seen as a public health disaster by academics. It brought overpopulation, overcrowding, and pollution on a wide scale. How could it be anything else? We have to keep in mind, though, that the Industrial Revolution was the forerunner of modern industrial society. Today, its pollution continues to contribute to despeciation (the loss of animal and plant species), global warming, and cancer (among many other diseases) but it has also led the way for modern industrial civilization replete with its diverse food supply, nice homes, trains, hospitals, and, yes, consumer products that improve our quality and length of life. The question is not so much whether modern industrial civilization is good or bad, but rather how we reduce the harms that it produces while maximizing the benefits.

Recently, many more severe incidents of waterway pollution in China have received notice. One factory spill effectively killed all life in the river that supplied water to Harbin, one of China's largest and most important cities. This benzene spill turned the river into a giant foamy, frothy mess. Chinese officials told citizens that they were shutting the city's water off for "routine maintenance" until the spill passed, but the water was probably still unsafe for some time (and by many accounts still is because so many pollutants were there to begin with) (see figure 1.4).

These examples highlight how industries bringing in economic growth and improvements in our standard of living also bring about new threats to human health through environmental degradation and occupational hazards. Certainly, even today, and even in wealthy countries, environmental problems cause concerns. But in wealthy countries, these problems have been mitigated with national regulatory policies that allow their citizens to enjoy the benefits of these technologies while reducing their harms (Schmidheiny, 1992). For example, cleaner, more efficient forms of power generation have meant that even coal-fired power plants produce significantly less harmful pollutants today than they did just a few decades ago. China is trying to move toward more sustainable development, too, as it becomes a wealthy country, but the potential scope of the environmental destruction in a country with 1.4 billion people adds a good deal of concern. There is hope, however, because industrialization in the modern era of green technology also offers the opportunity to leapfrog right over the problems of the industrial revolution if China is willing to make the investments (Schmidheiny, 1992).

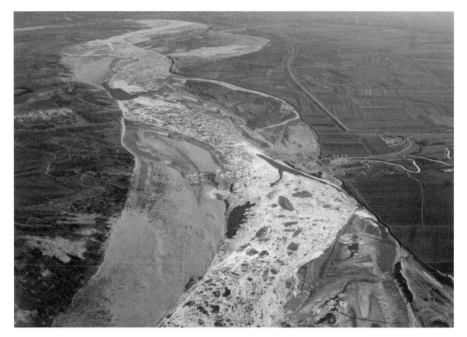

Figure 1.4. In 2005, a chemical plant explosion in Jilin, a province in northern China, led to a massive release of nitrobenzene into the Songhua River. The water became foamy and was too dangerous to drink. The spill at first was covered up by the Chinese government, but the truth was disclosed after large numbers of dead fish washed ashore in the large northern city of Harbin and residents began to panic.

Source: www.greendiary.com/polluted-water-may-affect-four-million-people-in-china .html.

Indeed, there is a global push to use technology to solve the very problems that technology creates. With advanced water and sanitation systems, it became possible to dispose of sewage and deliver clean water even in dense urban environments. These advances helped all but rid nations of diarrhea, greatly reducing the mortality of children under five (Gulland, 2012; Mayor, 2012). Greater nutrition also helped us stave off infectious disease, and mosquito control reduced malaria and other illnesses. These advances led to what is referred to as an **epidemiologic transition.** This occurs when infectious disease drops to the point that death among a nation's youth becomes a rare event and life expectancy greatly increases (Omran, 1971). This way, we see that the progress of human civilization has, in some ways and in some places, enabled the benefits of collective living—a reliable food source and protection from predators—without many of the downsides. Thanks to the epidemiologic transition, some nations enjoy average life expectancies that are approaching eighty-five years. This would have been unthinkable not too many decades ago.

EPIDEMIOLOGY IN PUBLIC HEALTH

Public health is built on a discipline called *epidemiology*, which we mentioned in the introduction to this textbook. *Epi* means *on top of* and *demos* means *people*. Thus, epidemiology could be the study of things that sit on top of people but that would be silly. In fact, it is the study of disease in populations. This disease can have roots in infectious agents, genes, the social environment, or some combination of these factors. As a result, epidemiology, and public health more generally, tends to be a science that combines genetics, biology, medicine, sociology, economics, political science, and urban studies, just to name a few disciplines.

THE AGE OF GLOBAL HEALTH POLICY

The epidemiologic transition also leads to large increases in the number of people alive on earth, posing yet another challenge. Previously we mentioned that collective living brought people together into villages and then cities and nations, opening the possibility of war.

It also brings new, improved ways of killing people. In the beginning of the twentieth century, technologies enabled us to bomb people from the air, killing dozens of people at a time from a single biplane. By the end of the twentieth century, we could do this from space (in the form of an intercontinental ballistic missile), with the potential to kill everyone on the planet. (On the bright side, there is a global treaty that keeps us from storing the weapons in space. In the event of nuclear war, this should prolong the survival of human civilization by up to six minutes.)

More people and better killing technologies, such as missiles, mean larger-scale and more violent conflicts. With dense collections of people, alliances between civilizations with similar goals were formed. This meant that wars could become quite large and devastating in scale, as evidenced by the World War I. In that conflict, new technologies such as airplanes and toxic chemicals were used as weapons with effects that were so devastating that international agreements were drafted to ban their use during warfare. These agreements gave rise to the notion of "civilized warfare," or wars in which attempts have since been made to limit the scale of human suffering brought about by new technologies, such as germs and chemicals.

Indeed, after World War I, it became apparent that global governance—the effective formation and application of policies across nations—would be needed to prevent a recurrence of the large-scale loss of life that came as a result. Still, efforts at improving governance did not go so well. The League of Nations, formed to unify the nations of the world, did not treat nations equally. Those that lost out opted out in anger. This opened the door to yet another worldwide conflict.

Well over sixty million people lost their lives during World War II, and countless others lost their homes and livelihoods as entire cities were leveled. Moreover, when atomic bombs were dropped on two cities in Japan, it became painfully clear that new technologies would outstrip our ability to regulate their use in conflict.

World War II created strong incentives for new institutions aimed at peacekeeping and financial cooperation. The leading economic powers formed new **intergovernmental institutions** such as the UN, which was primarily charged with creating dialogue between nations in order to stem wars. They also formed the International Bank for Reconstruction and Development, now commonly known as the World Bank, which was charged primarily with rebuilding Europe. Finally, the IMF was formed to reduce the chance of another global recession, one of the many major factors thought to precipitate the war.

The reconstruction of Europe was efficient and effective. Entire cities were rebuilt in just a few short years. To many, it seemed as if a new dawn of global governance had arrived. Once Europe was more or less completed, attention focused on poorer nations in Asia and Africa.

The thought was that global governance would be one of the final solutions to humankind's perpetual public health problems. With an effective global government, poor nations could be helped to develop, war could be ended with global police actions, and global institutions would thrive in a highly regulated environment. Of course, sadly, this is one innovation in the history of humankind that did not come to pass.

Still, they gave it a good shot. Following World War II, colonial powers began a slow process of decolonization. Poor nations were given autonomy and aid but were left with little by way of social institutions. As mentioned in the introduction to this book, institutions include banks, governmental agencies, and enforceable laws. Without these institutions, the nations were unable to absorb development aid. That is, there was nowhere to put the money and there were no agencies to give it to. The ability of a nation to effectively use aid is referred to as **absorptive capacity.**

If a country receives ten million dollars but has no banks to safely put the money in, the money cannot be stored. If there is no ministry of education to build local schools, the money cannot be spent. In sum, without adequate economic, social, or political structures in place to absorb and distribute the money, development will happen slowly if at all.

Let's take a look at one more example to drive the point home. To build a school, a region requires a department of education that is capable of managing construction, hiring teachers, and managing the schools. Efforts would be coordinated with other agencies, such as those of transportation, budgeting, and social work. For instance, the department of transportation would help ensure that there is a road to get to the school. These complex coordination efforts require top-down management. The president has to select ministers who are good managers. These ministers, in turn, have to select good managers in a complex array of departments below them. And these departments must all coordinate their efforts with one another.

Of course, the alternative is to conduct all of the development from the outside, bypassing local banks and ministry offices, but that means that these social institutions never get built so that the programs must be administered by whoever is giving the money. That is a pretty suboptimal situation when the management is coming from a very different cultural framework with very little local knowledge.

Further, the effectiveness of aid programs was compromised by political concerns. In the post–World War II era, the United States was by far the world's largest aid donor. But in that country, aid was framed in terms of national security. That is, it was mostly delivered as a counterbalance to the Union of Soviet Socialist Republics (USSR). By the 1950s, the Cold War was well under way. The United States and the USSR began to see some governments of poor nations run by sympathetic dictators as preferable to potentially unsympathetic democracies. Dictators were much easier to control and entice than democratic governments, after all. And neither the United States nor the USSR felt it could afford to lose any territory in the global struggle that pitted one political economy against the other. As one of many examples, in 1954, the United States overthrew a Jeffersonian-based democratic government in Guatemala in part because the government was left leaning (Schlesinger & Kinzer, 1982).

THE 1954 GUATEMALAN COUP D'ÉTAT

In 1944, Guatemala became one of the few countries in the world with a democracy styled after the United States (Schlesinger & Kinzer, 1982). This should have heralded the beginnings of a period of peace and economic prosperity that had the potential to spread to neighboring nations. In fact, despite the expected bumps along the way, Guatemala was doing quite well as an exemplar for what can be achieved when dictators are replaced with a representative government. When he was elected in 1954, President Jacobo Árbenz Guzmán responded to the demands of his still quite poor electorate with a series of programs designed to alleviate poverty. Among these was a proposal for land reform—a policy that some communist nations have employed. Although land reform takes many different shapes, it is at its essence a program that purchases or expropriates land from private or government entities and then gives the land to poor people to farm. In theory, this provides low-income families with autonomy, a means to feed themselves, and a strong economic asset that can be passed down from one generation to the next. Such an asset can also be used as collateral for loans to improve farming operations, to build a house, or to start another business. With a little prodding by a major corporation that held most of the land that was to be expropriated (at its declared tax value), the US government saw this as a push for communism in its backyard. The Central Intelligence Agency therefore began a successful campaign to depose President Árbenz, installing the ironically named Colonel Carlos Castillo Armas (*armas* being the Spanish word for *weapons*). This act ultimately led to a thirty-six-year civil war that ended the lives of perhaps hundreds of thousands of Guatemalans (Gleijeses, 1992). In addition to the direct bloodshed, it greatly limited Guatemala's ability to build a public health infrastructure or to otherwise develop economically. To this day, Guatemala is one of the poorest nations in the Americas, and its life expectancy of seventy-two years ranks it in the bottom third of all nations worldwide.

At the start of the 1960s, the Kennedy administration in the United States set out to win the hearts and minds of people in poor nations (democratic or otherwise) with a good deal of development aid. If the problem with development was too little aid, the 1960s should have solved that problem. Wealthy nations and the citizens of wealthy nations contributed to this agenda, leading to a decade of unprecedented giving.

However, by the end of the decade, only modest economic or human development had actually taken place. It had become increasingly evident that it is difficult to impossible to speed poor nations through the cycle of development in the same way that Europe was redeveloped after World War II.

Economic development—the growth of national economies—was slow in the 1960s. This is in part because, even after decades of development work, poor nations still had weak institutions. Thus, without the presence of good banks, even in the absence of thieving dictators, the money could not be easily spent. Another interrelated problem was that the Cold War continued on at full steam so the United States and the Soviet Union maintained strong interests in maintaining puppet governments around the world, virtually all with poor management skills.

A final possible problem, one that was only somewhat recognized at the time (and is still contentious), is that aid may itself pose challenges to development. This can occur because providing a reliable source of funding incentivizes corrupt people to go into government (so that they can steal it). Some also argue that aid creates dependence on outside help. This way, there is little incentive to build the complementary institutions required to ultimately form a mature and stable functioning government (e.g., a system of taxation). We will cover this hypothesis in more detail in chapter 3.

Human development was slow in part because almost none of the money given away was actually going to alleviate poverty. Human development, as measured by the UN Human Development Index (HDI), focuses on the growth in life expectancy, literacy, and standard of living (purchasing power) in a nation. (At the time of press, there were efforts to expand this measure beyond just these three measures.) Rather than focusing on schools or other institutions that directly benefited the poor, aid was mostly going to large infrastructure projects, such as dams, that were intended to help these countries move along economically. There is logic to this. Dams can provide needed electrical power for job-creating factories. But human development requires more than electricity. Without investing in schools, it becomes impossible to provide the education needed to ultimately transition an economy into one with skilled jobs that offers a living wage. Thus, the world of the poor entered the 1970s with only modest improvements in literacy, life expectancy, and economic growth.

The good news is that some nations, especially in Asia, did plant the seeds for future growth, investing in schools and agriculture in the post–World War II period. (Yes, a good education can be accomplished without electricity from dams.) The agricultural efforts were more or less led by a man named Norman Borlaug who helped usher in the **green revolution** (Evenson & Gollin, 2003). The green revolution involves investments in hearty grains and the use of cutting-edge crop technologies, particularly for poor nations. These benefits were slow to come, and, sadly, although these efforts were slowly building through the start of the 1970s, the world saw another governance setback that helped derail some of the progress in education and agriculture that had been realized up until then.

THE FALL OF GLOBAL GOVERNANCE

The 1970s saw the formation of the Organization of the Petroleum Exporting Countries (OPEC) (Barsky & Kilian, 2002). These were generally poor Middle Eastern countries. However, they were able to coordinate spikes in oil prices worldwide (primarily with the intent of punishing the United States for assisting Israel). The plan worked, but it also hurt low-income nations that could not afford the high oil prices. Moreover, the OPEC countries did not have mature economic institutions, such as banks, and their governments had to deposit their newfound riches in the banks of the Western countries they meant to punish.

Of course, poor nations needed cash to pay for the higher fuel costs. Western banks, overflowing with petrodollars, then lent the money back to poor nations with interest. The result of this vicious cycle was skyrocketing debt in poor nations. Because fuel costs were so high, price inflation was running rampant. Central banks raised interest rates (thus encouraging people to save money instead of spend) to dampen inflation. This, in turn, meant that poor nations had to spend even more on their loan costs. Soon, it became nearly impossible for some nations just to pay the interest on all of the loans that they had taken out.

In the 1980s, Ronald Reagan and Margaret Thatcher were respectively elected to power in the United States and the United Kingdom. Their administrations enacted what is now known as the *Washington Consensus,* or a set of economic mandates attached to aid dollars by multinational organizations, including reducing expenditures on government services (e.g., education, health, and transportation), privatizing government agencies, and removing trade barriers (Williamson, 1993) (see figure 1.5). This set of ideas was named the *Washington Consensus* because its two main intergovernmental actors, the IMF and the World Bank, sit across the street from one another in Washington, DC. A third important actor, the United States Treasury, is also close by.

As mentioned in the introduction, the IMF and the World Bank's mandated **structural adjustment programs** (SAPs) were a set of rules (called *conditionalities*) that poorer countries were forced to adopt if they were to receive loans or aid from these agencies. These rules were designed to "adjust" the loan recipient country's debt burden by reducing government regulations and expenditures. By reducing expenditures on schools, health care, transit, and other government programs, poor nations should, in theory, be better positioned to pay off debt. By reducing regulations, such as environmental protections, paperwork needed to do business, and so forth, business would start more easily and the economy should run more efficiently and therefore generate more revenue for paying off debt. These structural adjustments often also

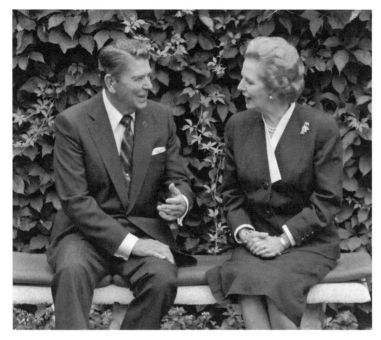

Figure 1.5. President Reagan meeting with Prime Minister Margaret Thatcher at the Hotel Cipriani in Venice, Italy, 6/9/1987.

Source: Photo courtesy of the Ronald Reagan Library. Available online at http://www.reagan.utexas.edu/archives/photographs/large/C41109-27.jpg

included currency devaluation, wage suppression, business deregulation, and lower taxes on imported goods.

Currency devaluation means that the nation's currency becomes less valuable than other nations' currencies, such as the US dollar. This makes everything that the country produces much cheaper to those in other nations. (Those of you who have traveled to poor nations and have been awed at the purchasing power of your currency have reaped the benefits of some of these SAPs.) But SAPs also tended to be formulaic. So a country that relies on imports, such as Jamaica, would be expected to lower the value of its currency even though this would mean that imports would become more expensive.

Therefore, in many cases, these SAPs led to recessions and dramatic increases in poverty from which some countries have not yet fully recovered. Structural adjustment did help to reduce the debt burden, which by the 1980s led to a net flow of money from poor nations to rich nations in the form of interest payments. However, because it often forced governments to cut back on necessary public goods and spending as well as wasteful spending, it also caused the virtual disappearance of the middle class, most of whom were government employees, in poor nations (Gaidzanwa, 1999; Moghadam, 1999).

The criticisms of the Washington Consensus do not end there. Joseph Stiglitz, a Nobel Prize–winning economist, points out that the economists making decisions at these institutions often saw the world in terms of mathematical and theoretical relationships, without adequately examining what is truly happening on the ground. As a result, they recommended that countries withhold subsidies for fertilizer and seeds for their farmers, completely ignoring that the United States and Europe provide heavy subsidies for agriculture. Thus, for one, the Washington Consensus asked countries to compete in an idealized world. In reality, the playing field was far from level. This can result in failed crops and hungry people when agriculture is a nation's main source of income. Most African residents live on less than US$2 a day, even as the average European cow receives approximately US$2.20 in subsidies each day (CFR, 2005).

The 1990s saw the end of the Cold War and thus there was less incentive for the United States and its allies to provide official direct assistance (ODA). This, coupled with the burgeoning HIV/AIDS epidemic (worsened by the impact of structural adjustment on public health infrastructure), resulted in declines in life expectancy in many African nations. In 1988, South Africa boasted of a per capita gross domestic product (GDP) of US$7,966, and a life expectancy of sixty-one years. Two decades later, their per capita GDP had improved a little bit and stood at US$9,429, but the average life expectancy had plunged to fifty-two years. But the decade also saw the stellar rise of formerly impoverished nations in Asia, a rise mostly attributed to investments in agriculture and education.

The 2000s saw the rise of humanitarian aid, with the world's two richest men—Warren Buffet and Bill Gates—pooling resources to form the largest charitable organization yet, the Bill & Melinda Gates Foundation. Other forms of private giving increased, but so did government aid. China's powerful manufacturing engine, coupled with unparalleled consumer spending in the United States, led to an enormous rise in the prices of raw materials such as oil, copper, and iron. But it also led to soaring economic growth in the places that supplied these goods, particularly Latin America and Africa. China, eager to fuel its manufacturing engine, turned to poor nations that were rich in mineral resources, often exchanging government aid for access to these resources (Michel, Beuret, & Woods, 2009). Moreover, China has been willing to go where few aid agencies dare, tapping into war-torn areas and highly corrupt governments alike. Thus it has served as a model and as an investor, ushering many nations into double-digit economic growth.

With all this money flowing into poor nations, particularly from China, the IMF—with all of its stipulations for aid—fell out of favor. In 2006, Turkey was its main debtor, and the only large one in its portfolio. This led some to jokingly call the IMF the TMF, or Turkish Monetary Fund. Interest payments declined to the point that the fund had to sell off some of its gold assets. Then, in 2007, a real estate crisis struck wealthy nations, and they in turn became in need of structural adjustment. European nations received loans from the IMF, and the IMF was back in business. Ironically, during this crisis, few wealthy nations took up structural adjustment to the extent that they required poor nations to structurally adjust in the 1980s. Instead, they mostly printed money and embarked on economic stimulus programs. Yet it is good that they did not. Stimulation in many cases proved to be a good thing, because if wealthier nations such as China and the United States had not stimulated, the entire world economy might have ended up looking like the low-income nation economies did in the 1980s.

Despite the Great Recession, mostly the new millennium brought good news with respect to health worldwide. For one, we have witnessed effective public health campaigns directed at combating the tobacco and lead industries that have robbed humans of countless years of life and intellectual capacity. With these lessons, public health officials are moving against manufacturers of unhealthy foods, the coal industry and other heavy pollutants, and other industrial threats to human health. As with most advances, industry will move on to prey on less-developed countries, until those countries, too, can build effective institutions and regulatory agencies to address public health challenges. Reductions in smoking rates in rich nations and increasing aid in very poor nations are two of the many factors contributing to the constantly brightening health picture worldwide at the time of the publication of this book at the end of 2013.

The improvements in global health coincided not just with the economic rise of low-income nations, innovative ways of tackling old public health problems, and new investments in global health, but also with an ambitious set of goals forwarded by the UN called the **Millennium Development Goals**. Even with the global financial crisis of 2007, the economic rise of poor nations and improvements in basic sanitation, education, and immunization programs put some of these goals within reach.

THE MILLENNIUM DEVELOPMENT GOALS

Recognizing that modern health problems arise from policy failures, the UN set out to generate a set of goals that might be realistically achieved to move global health and development forward. These Millennium Development Goals were devised at the Millennium Summit in 2000 and were targeted at the poorest nations on earth, to be completed by 2015.

THE MILLENNIUM DEVELOPMENT GOALS

The Millennium Development Goals comprise a set of eight goals:

Goal 1: Eradicate extreme poverty and hunger.

Goal 2: Achieve universal primary education.

Goal 3: Promote gender equality and empower women.

Goal 4: Reduce child mortality rates.

Goal 5: Improve maternal health.

Goal 6: Combat HIV/AIDS, malaria, and other diseases.

Goal 7: Ensure environmental sustainability.

Goal 8: Develop a global partnership for development.

Each set of goals contains a number of targets. For instance, the first goal, to eradicate extreme poverty and hunger, has the following targets:

Target 1.A: Halve, between 1990 and 2015, the proportion of people whose income is less than US$1 a day.

Target 1.B: Achieve full and productive employment and decent work for all, including women and young people.

Target 1.C: Halve, between 1990 and 2015, the proportion of people who suffer from hunger.

Although the goals may have seemed unrealistic at the time that they were formulated, progress has been made. Much of this is probably attributable to the huge economic success of China between 2000 and 2013, which lifted over four hundred million people out of extreme poverty within its borders alone. The extended reach of the Chinese miracle, with tentacles reaching as far as Africa and South America, has probably helped these nations' economic prospects, lifting many hundreds of millions more out of poverty. In fact, most of the fastest economically growing nations on earth in 2013 were also among the poorest nations. A number of these poorer nations also used this windfall to implement massive social welfare and health programs in the first decade of the twenty-first century. It may well be that by the time you are reading this, extreme poverty is on track to disappear in some places. (Alternatively, you may be laughing at how naive that kind of a statement is. Publishing moves slowly but the world changes quickly.)

Indeed, many questions remain. Will China's growth be sustained? (Many feel that this is unlikely.) Will it end up speeding up climate change to the point that many people are displaced, thus worsening misery? Will rising inequalities and authoritarian policies lead to social turmoil, as in nations that participated in the Arab Spring? Will China's rise mean a sustained period of relative peace, as is currently the case? Will state ownership and mismanagement lead to a spectacular global financial collapse?

AN ALTERNATIVE HISTORY

What you have read so far has been more or less told in various ways in books covering global public health (Black, 2002; Moyo, 2009). But we would like to tell an alternative history, one that looks a little rosier.

First, let us stop for a moment and imagine that after World War II development had been successful. When people spoke of development back then, they meant *economic* development. Imagine for a moment that sub-Saharan Africa had been as easy to build with development aid as was post-WWII France. We would now be living in a world with potentially more than six billion people with US habits—driving cars, using air-conditioning, generating a ton of trash, and eating an average of 273 pounds of meat each year (USDA, 2012).

This successful development agenda could have meant that we would have developed technologies that allowed us to survive in a world full of billions of consumers. Economic development, after all, brings unimaginable technological advances that can have a positive and negative transformative effect on well-being and the environment in which we live (Schneider et al., 2011). It could also have led to slower population growth. As people urbanize and become more educated, reproduction drops dramatically (Lewis, 1955).

But this alternative development scenario could also have meant Armageddon. Had the development agenda of the 1940s been successful worldwide, the Eastern seaboard of the United States and much of South and Southeast Asia could have been entirely underwater due to environmental change. This would not only have meant the loss of major cities, such as New York City, but it would also have meant that populations would have had to adapt very rapidly to such changes, in part by migrating across what are now mostly sealed borders.

Previously, we mentioned that human development—the growth in literacy and life expectancy—was slow in the 1960s. That is mostly true but is not entirely the case, as we alluded to previously when we mentioned the green revolution. Recall that in much of Asia and parts of Latin America, nations began investing in schooling and new agricultural techniques in the 1960s (Evenson & Gollin, 2003).

The green revolution involved the use of more hearty grains coupled with modernized farming techniques, including hybridized seeds, synthetic fertilizers, pesticides, and new management strategies. This produced a large immediate payoff in terms of economic growth (from selling the crops), health (from better food supply and from eating the crops), and schooling (now governments could afford schools and the children's bellies were full). It also helped ease fears of global food shortages that might arise from the skyrocketing number of humans on earth. The investments in education then kicked in decades later, allowing many nations to greatly improve their healthy life expectancy and sustain reasonable economic growth. These changes in life expectancy can be easily visualized by visiting www.gapminder.org and exploring the past century's life expectancy and GDP per capita paths in Malaysia, South Korea, and most of the other nations in the neighborhood.

HOW PUBLIC HEALTH RESEARCHERS MEASURE THINGS

Gapminder.org provides us with a sense of overall trends in the associations between development indicators such as income and health over time. This is an example of correlational data. The term emphasizes the idea that we can infer and test whether some association, correlation, or relationship between two variables (such as per capita GDP and life expectancy) exists but not whether one variable causes or leads to the other, what the complex causal pathways and dynamics between these two variables are, how these variables interact, and what else might be going on. This sort of trend analysis, using large datasets, is probably the most common approach. But it is also the weakest study design in public health. Humans have a tendency to draw conclusions from what they see in data. For instance, coffee was first found to be highly correlated with heart disease and lung cancer in early research studies. Can you guess why? Well, it was not the coffee, so you can rest assured (even if you now have the coffee jitters!). It was the fact that coffee drinkers are more likely to smoke cigarettes. Thus, the dictum "correlation is not causation" must be considered when reading studies in your local newspaper.

An alternative to the correlational study design is an **experimental study.** In an experimental study, scientists manipulate the environment to make sure that they are measuring what they think that they are measuring. For instance, you might start by randomly assigning one group to drink coffee and another group to drink water every morning and follow them to see who gets heart disease and who does not. In this case, smokers are just as likely to end up in one random group as the other. So, using a randomized trial, smoking cannot be the hidden or underlying **confounder**, or confounding variable in the study. (In this example, smoking is the real link between coffee consumption and higher rates of heart disease.)

If we measure progress in terms of life expectancy growth, we see that, up until the AIDS epidemic, the growth in this life expectancy has been fairly steady even in parts of the world that had been completely written off by development economists. Data on literacy rates only go back a decade and a half, but even here, we have seen significant progress. Between 1991 and 2002, Burkina Faso has gone from a literacy rate of around 13 percent to around 24 percent. Between 1987 and 1997, Malawi's literacy rate has increased from 49 percent to 64 percent. Botswana has progressed from 69 percent to 81 percent between 1991 and 2003.

Recently, national governments in some countries such as Malawi have begun to ignore the international economic development experts and to instead follow their own common sense. Malawi's government has begun to subsidize fertilizer and seeds, allowing for a miniature green revolution in that nation. These subsidies are essential for local farmers to grow crops because fertilizer and seeds would be unaffordable at market prices. (See the following box for an explanation of why subsidies might be a good or bad idea.) Internal investments, coupled with the efforts of many smaller aid agencies and **nongovernmental organizations** (NGOs), have begun to improve educational opportunities for many poor people.

These statistics suggest that development progress is being made, just as long as we measure outcomes in terms of human development. Still, some NGOs are so poorly coordinated that they are doing more harm than good. Some of these changes in practices might not catch on, and governments can quickly go into decline. But if our ultimate goal is to improve well-being—as measured by literacy and a rising life expectancy—the development agenda is, and has been, on the right path even though researchers disagree on precisely how or why.

WHY DO SOME DEVELOPMENT EXPERTS DISLIKE SUBSIDIES?

The primary argument against subsidies for fertilizer, soil, crops, and so forth is that, in theory, the free market will raise all boats more quickly than government programs. Some argue that it is inefficient to take money from individuals and businesses and then spend this money on something else using inefficient and noncompetitive government agencies. Some of this money can disappear in paperwork, red tape, or corruption, particularly in poor nations. This approach effectively wastes the money of those who are productive so that fewer goods are produced overall. Finally, by subsidizing agriculture, farmers might not do everything they can to become competitive; at their worst, subsidies, similar to other welfare benefits, act as a disincentive for work and a disincentive to think creatively about innovative ways of solving problems.

The arguments for these subsidies are that the existence of corrupt officials or fears of disincentives should not serve as an excuse for intergovernmental agencies to abandon aid for the poor. Some argue that in desperate situations, subsidies for food production are not the same as subsidies for luxury goods. They argue that the lives of millions of poor people should not be collateral damage in a political argument about the efficiency of their leaders. Moreover, by subsidizing seeds, it becomes possible to encourage farmers to modernize the crops to those that require less water and less fertilizer. This argument aside, the private sector will not sell fertilizer or seeds at a loss. If farmers had to buy fertilizer and seeds at market rates in places like Malawi, they wouldn't have enough money to eat. Farmers may eventually need to learn to become more competitive, but they first need the sort of nurturing that so-called infant industries in industrialized nations received decades before. Often, farmers in poor countries barely have the funds to feed their families, especially during years when the yield is low. In short, farmers in poor countries would never become economically productive and competitive without receiving some aid and training to kick-start their efforts. And they must compete against highly subsidized and mechanized corporate farms in wealthier countries. Without fertilizer or seeds, poor farmers will rarely have a successful crop, so one bad year can lead to a downward cycle of perpetually declining yields. A more rational policy might be to make policy not by economic theory alone but via a much more participatory discussion that takes into account the situation on the ground.

LOVE AND HEALTH IN MODERN TIMES

Today, the development landscape can be thought of as a museum of the entirety of human history with exhibits arranged by geographic region. In one section of this museum, the Congo, we see some tribal societies struggling to ensure that half of all children born survive to age five. This, amid raging infectious disease, war, and hunger. However, the Congo is also surrounded by rising prosperity, as shown by sub-Saharan Africa becoming the next economic miracle. (China, now laced with high-speed rail and buildings built by some of the world's greatest architects, looked quite similar three decades ago.) In other sections in the United States of America and China, we see struggles to overcome problems associated with human hierarchies, industrial waste, and poor regulation. In these sections, politics (in the United States) and the desire for economic growth (in the United States and China) take precedence over what others might see as "rational" social policies—those that accept slower growth in exchange for stricter pollution controls, higher taxes to pay for education, occupational safety standards, and heavy investments in public transit. (In all fairness, China has made some of the heaviest investments in public transit of any nation, and the United States has fairly decent occupational safety standards.) In yet another section of this museum of human history, the Netherlands, we find reasonable work weeks, social safety nets, and previously unimaginable life expectancies, but also struggles to cope with an aging population in the face of a society resistant to allowing younger immigrants and increasing family size. Finally, in a series of strange new additions to this museum, small, mostly nondemocratic societies are popping up in which highly socially regulated societies challenge Norway for dominance in world health rankings. One section, Singapore, offers not only extreme public health measures, but also heavy regulations on potentially unhealthy human behaviors, such as mandatory death penalties for drug trafficking. Here, we see that other aspects of well-being, such as democratic participation, take a back seat to social order.

In low-income nations, we await various significant health events. The first is the aforementioned epidemiologic transition, in which infectious disease and hunger are brought under control and the population's life expectancy begins to increase. This is typically followed by a **demographic transition,** in which birthrates decline. These transitions are best illustrated by population pyramids, such as the ones in figure 1.6, showing different stages of population and demographic change.

The first pyramid is typical of nations prior to their epidemiologic transition. The second is typical of a nation following the epidemiologic transition, the third for one undergoing a demographic transition, and the final, a country after a demographic transition.

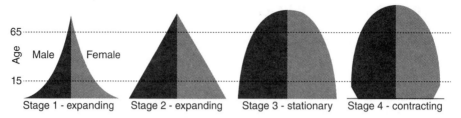

Figure 1.6. Population pyramids typical in various stages of development.

These transitions coincide with responsible governance. If industry is poorly regulated and the country becomes extremely polluted or the government fails to continue to invest in beneficial social policies, then the health and quality of life benefits associated with the epidemiologic and demographic transitions can be mitigated.

Thus, we strive for healthy development that moves nations from a low life expectancy to a high life expectancy. However, each of these sections of the world's new museum suffers from its very presence in the same museum building. These include the widespread availability of cheap, tasty sources of empty calories, the inability to protect borders from pollution or new strains of infectious disease, and the spread of new and old war technologies. Although the process of development mostly follows historical trends, these truly *global* health risks transcend borders and pose new challenges for public health. They also point to a need for effective forms of global governance. These new risks are all in keeping with the notion that, as humans manage to tackle threats to health, the solutions to old problems inevitably produce new ones.

From this new landscape, new and challenging questions arise. Namely, how do we regulate human behavior but maintain freedom and quality of life? How do we deal with skyrocketing birthrates in some areas of the world and plummeting rates in others? How do we manage the increasing prevalence of floods and droughts, coupled with rising sea levels? How, exactly, do we maintain a robust and vibrant free market economy and foster this market so that it maintains, rather than harms, human longevity at the same time? How do we cope with populations that are too young in some places and too old in others? How do we manage the massive movements of humans across borders as they seek to equilibrate economic and demographic inequalities?

The answers to some of these questions are easy. Increased immigration has not only helped solve economic problems in nations such as the United States, but it has also helped solve demographic and health problems. That is because immigrants tend to be slightly younger, have higher birthrates, and are healthier than native-born Americans (Muennig & Fahs, 2002; Muennig et al., 2012).

SUMMARY

Even this brief history holds some important lessons about global health policy. Most important, we need clear, coordinated global policies and strong leadership to manage global issues. This obviously has not happened at a global level. As this is being written, various large-scale conflicts are well in progress. There is a constant threat of nuclear attack, within countries such as the United States and between nuclear-armed nations such as India and Pakistan. The world remains ill-prepared for an infectious disease pandemic. There is no clear path to addressing global climate change. Industrial pollution is causing air quality problems not only for industrializing nations but also for their neighbors. Deforestation and despeciation are running rampant and unchecked. Much of this can be attributed to ineffective, toothless global institutions, such as the UN or WHO.

But even if such organizations were to transform themselves into effective governing bodies with actual political power, we still are not sure what those policies need to look like. For instance, we need to decide what we mean by development. Does development mean economic development to the point that we have replicated US GDP and consumption patterns in all 191 (or more) nations on earth? If so, then the world will face entirely new public health threats, such as massive environmental destruction. Or does it mean striving for the policies that will prolong our lives and improve our health, such as universal primary school education and vaccination? When do economic development and human development go hand in hand? When do they not?

KEY TERMS

absorptive capacity	green revolution	Millennium
confounder	human development	Development Goals
demographic transition	Industrial Revolution	nongovernmental
economic development	intergovernmental	organizations (NGOs)
epidemiologic transition	institutions	social hierarchies
experimental study		social institutions

DISCUSSION QUESTIONS

1. How would you define *global health?*
2. What is the best way to achieve an epidemiologic transition?
3. Who are some of the main actors and institutions that currently help to set global health policy?
4. What are some of the key events in the late nineteenth and twentieth centuries that affected global health? How did they do so?

5. What kinds of regulations should we put on markets in the name of health, if any?

6. Is global warming a public health threat? How so?

FURTHER READING

Sachs, J. D. (2012). Malawi and anti-hunger programs. *New York Times*, April 19. Available online at www.nytimes.com/2012/04/20/opinion/how-malawi-fed-its-own-people.html

REFERENCES

Ashton, T. S. (1997). *The industrial revolution 1760–1830*. Oxford: Oxford University Press.

Barsky, R. B., & Kilian, L. (2002). Oil and the macroeconomy since the 1970s. *Journal of Economic Perspectives, 18*(4), 115–134.

Black, M. (2002). *The no-nonsense guide to international development*. Scranton, PA: Verso.

CFR. (2005). *The WTO's troubled "Doha negotiations."* Available online at www.cfr.org/wto/wtos-troubled-doha-negotiations/p9385—p3

Denham, T. P., Haberle, S. G., Lentfer, C., Fullagar, R., Field, J., Therin, M., et al. (2003). Origins of agriculture at Kuk swamp in the highlands of New Guinea. *Science, 301*(5630), 189–193.

Diamond, J. (1998). *Guns, germs, and steel*. London: Random House.

Evenson, R. E., & Gollin, D. (2003). Assessing the impact of the green revolution, 1960 to 2000. *Science, 300*(5620), 758–762.

Gaidzanwa, R. B. (1999). *Voting with their feet: Migrant Zimbabwean nurses and doctors in the era of structural adjustment*. Uppsala, Sweden: Nordic Africa Institute.

Galvani, A. P., & Slatkin, M. (2003). Evaluating plague and smallpox as historical selective pressures for the CCR5-Δ32 HIV-resistance allele. *Proceedings of the National Academy of Sciences of the United States of America, 100*(25), 15276.

Gleijeses, P. (1992). *Shattered hope: The Guatemalan revolution and the United States, 1944–1954*. Princeton, NJ: Princeton University Press.

Gulland, A. (2012). Child mortality falls, but 19,000 under 5s still die every day. *BMJ, 345*, e6229. doi: 10.1136/bmj.e6229.

Lewis, W. A. (1955). *The theory of economic growth*. London: Allen & Unwin.

Lowry, R., Wechsler, H., Galuska, D. A., Fulton, J., & Kann, L. (2002). Television viewing and its associations with overweight, sedentary lifestyle, and insufficient consumption of fruits and vegetables among US high school students:

Differences by race, ethnicity, and gender. *Journal of School Health, 72*(10), 413–421.

Mayor, S. (2012). Child mortality is falling but some developing regions will miss millennium targets. *BMJ, 345*, e5801. doi: 10.1136/bmj.e5801.

Michel, S., Beuret, M., & Woods, P. (2009). *China safari: On the trail of Beijing's expansion in Africa*. New York: Nation Books.

Moghadam, V. M. (1999). Gender and globalization: Female labor and women's mobilization. *Journal of World-Systems Research, 5*(2), 367–388.

Moyo, D. (2009). *Dead aid*. New York: Farrar, Straus and Giroux.

Muennig, P., & Fahs, M. (2002). Health status and hospital utilization among immigrants to New York City. *Preventive Medicine, 35*, 225–229.

Muennig, P., Wang, Y., & Jakubowski, A. (2012) The health of Chinese New Yorkers: Evidence from the New York City Health and Nutrition Examination Survey. *Journal of Immigrant and Refugee Studies, 10*, 1–7.

Myers, M. L., & McGlothlin, J. D. (1996). Matchmakers' "phossy jaw" eradicated. *American Industrial Hygiene Association Journal, 57*(4), 330–332.

Omran, A. R. (1971). The epidemiologic transition: A theory of the epidemiology of population change. *The Milbank Memorial Fund Quarterly, 49*(4), 509–538.

Parkin, D. M., Bray, F., Ferlay, J., & Pisani, P. (2005). Global cancer statistics, 2002. *CA: A Cancer Journal for Clinicians, 55*(2), 74.

Schlesinger, S., & Kinzer, S. (1982). *Bitter fruit: The story of the American coup in Guatemala*. New York: Doubleday.

Schmidheiny, S. (1992). *Changing course: A global business perspective on development and the environment*. Cambridge, MA: MIT Press.

Schneider, U. A., Havlík, P., Schmid, E., Valin, H., Mosnier, A., Obersteiner, M., et al. (2011). Impacts of population growth, economic development, and technical change on global food production and consumption. *Agricultural Systems, 104*(2), 204–215.

Trichopoulos, D., Li, F. P., & Hunter, D. J. (1996). What causes cancer? *Scientific American, 275*(3), 80–84.

USDA. (2012). *Cattle and beef*. Economic Research Service. Available online at www.ers.usda.gov/topics/animal-products/cattle-beef/statistics-information.aspx

Williamson, J. (1993). Democracy and the "Washington Consensus." *World Development, 21*, 1329–1336.

CHAPTER 2

Case Studies in Development and Health

KEY IDEAS

- More money does not necessarily buy more health in international development.
- How policy makers allocate resources and use a nation's wealth matters most.
- The case studies on China, Kerala, and Chile highlight some of the strengths and weaknesses of focusing on economic development relative to focusing on healthy development.

Wanda lives in the United States, in what is often dubbed the wealthiest country in the world. She has a good job she believes in: she is a community organizer who helps local residents work on social justice campaigns in New York City. She has many friends, lives in the neighborhood she grew up in, and is recognized as a community leader. As part of her work, she has gotten to have one-on-one meetings with policy makers such as Mayor Michael Bloomberg. Her neighbors and friends respect her.

As someone who works for an NGO (remember, this stands for *nongovernmental organization*), Wanda has a lot of knowledge about politics and bureaucracies so she knows how to get the resources she needs. She possesses quite a bit of so-called **social capital,** or rich networks of friends and connections in her field of work with strong norms of sharing tips and resources (Putnam, 1995). She is not rich but she earns enough to care for herself, and her job provides her with ample vacation time (at least compared to most

31

Americans), flexibility, and benefits such as health insurance. Plus, she has all of the rich cultural resources of New York City—the famous museums, world-class universities and research centers, diverse immigrant neighborhoods, and good restaurants at all price points. As compared to the rest of the country, New York City also has a more comprehensive welfare infrastructure—with a greater constellation of public transit routes, community centers, food programs for the poor, free English classes for immigrants, free outdoor concert series by musicians and orchestras from around the globe, and so on—than probably any other area in the country.

WHY IS SOCIAL CAPITAL GOOD FOR YOU?

Having social capital means that you are well connected to others around you. If you are stressed or lonely, others can provide comfort. If you need money, others can give it or loan it to you. If you need a doctor, others can give a referral. For this reason, people who belong to community groups, churches, or other organizations that provide a lot of social connections tend to have better health (Kawachi, Subramanian, & Kim, 2010). So do people who spend time with their friends or family rather than watching television at night. But, of course, social capital can also be bad for you or for others. Take, for instance, friends with whom you go out to smoke and drink. People who belong to criminal organizations such as the Ku Klux Klan or the triad gangs of Hong Kong and China may harm themselves and others around them (Kim, Subramanian, & Kawachi, 2006). So, we have to be sure we define what we are talking about when we talk about social capital. Political scientists such as Robert Putnam, famous for his book *Bowling Alone* (the title refers to a decline in all sorts of group activities, including bowling leagues, in US public life after World War II), tend to emphasize more positive aspects of social capital. Sociologists such as Pierre Bourdieu, famous for books such as *The Forms of Capital*, tend to emphasize the ways in which nonmonetary resources such as social capital also largely reproduce and perhaps exacerbate class structures. After all, the so-called old boys' clubs and their golf games might benefit those who are already wealthy, but such hubs of rich social capital exclude almost everyone else.

The life expectancy for Hispanic females like Wanda in the United States is eighty-one, in between the immigrant (foreign-born) Hispanic female life expectancy of eighty-four and the average US female life expectancy, regardless of race or immigrant status, of seventy-nine (Singh & Miller, 2004). But much as Wanda's parents died at a much younger age than their parents, life expectancy among females in some local areas of the United States is declining. This is an unprecedented phenomenon in a wealthy country that is not undergoing political turmoil, facing famine, or experiencing an epidemic disease. No one knows why this is, but maybe we can get some clues from other nations.

Although we mention many different nations throughout this book, we chose the examples of Chile, China, and the state of Kerala in India as case studies to highlight. We did this because each of these states provides a good example of what happens to health when a government invests heavily in social programs and what happens when the market is left to its own devices. Although China has been nondemocratic since 1949 through the time of publication of this book in 2013, it made a large shift from investments in public health, medical, and other social programs to a predominantly market-based approach in 1979. Around 2000, it shifted its course back and began to once again invest in social programs. This provides us with a sort of internal comparison group to look at the effects of less-regulated markets versus health investments. The state of Kerala in India has been democratic for a long time. However, communists were elected to power for long stints punctuated by somewhat more market-oriented governments. This has also changed the funding landscape for health and social programs over time. Finally, Chile has also experienced democratic and nondemocratic leadership over an even longer period and has had intervals of emphasis on social investment and intervals that emphasized a free market approach to development. These examples all highlight precisely why this health textbook reads so much like a policy textbook. We hope to use these examples to very clearly delineate a precise answer to the question of whether democracy matters and whether social investments matter for health. That is, we hope that each and every student reading this will emerge with a very clear and firm answer to this question. As a hint, that answer is: it depends.

THE PUZZLE OF "GOOD" DEVELOPMENT FOR HEALTH

Figure 2.1 shows what is known as a **Preston curve**, named after the famous demographer Sam Preston. In this figure, we see that there is a strong relationship between per capita GDP and life expectancy up to about US$4,000 per year (Acemoglu & Johnson, 2006). After this point, we see what economists would call *diminishing returns* to each marginal increase in GDP, and in general, the overall correlation between increased GDP and increased life expectancy becomes much weaker. Eventually, it disappears altogether. (This

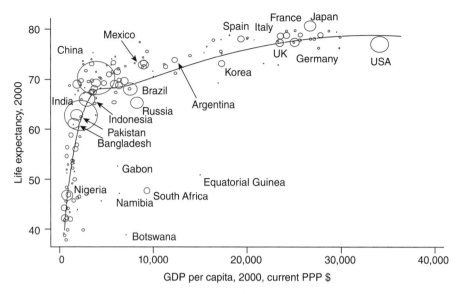

Figure 2.1. The Preston curve: Life expectancy versus GDP per capita.

Note: Circles are proportional to population, and some of the largest (or most interesting) countries are labeled. The solid line is a plot of a population-weighted nonparametric regression. Luxembourg, with per capita GDP of $50,061 and life expectancy of 77.04 years, is excluded.

Source: Deaton, A. (2003). Health, inequality, and economic development. *Journal of Economic Literature, 41*(1), 116, Fig. 1.

is mostly—as Wanda in the case study attests—thanks to the United States pulling down everyone else.)

Some countries down in the sub-US$4,000 earning range have life expectancies similar to those seen in developed nations. For instance, Costa Rica (nominal per capita GDP US$7,000 and purchasing power parity [PPP]-adjusted per capita GDP US$11,000) and Chile (US$10,000 nominal and US$15,000 after adjusting for PPP) have life expectancy values that are a bit better than the United States as a whole (per capita GDP US$47,000), despite being low GDP countries. Most notably, most citizens of Cuba earned about US$30 per month, or a dollar a day, in 2012. So, how does this island nation have a life expectancy similar to the United States? The answer could lie in how the money is spent.

Cuba has historically invested much of its very limited national wealth in food, water, education, and health care. This prioritization of social goods may account for why it has been able to maintain a reasonable life expectancy.

These variables might be the only factors in global life expectancy values that raise a nation's life expectancy into the seventies or even eighties.

Among the higher-earning countries, most of which have already made these investments, there is little to no relationship between life expectancy and per capita GDP (Preston, 1976). That big kink in the curve (right next to where Indonesia is on the graph) disrupts the so-called **wealth-health gradient,** whereby a higher income or GDP per capita earns you (whether an individual or a nation) a higher life expectancy. The wealth-health gradient tends to exist within nations, but not so much between them, especially among nations with more than US$5,000 a year in GDP per capita.

The Preston curve thus presents two major questions. First, why do countries tend to get less bang for their buck (or peso or yen or whichever currency they hold) when per capita GDP surpasses US$4,000 per annum? Second, why are some countries below the trend line and others above it? For example, why is Mexico's life expectancy more than twenty years longer than South Africa's?

Wanda, the woman we interviewed for this book, is Puerto Rican and of African descent. She first moved to the mainland United States at the age of eight, after her mother caught her father cheating on her. Wanda, Wanda's mother, and Wanda's sister Sandra made a new home for themselves in New York. At first, this was not so easy. Wanda had an uncle who worked as a building superintendent in the Bronx, so they tried to live there at first. However, this was 1975, and the city was suffering from a massive fiscal crisis. Conditions in the borough were so bad that some landlords deliberately set buildings on fire, sometimes with tenants still in them, in order to collect insurance money. For the landlords, this was more lucrative than collecting rent. That moment in history was most famously captured when the Yankees played at their Bronx stadium during the 1977 World Series. A skyline of smoke was visible throughout the game, which was televised nationwide. The presiding sportscaster announced, "Ladies and gentlemen, the Bronx is burning."

So, between 1975 and 1989, Wanda and her family moved eight times, eventually resettling in the Bronx. Wanda's mother was quite strict but also incredibly loving, and she made sure that her daughters worked hard in school. Wanda recalls her high school experience with ambivalence, however. She had some good teachers, but the school was so rife with marijuana dealing that it had been nicknamed *the drugstore*—a term not meant to refer to a friendly, neighborhood pharmacy. After high school, Wanda got a business administration certificate from a local, for-profit sixteen-month program. She then worked as an administrator for an insurance company for a while, became more involved as a volunteer in local NGOs, and eventually turned to the nonprofit sector, where she has been ever since. In 1989, when Wanda was twenty-three, Wanda's mother passed away from a heart attack. Her mother was forty-three years old when she died. Wanda is overweight, even though she is an avid *cumbia* and salsa dancer. She recently bought a bicycle for US$30, but she has not gotten many chances to ride it just yet.

Wanda's case may help us understand why the United States is relatively unhealthy despite its wealth. In one of the wealthiest cities in one of the wealthiest countries on earth, Wanda lives and works in what most people in wealthy nations consider poverty. She lives in the Bronx, where the per capita income is US$17,464, less than half of that of the city as a whole. The median *family* income is still just US$38,923, and the mean family income is US$52,327. In the South Bronx, where she works, 40 percent of households live below the poverty line—around US$22,000 for a family of four in 2011.

By means of comparison, Manhattan, the city's wealthiest borough adjacent and directly south of the Bronx, boasts a per capita income of US$60,596, a median family income of almost US$76,470, and a mean family income US$166,997. More than 84 percent of residents have completed high school and more than 56 percent are college graduates. In Manhattan, only 14.3 percent of households live below the poverty line.

In 2009, Wanda's asthma had gotten so bad that her doctor prescribed her an inhaler. She has been trying to eat healthier, to turn away from the starch-heavy comfort foods of her Puerto Rican childhood, and to abandon the recipes she knows by heart. She got excited when she discovered that the Costco warehouse store she drives to has olive oil and produce. The local neighborhood stores tend to carry few vegetables, if any. Ironically, most of the city's organic produce—especially the produce that gets served at US$40-per-entrée restaurants downtown—first stops in the South Bronx at a food distribution center. In order to access the distribution center, you have to pay an entry fee per person and per car, so Wanda doesn't go unless she makes it a field trip for all of the neighbors.

Sometimes, it is a struggle to keep stress levels down. Community organizers work long hours, and in the past, staff meetings took place at 9 PM, sometimes at local bars, surrounded by smoking (until Mayor Bloomberg banned it in 2002) and drinking. On top of these work conditions, it is difficult not to draw boundaries when helping others in challenging situations. In 2010, Wanda's half-sister (the daughter of Wanda's recently deceased father in Puerto Rico) lost custody of her four children, ages four, five, seven, and eleven. Wanda, who is not close to this half-sister, called the government social worker in Puerto Rico to check up on the situation. To her dismay, she was immediately offered custody of the three oldest children. They arrived in the Bronx in a matter of weeks. Wanda quickly enrolled them in school and worked to provide them with a new, loving home.

IS STRESS REALLY BAD FOR YOU?

We talk about people going gray from stress, aging, getting sick. But is it an old wives' tale? As it turns out, probably not. In experimental studies in animals (though we will explore the external validity problem in chapter 3) and in observational studies of humans (and we will explore the internal validity problem in chapter 3), stress seems to be harmful. For one, it seems to cause the body's regulatory mechanisms—internal "thermostats"—to go haywire. This creates problems with the immune and endocrine systems, among others. It also seems to cause genetic changes, including damage. In one study, women in the highest stress group showed signs that their immune cells were ten years older relative to women in the normal stress group of the same age (Epel et al., 2004).

Public health researchers have also begun to differentiate among different types of stress, their effects on health, and the social policies that should be considered in response. When the basic necessities of life are covered or when systems of social insurance exist in cases of disaster, stress is short-lived. It most certainly exists in times of crisis or when an individual opts to enter a volatile occupation like that of a stockbroker but it may not take the same toll as long-term and chronic stress does on families in dire poverty.

"I want to make sure I'm here for the long haul," like the elders who made a difference in her own early childhood in Puerto Rico, Wanda declared. She reminisced that, back then, she knew where everybody would be on Sundays—with their families. Her great-aunt lived until ninety-seven, her grandfather until eighty-seven, and her grandmother died of cancer at age seventy-nine. They led much longer lives than their children, outliving some of them. "Here, there are no elderly people," she said. "And the people in my building don't talk to one another."

What has played, and what will play, the greatest role in shaping Wanda's health—her personal habits, family, how she grew up, her neighborhood, her city, or her country? How does globalization shape her life now? Do Wanda's gender, race, and ethnicity affect her health? Can we really disentangle and separate out each of these factors or are they all jumbled up together?

THE NEXT SUPERPOWERS? TAKING A CLOSER LOOK AT MIDDLE-INCOME COUNTRIES

Throughout this book, we will reference two case studies of middle-income economies and one low-income economy: China, Chile, and the state of Kerala within India, respectively. According to the World Bank, low-income countries are those where the gross national income (GNI) per capita is below about US$1,000, and high-income countries are those where the 2008 GNI per capita is above US$12,000. Middle-income countries are all those in between.

A ROSE BY ANY OTHER NAME

The **global south, least-developed countries,** and **industrializing nations** are the most common among terms used to refer to those countries that are poorer. Some define these nations as those with a score of less than 0.8 on the UN HDI (see the website http://hdr.undp.org/en/statistics/hdi). Others use per capita GDP (see http://data.worldbank.org/about/country-classifications). The term *global south* arose because most of these countries are in the southern hemisphere. Two important exceptions, Australia and New Zealand, are the only countries in the southern hemisphere with an HDI higher than 0.8. The countries with very high HDI scores are called the **global north** because most of them are in the northern hemisphere.

For the most part, we will try to be a bit more precise and identify whether the countries we discuss are low income, middle income, or high income. But this can be confusing, too. For instance, at the time of publication, about one-third of those living on less than US$2 per day lived in middle-income countries with relatively high per capita GDP but dramatic income disparities.

We give precise definitions for each of these categories in the main text introducing our case studies: China, Kerala, and Chile. We focus on income because it is too difficult (and problematic) to label countries *more developed, underdeveloped,* or *less developed.* How do we know what the perfect level of development is anyway? As we have already discussed, development can mean lots of things—economic development and high income and GDP, human development and high life expectancy and education rates, happiness, well-being, or something else.

You may have also heard the terms *first world, second world, third world,* and *fourth world.* These are a bit dated because they refer to Cold War–era designations. Still, you might find these terms in the global health literature, so it might be good to have these definitions in mind: the first world consists of the highly industrialized countries that also consist of the global north. The second world traditionally consisted of centrally planned communist countries in the former Soviet Union. Some of these countries, such as Slovenia, are now classified as wealthy nations. The third world originally referred to those countries that did not align with either the United States or the Soviet Union during the Cold War, and then it referred to countries not in the first or second worlds. It became a phrase that implied "poor countries," but this was not always well defined. The fourth world refers to the six thousand indigenous groups and roughly six hundred million people who may or may not identify with the nation-states recognized by the United Nations.

Why are we focusing on middle-income countries? We do so because they represent a great hope (and a great puzzle) in global health policy. They have begun the epidemiologic and demographic transitions, but no one knows whether they will replicate the paths first traveled by current industrialized countries (such as Sweden, Japan, or Canada) or if their paths to development will be completely new ones. They have passed the turning point along the Preston curve (see figure 2.1) so we suspect that simply pouring money or increasing GDP is unlikely to guarantee anything unless the revenues from this growth are invested in human development. They could become the next power players, or even global powers, or they could stagnate as struggling economies. Middle-income countries also matter in terms of pure scale. There are forty-three low-income countries left in the world. Although there are sixty-six high-income countries, only twenty-seven are members of the Organization for Economic Co-operation and Development (OECD). Non-OECD high-income countries provide some clues for alternative models for industrial development; these mostly lie in the oil-rich Middle East. Middle-income countries constitute the biggest category of economic development right now, with 101 countries. The People's Republic of China alone has a population of almost 1.4 billion people and India around 1.2 billion in 2012. (Together, these two countries account for more than one-third of the world's population.) The next largest country, the high-income United States, looks like a peon by comparison, with just 310 million people. In fact, many of China's smaller cities, such as Suzhou, have populations that are ten times as large as that of San Francisco.

It might seem odd that a state in India, Kerala, is one of our three case studies. After all, there are many countries with similarly impressive health and education outcomes, such as Cuba or Costa Rica. We partly chose to profile Kerala because it boasts a larger population than these other countries. With almost thirty-two million people, it would rank as the thirty-eighth most populous country in the world if it were one, just two notches below Canada. In contrast, Cuba has roughly eleven million residents and Costa Rica just four million. Kerala also better illustrates the complex relationship among economics, governance, and health that we focus on in this book. Why has Kerala historically thrived with respect to health when almost all other states in the same country—most with much higher income—have floundered?

All three case studies have market-oriented economies, and Chile and Kerala boast of democratically elected governments. From time to time, we will include examples from other countries; it will be useful, for instance, to take a look at some of the policies that garnered Costa Rica third place on the Environmental Performance Index in 2010, after Iceland and Switzerland, which are both much wealthier countries. We will also include examples from much poorer countries, such as the Democratic Republic of the Congo. That nation underwent elections and has made some progress away from being the grave human rights disaster site it was just a few years ago.

GROWTH-MEDIATED MODELS

China provides an example of a country with what Jean Drèze and Amartya Sen call a **growth-mediated economy,** at least since reforms in the 1980s (Drèze & Sen, 1989). Before the 1980s, China was a communist, totalitarian country with a central political party making decisions about which goods and services should be produced and at what scale.

Deng Xiaoping, who became chairman of the Chinese National People's Congress in 1978, launched a model of "socialism with Chinese characteristics" that year. His plan was to gradually open the internal economy to markets and increase foreign trade. Unlike countries such as Russia, China moved to a free market economy in a gradual, experimental fashion. The experiments were local and proved successful at increasing economic growth. According to free market principles, government should also stay out of the way (thus the nickname *laissez-faire economics*), save for regulating against fraud and force and upholding property rights (Friedman, 1982). In an ideal free market, buyers and sellers mutually consent to prices without any coercion or government intervention so that aggregated supply meets aggregated demand, at a "general equilibrium." Free markets work best when they meet a certain set of criteria, such as the existence of many firms competing to supply or buy goods and consumer access to good information about the costs, benefits, and potential consequences of all available options.

Of course, real-life markets—even ones that aim to be "free"—are much more complicated. Copyright laws on everything from pharmaceutical drugs to pop songs downloaded via the Internet are often considered probusiness when they extend patent rights and demand more governmental intervention, not less.

For the purposes of this book, three characteristics of "free market" policies stand out because of their economic or health implications. First, they aim to reduce costs associated with participation in the market by firms and businesses. For instance, "freer" markets would not only offer low taxes but also make it easy to open a business without much government interference. Second, as a result of less government interference, free markets provide relatively loose regulations protecting workers, consumers that buy the products produced by the free economy, and the environment. Third, they are more concerned with efficiency than with fairness in the allocation of goods. This means that large wealth inequalities are a frequent consequence of efficient free market policies.

No modern nation adheres entirely to free market principles. By "growth-led models," we usually mean that worker, consumer, and environmental protections are less emphasized. The success (measured in terms of economic growth) of the growth-mediated model depends on wide distribution of economic activity, especially in employment. If a large enough percentage of the country's residents participate in the economic boom, they can share the rewards and other aspects of economic development that we associate with high-income countries—public infrastructure such as good roads and bridges, hospitals, and so on—which rise alongside personal income.

SUPPORT-LED MODELS

In contrast to China, the state of Kerala in India has mostly stuck to what Drèze and Sen call a **support-led model** of economic development. Instead of postponing social investments until after economic growth has occurred, the state invested heavily in health care and education while placing relatively high taxes and regulatory burdens on businesses. Sen argues that although these sorts of programs feel quite expensive in industrialized countries, they are more affordable than many policy makers assume in lower-income countries because schools, clinics, and so on are so labor- rather than technology- or capital-intensive (Sen, 1999). Labor tends to be cheap in poor countries so these services, in turn, are cheaper to implement than they are in rich nations. Nevertheless, support-led models are associated with less economic growth than growth-led models.

An emphasis on primary and secondary school, supplemental nutrition programs, and safe drinking water can all have huge economic benefits. In the case of China, the transition to a growth-led model came on the heels of decades of investment in these policies, making it easier to make the leap to a growth-led model.

On the pantheon of support-led policies, education holds a special and central position. It is often argued that, in a global economy, education investments are essential if future economic growth is to be maintained. For instance, it builds **human capital,** which can be thought of as a nation's stockpile of knowledge, personality attributes, and skills. These goods make it possible for people to understand how to keep themselves healthy, to invest, to create jobs, and so forth. It probably also makes people better workers. Education is also essential to citizen participation in public debates, information exchanges, and goal setting. Generally, education is also the most reliable indicator of a country's support-led policies (Evans, 2006).

BANGLADESH, A DEVELOPMENT "BASKET CASE"?

Henry Kissinger referred to Bangladesh as one of development's "basket cases." By this, he meant countries that could never reach a full state of economic development no matter how much aid one throws at them (*Economist,* 2012). Although Bangladesh has remained a poor country—significantly poorer than its neighbor, India—aid does seem to be working its magic. It has achieved a steady growth in educational attainment and public health improvements, reaching higher rates of female education, female literacy, and infant immunization than India, even while falling further behind India with respect to per capita income. These improvements in education and public health may explain why it has been able to surpass its neighbor in life expectancy by four years.

But support-led models also slow economic progress down in some ways by making it more difficult to start and run a business. Some entrepreneurs simply will not invest or will move to places where it is easier to do so. Although there are many poor countries with very high life expectancies because they have invested in clean water, sanitation, education, and nutrition programs, most people also want the chance to enjoy the benefits of capitalism. Large populations in communist-era China or Cuba expressed dissent over the scarcity of consumer goods, even as they reaped the benefits of strong social infrastructure. (Cuba and China are somewhat odd cases because they are also authoritarian states. Even in democratic Kerala, constituents implore their elected officials to balance economic growth with social mandates such as good, affordable health care and worker protections.) So, in the ideal, how do policy makers decide where to draw the line between support-led and growth-led models?

TOWARD A HAPPY MEDIUM?

Although there are no perfect, real-life "growth-mediated" and "support-led" models, China, Kerala, and Chile provide some perspective on the public health benefits of different development investment strategies. One point to remember is that public health policies are major determinants of the speed at which a country undergoes an epidemiologic and demographic transition. Recall that most of the gains in life expectancy globally since the mid-eighteenth century have come from tackling infectious disease and poor nutrition. This leads to an epidemiologic transition when infectious diseases are largely conquered with public health measures. The epidemiologic transition is followed by a demographic transition, which occurs when the population has a sufficiently low infant mortality rate that women bear just a few children on average, and the population begins to age until it starts to either shrink or accept immigrants from nations that have not yet undergone an epidemiologic transition. At some point in the twenty-first century, the global population may begin to decline when virtually all nations seem to be headed toward an epidemiologic transition. *Therefore, public health investments made by governments are probably leading to the global changes that will allow us to survive as a human race.* (If we do survive, that is.) Economic development appears to be important in this regard because it allows governments and individuals alike to invest in necessities such as toilets, food, and vaccines.

Another point of these case studies is that, once these transitions are completed, one must ask whether they can be sustained. That is, although economic growth can help us solve our public health problems, we must be careful to ensure that the money earned from economic development is spent wisely. One definition of **sustainable development** is "development that meets the needs of the present without compromising the ability of future generations to meet their own needs" (WECD, 1987, p. 43). The goal behind sustainable development is to create a policy environment that allows people to lead a healthy, enjoyable life with minimal environmental impact. One assumption behind sustainable development is that, eventually, countries that focus on rapid economic growth at the expense of other social goods, such as the United States and China, will eventually be unable to support the needs of their populations. In short, the thought is that nations with "unsustainable" social policies will self-destruct unless broad policy changes are made (or new technologies mitigate the impact of more destructive ones) (see figure 2.2).

A final point of these case studies is to help readers understand that most social policies, not just those dealing with medical systems and food, affect one's health. Investments in sewage systems, clean water, and vaccinations ultimately need to be accompanied by investments in schools, product safety, and occupational regulations. Further, all policies have unintended side effects,

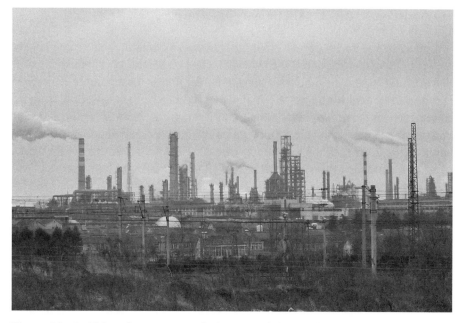

Figure 2.2. In China, the export revolution started during the transition to a predominantly capitalist economy led to massive environmental destruction, causing broad effects on ecosystems and adversely affecting the quality of life of hundreds of millions of Chinese citizens.

Source: Wikimedia Commons/Vmenkov.

good and bad. Roads can greatly speed economic development and improve access to schools and clinics, but they also increase pollution and traffic fatalities and can even facilitate the spread of infectious diseases such as HIV/AIDS. (For instance, truckers can visit lovers or brothels along their regular routes.)

After three decades of growth-mediated policies, China ended up with a robust economy that raised hundreds of millions of people out of poverty, but it did so at the cost of widespread environmental destruction, massive displacement of its people through unregulated development projects, and rising so-called "cancer villages," with unusually high levels of pollution and disease. Kerala achieved near universal literacy and became the envy of India with respect to indicators such as infant mortality and life expectancy, but it did so at the cost of economic stagnation and, as a result of poor job opportunities, a vast migration of its educated people out of the state. Chile invested heavily in public health and education, and also enacted market reforms that lifted its economy to enviable income and life expectancy levels, but it did so haphazardly and at a great cost of lives during periods of political upheaval.

Similar to China, Kerala also saw a massive displacement of its people. China's families were displaced by rising waters behind dams and the bulldozers of developers. Kerala's people, however, were displaced by their own quest for skilled labor opportunities. Because their human capital skills could not be used at home, they ventured to the Middle East, the United Kingdom, the United States, and to other states within India. Still, the Kerala model may be the primary hope for the poorest countries with little or nothing to sell in the global economy because they have little in the way of natural or economic resources. In this section, we take a look at each locale's history, governance, economic philosophy, and public health investments.

CHINA'S EXPLOSIVE GROWTH

Gleaming bullet trains bound for Shanghai whisk passengers at an average speed of 217 kilometers per hour through Wenzhou's thick, gray skies. Through the haze, one sees extreme poverty and crumbling houses. Pristine Mercedes models dodge rusty rickshaws as they blast through intersections filled with rubble, not pausing for the red stoplight. The patchwork farms on the outskirts of Wenzhou are seeded and picked by hand by workers earning a few dollars a day, even as factory owners and real estate investors in the city join the world's burgeoning billionaires. Today's China paints a picture of great hope and promise interwoven with suffering and despair. It is a nation that has placed humans in outer space but has yet to ensure that its doctors have soap to wash their hands after using the hospital's filthy bathroom. It is the perfect case study for the growth-led model in many ways. But that, like the rest of China, is changing as well. As you read this, enormous investments are being made in the health and welfare of the Chinese people.

Shortly after the Communist revolution of 1949, China embarked on experimental public health efforts. In 1965, China institutionalized these efforts, mobilizing large groups of citizens to tackle infectious diseases and installing basic medical providers in virtually every community across the unimaginably large and overpopulated nation.

These medical providers, known as **barefoot doctors,** tended to have just six months or so of medical training and only about seven years of education of any sort. Yet it does not take a good deal of training to set bones, to administer vaccines, or to correctly diagnose and treat common ailments (see figure 2.3). Schools also received a boost from the Communist Party. In postrevolutionary China, literacy improved steadily from pathetically low levels.

Infectious disease was attacked with large-scale public health programs. These involved not only simple sanitation measures but also disease eradication efforts. For instance, schistosomiasis, a parasite that spends part of its life

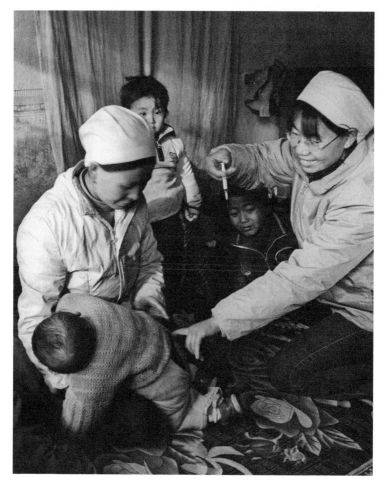

Figure 2.3. A woman helps one of China's barefoot doctors with nursing duties in Luo Quan Wan village.

Source: Copyright © Yves Gellie/Corbis.

in snails, was eradicated by a public works program that rid the rivers of the snail that hosts the parasite.

China's communist years did see some of the greatest public health disasters in the recent history of human civilization. The "Great Leap Forward," for instance, was a national policy aimed at mobilizing China's massive workforce to produce large quantities of steel. Unfortunately, farmers are not steel workers and the steel was of extremely low quality. And making it required pulling workers out of agriculture and other life-sustaining industries within their largely closed economy. The massive starvation that followed caused a ten- to twenty-year drop in life expectancy. The Maoist government also tortured and publicly humiliated entrepreneurs or suspected traitors, further endangering population health and well-being.

Still, China saw large and consistent improvements in life expectancy through the communist years. This was because the government made large investments in sewage, sanitation, education, and basic health care. As a result, it probably underwent an epidemiologic transition somewhere in the 1960s or 1970s. Interestingly, this happened despite relatively weak progress in nutrition.

In the 1980s, China began to transition to a capitalist model. This model involved creating special enterprise zones (SEZs), in which capitalism could flourish in a confined and controlled environment. The SEZ's policies encouraged foreign direct investment, streamlined processes for starting businesses, and implemented competitive taxation rates. The most successful of China's five original SEZs, Shenzhen, grew from a fishing village of twenty-five thousand to a city of ten million in just two decades.

China's economic reforms also dismantled the commune system, which was the source of community and health care for the average Chinese person. Under the traditional system, rural dwellers were mostly organized into small groups called *communes*. Each commune had one of the barefoot doctors associated with it, and the barefoot doctor was funded by local and central sources. Under the reforms, the barefoot doctors mostly disappeared (or became private doctors focused on curative rather than preventive care) alongside the communes.

Public health programs also generally went by the wayside. School fees, and even fees for vaccinations, were required in some places. The gains of the previous thirty years slowly yielded to outbreaks of infectious disease and great hardship for some of China's poor. For the newly rich, however, it created the opportunity to move from a future of cramped dormitory life to four-story mansions, replete with koi ponds running under glass floors, tennis courts, and a pool.

Toward the end of the twentieth century, for the first time in many years, large numbers of Chinese went without health care. At the same time, the rising class of entrepreneurs enjoyed access to medical technologies previously reserved only for the highest-ranking party officials.

Local officials began to own and operate businesses. These officials worked with other business owners to build factories and power plants that spewed effluent into waterways used for drinking water. In some cases, the officials did not own the businesses, but they did receive kickbacks from polluters to skirt rules. Some of the rural poor were relegated to sifting their water from toxic sludge before boiling it and drinking it. Unsurprisingly, villagers along some of these waterways were reported to have mostly died young of cancer or other complications of industrial pollutants, such as liver failure.

One classic example of one of the industrial pollutants now common in China is lead. Lead is a heavy metal that primarily causes brain damage, sapping youth of their future as professionals in China's rising capitalist society (Muennig, 2009; Schwartz, 1994). Although regulations technically forbid human settlement around smelter plants, these were largely ignored because factory owners wanted workers in close proximity to their workplace. Childhood lead poisoning cases soared as a result.

Air pollution has become so bad in China's many urban centers that only rare, highly favorable atmospheric conditions yield days when it is safe to go outside. Because people essentially must go outside, lung diseases such as pneumonia have reached epidemic proportions (Xu, Gao, & Chen, 1994). Wealthier Chinese are protected by air-conditioned private cars and offices with filtered air. The poor still ride bicycles to work—something we would associate with a healthy lifestyle in industrialized nations but which is a dire threat in China's urban centers (even more so now that cars vastly outnumber bicycles).

Important regulations, such as occupational safety or consumer protections, have, in some instances, taken a backseat to economic growth. In others, they fall prey to corrupt local politicians who fear such regulations will cut into profits. In fact, such regulations do increase the cost of doing business. Some argue that they must be ignored if the nation is to maintain its 10 percent economic growth rate (an average of values between 2003 and 2013), and others argue that pollution will cost future growth prospects (BBC World Service, 2008; Neidell, 2004; Xu et al., 1994). Peasants routinely fall to their deaths from construction sites, are crushed in mining accidents, or die from tainted medicines and foods. These deaths too often go unnoticed within a country that controls what does and does not go into the media. Although some are reported, many of these incidents are picked up only by foreign journalists who happen to stumble on them or by webizens who risk prosecution for reporting them.

Even with press restrictions, these ecological and safety problems have led to unrest. As more citizens risked arrest and detention in "black prisons" to protest China's environmental, health, and public safety problems, the central government began to take notice. ("Black prisons" are extralegal centers used by Chinese security forces to detain, without trial, citizens who travel to regional or central government offices to address grievances they could not resolve at the local level.) In 2006, Hu Jintao declared a new period of "harmony," in which social safety net programs would be reinstituted and the environment would be given serious attention. Unfortunately, these programs to date have been difficult to implement because the local officials in control of polluting factories have chosen largely to ignore them.

Still, the government is actively working to overcome these problems, and it is pushing ahead with a variety of national programs in health, housing, and education. One such reform surrounds an attempt to reinvest in rural health programs. Each locality has been given matching funds for health care and has been asked to design its own unique health program. These funds amount to US$2.50 per person in 2009 dollars. The state and the patient must come up with another US$2.50 and US$1.25, respectively. These programs, although totaling only US$6.25 on the high end (a figure that has since increased), have added financial relief for catastrophic illness in rural areas. Some localities, such as Daxing near Beijing, have had great success in implementing minimal basic health programs (personal communication).

China is fortunate in that it completed its epidemiologic and demographic transitions before undertaking market reforms. Indeed, these transitions have provided a jumping-off platform for its remarkable economic success. The question now is whether its economic growth has been so unchecked that China's larger environment will survive. Unless there are significant breakthroughs in environmental technology that China can afford to use, China's environment might eventually collapse, creating major public health problems for its citizens.

KERALA'S QUALITY OF LIFE

Kerala is a state in southern India with around thirty million people packed into a relatively small area. It is a poor state, ranking toward the bottom of India's per capita GDP rankings (Parayil, 1996; Ratcliffe, 1978; Veron, 2001). Nevertheless, it ranks at the top in terms of life expectancy, public health infrastructure, and literacy. It also has among the country's (and the world's) lowest infant mortality and birth rates.

Although most states within India are predominantly male—a combined result of sex-selective abortions and giving female children less food or resources when money runs short—Kerala has a male-to-female ratio comparable to most European nations. In fact, many measures of health and education are in the ballpark range of much wealthier nations.

To many, these positive statistics are shocking. After all, health and wealth are supposed to be two great things that go great together. Certainly Costa Rica, Chile, and many other low- or middle-income countries have achieved high levels of literacy and life expectancy with relatively little economic power, but these nations are by no means quite as poor. Cuba is neck and neck with the United States on measures such as life expectancy, but it devotes a huge proportion of its resources to education and health. Kerala, in contrast, is something of a miracle, at least at first glance. After all, many in Kerala lack even basic necessities, such as cooking ware or bedding.

How has Kerala achieved this? One clue lies in its long history of education funding. In the early part of the twentieth century, local royalty ceded to the demands of its people for more schools. Girls were not shunned for wanting to read or learn math. By mid-century, Kerala's literacy, life expectancy, and male-to-female ratios were already among the best in India.

In 1959, a democratically elected communist government began wider-scale schooling programs and coupled them with public health initiatives. In 1988, early efforts culminated in a massive attempt to mobilize as many educated Keralans as possible to teach even previously out-of-reach villagers how to read and write. Many texts were translated into local languages, such as Malayalam. Before long, the percentage of literate Keralans had climbed and Kerala had broken away from Indian averages, instead chasing much richer nations in terms of literacy and longevity.

Kerala makes for an interesting case study because it is poor and has achieved greatness in measures of human development. However, it is also famous because it has enacted "communist" or "socialist" policies in the context of a democracy. It even has environmental protections in place that are stronger than one typically sees in a low-income region. For these reasons, Kerala has been touted as a model for sustainable development (Heller, 2012; Parayil, 1996).

The main countries that have come close to achieving similar sustainable development goals are Scandinavian ones. Norway, for instance, ranked first on the HDI and Global Peace Index in 2007 (albeit aided by massive crude oil reserves). Scandinavian countries have invested heavily in health and education and have stringent environmental regulations. By minimizing environmental degradation and maximizing the well-being of future generations, these countries are seen as much more likely to remain viable over many generations. Thus, the Kerala model has been proposed as a sort of "Scandinavia light" for poor countries.

Does Kerala help us understand what makes for healthy, sustainable development? Certainly, much of Kerala's success comes on the back of literacy and public health policies. But it also partly arose from a relatively cohesive, somewhat matrilineal society dominated by *aliya kattu*, a property inheritance system in which female children inherit the majority of a mother's belongings. So it may be impossible to disentangle the state's underlying culture from its successful policies.

Indeed, political scientists have debated for years whether homogenous or more cohesive societies are more likely to enact health-producing social policy, so we will never really know for sure how much of which is responsible for health (Orloff & Skocpol, 1984; Skocpol, 1979; Weir, Orloff, & Skocpol, 1988).

Some researchers contend that Kerala boosters may have overstated their case (Veron, 2001). With all of the regulations in place, the Kerala government has recognized its need to improve the way that the government functions. Most of the state's low level of environmental destruction, for example, may partly be attributed to its lack of industry. The same might be said of Kerala's nondemocratic cousin, Cuba. In the case of Cuba, it is poverty and economic isolation more than good intentions about a green revolution or sustainable development that initially led to an uptake in organic farming. In fact, the nation's agricultural profile is now retreating and looking toward a more capitalism-based farming model.

Nevertheless, Kerala and Cuba demonstrate that a nation does not have to be rich to be well educated and healthy (see figure 2.4). Poignantly, Kerala has been able to achieve impressive outcomes without coercion or human rights violations. As with any case study, readers should keep in mind that

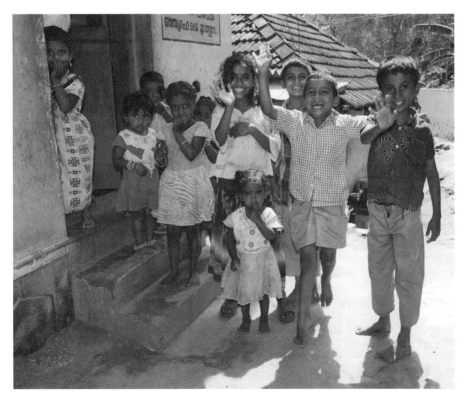

Figure 2.4. Children outside a school in Kerala.

Source: Christopher Michel Photography. Available at www.flickr.com/photos/cmichel67/4077411904/.

these examples serve to illustrate only what *might be* the cause of better health rather than what *is* the case for better health.

CHILE AIMS FOR A BALANCING ACT

Chile has a long history of having a largely bifurcated society, especially in terms of class and political ideology. On one side, there are many Chileans who oppose more expansive support-led reforms and who hope for a low-tax, high-performance economy. (Recall that "support-led" refers to policies that favor social welfare over economic growth.) On the other side are a large number of progressive Chileans who demand social investments in the name of social justice. These two competing forces have created a rich experiment in economic versus social reform that gives us a sense of how these competing investments may have affected Chilean life expectancy (figure 2.5).

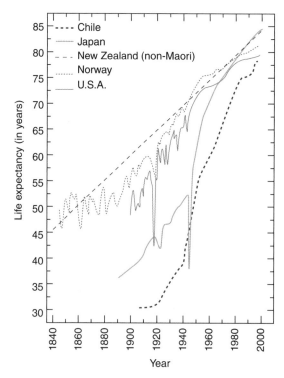

Figure 2.5. Life expectancy of women in Chile relative to Japan, the United States, New Zealand, and Norway.

Source: Oeppen, J., & Vaupel, J. W. (2002). Broken limits to life expectancy. *Science, 296*(5570), 1029. Retrieved from www.sciencemag.org/content/296/5570/1029 .summary.

The solid line in figure 2.5 represents the moving average of female life expectancy over time. Chile had extraordinary increases in life expectancy through around 1980, which then again started to rise quickly in the late 1990s.

In the 1920s and for much of the 1930s, right-leaning parties dominated Chilean politics (Collier & Sater, 1996). This was in no small part due to the electoral laws allowing only literate men to vote. Because the majority of the country was poor and illiterate, this meant that only the elite class, which previously held power as dictators, would be elected into office. The slow rise of a middle class did lead to a slow trickle of reformers into office, including the office of the presidency.

The right-wing dominance was interrupted, however briefly, by the Great Depression, leading to some reforms. For instance, limited suffrage was granted to women in the early 1930s (Pernet, 2000). Then, in 1938, an unsuccessful military coup by the socialists was brutally suppressed, leading to a backlash. This coup and backlash angered Chileans to the point that Pedro Aguirre Cerda was voted into office (Collier & Sater, 1996). Aguirre Cerda's left-leaning administration focused on education reform, building thousands of schools. It also invested heavily in public health measures, slowly bringing sanitation, cleaner water, improved nutrition, and vaccination programs to the masses.

Most important, the administration enacted electoral reforms that largely entrenched left-leaning parties in the Chilean political machine. For instance, they not only removed restrictions on whether women or those with less education could vote, but they also made voting compulsory. This had the effect of bringing the poor masses into the political process and helping to ensure future leftist victories.

During this period, the government continued to make heavy investments in health, public health, and education. These investments accelerated until the welfare state consumed much of the economy. Land reforms (including expropriations of large land holdings and subsidies for small farms), coupled with heavy investments in education and health, led to dramatic increases in life expectancy among the poor. The country entered its demographic transition in the 1940s, rapidly climbing from a life expectancy of around thirty years in 1920 to sixty years by 1960—nearly one year of life expectancy gained per year of time passed.

However, all of this did little for the Chilean economy. Despite its abundance of health and mineral wealth (especially copper), Chile's economic growth was quite slow. Then, in the 1970s, President Salvador Allende attempted to open clinics twenty-four hours a day and pushed through a number of far-reaching social programs. He also gave huge raises to public sector employees. This huge boost in government spending led to soaring economic growth, rapidly followed by hyperinflation, debt, and economic chaos.

A PRIMER ON THE ECONOMICS OF DEVELOPMENT

Most nations are in control of how much currency is in circulation. As a result, there is a huge temptation to simply print (or create in digital form) currency to pay off a nation's debt. When this happens, though, the supply of the nation's currency increases. Unless the economy is shrinking and the currency is deflating anyway, printing money will lead to inflation.

Something similar happens when wages are increased. More money in people's pockets leads to more spending, which leads to more economic growth and, ultimately, inflation. This can cause an **inflationary spiral**—a condition in which the cost of goods increases so it becomes necessary to raise wages, which then also contributes to increases in the cost of goods.

Inflation also reduces the value of the currency relative to other nation's currencies (as we all learned in economics, an increase in the supply of something reduces the cost of that thing). When the value of a nation's currency falls relative to others, it becomes cheaper to buy things that the country produces, so its exports tend to increase. This can give a huge boost to a nation's economy, but it also makes foreign goods more expensive. The combination of economic growth (which creates inflation overall) and higher prices for imports (which creates inflation in some goods) can result in a situation that quickly spirals out of control. Therefore, reducing a currency's value can also have a huge inflationary effect, particularly in countries that rely on critical imported goods such as food.

This is important for health because falling into poverty is not good for the average citizen. For instance, it can affect a family's nutrition, ability to buy medicines, and quality of the housing.

The economic crisis endangered the survival of the Allende administration. In addition, the US government used operatives to assassinate Allende's supporters in the Chilean military and worked in conjunction with his detractors to stage a coup in 1973 (Collier & Sater, 2004).

The years between 1973 and 1989 were marked by decentralization (public schools, for instance, went from being nationally funded to being governed and funded by local municipalities) and defunding of social services. Thousands of people "disappeared" in the coup (and were never recorded as official deaths), tens of thousands were interned and tortured, and an additional two hundred thousand or so fled into exile (Ensalaco, 2000). Even setting these disappearances aside, Chile experienced a slight slowdown in life expectancy during these years (Oeppen & Vaupel, 2002), even as it realized a large boom in economic growth by the 1980s. Augusto Pinochet, the brutal dictator installed in the 1973 coup, called a general election and was defeated. In 1990, a center-left coalition was elected to office.

Chile potentially serves as a counterfactual to the Cuba, China, and Kerala examples because it has excellent health and educational outcomes coupled with low fertility but a very different history. Even though Chile is a bit better off and Chilean life expectancy data are fairly reliable over much of the twentieth century, it is still difficult to guess how changes in Chilean policy might have affected life expectancy. Education enhancement probably takes years to affect life expectancy or fertility rates, for instance, so any rapid changes in governance are difficult to map to either of these important outcomes.

If we humor this notion that social programs and democracy could be linked, we see that life expectancy skyrocketed after the reforms of the 1930s and leveled off after these social programs were defunded in the late 1970s and 1980s (the periods of fastest economic growth; see figure 2.5). It increased again after social democracy returned in the 1990s.

The real reason we have included the Chilean case study, though, is to show that a nation need not be a totalitarian communist state nor impoverish itself with social spending to achieve a long life expectancy. With relatively modest means, it has achieved a life expectancy that is equal to that of the United States (about seventy-eight years for both countries).

Unlike the Keralan or Cuban cases, Chile's development has been far from environmentally sustainable. Environmental protections have only recently become front and center in Chile's official policy. These environmental policies also tend to be a bit weak. Of course, Chile is destroying its habitat at a slower rate than China.

A note: You also may have noticed that our brief descriptions of the different models focused most on the governments' economic policies with only short mentions of politics, even though we included labels such as *capitalist, socialist,* and *communist.* Why? One reason is that it is really difficult to place a concise but accurate label on a country. How can China be a "communist country," for instance, after decades of dismantling communes and public enterprises? How can a Chilean "socialist" president aggressively pursue market-oriented policies? Even Cuba is slowly giving way to a model that looks a lot like China's. The relationship among public health, development, and politics is a complicated one, and we will hold off on focusing on that piece of the puzzle until chapter 6.

SUMMARY

Although most of the world's wealthiest nations (with respect to per capita GDP) rank among the top nations worldwide in terms of life expectancy, there are some exceptions. Likewise, although most of the poorest nations rank toward the bottom, some of these nations and states rank closer to the top. Many experts believe that health and life expectancy are less dependent on whether a nation is rich but rather on how the nation spends its money. Cuba and the state of Kerala within India provide two examples of how the right social policies may improve population health. If we take a historical perspective, Chile's story also suggests that health can be gained or lost depending on the investments made. China appears to have initially damaged its prospects for rapid gains in life expectancy during its conversion to a capitalist model of development. As of now, though, it seems to be on track to repairing this damage as it invests in transit, health care, and healthy cities. This brings us to the next unit, which focuses on policy as a means to better health.

KEY TERMS

barefoot doctors
global north
global south
growth-mediated economy
human capital

industrializing nations
inflationary spiral
least-developed countries
Preston curve
social capital

support-led model
sustainable development
wealth-health gradient

DISCUSSION QUESTIONS

1. What is the Preston curve? What puzzles does it present for global health policy makers?

2. What does a growth-mediated model of development look like? What are some of its strengths and weaknesses?

3. What does a support-led model of development look like? What are some of its strengths and weaknesses?

4. Based on the very short summaries you have read thus far, what do you think the key characteristics of China's current development situation might be? Its key challenges? What about for Kerala and Chile?

5. Think about another middle- or high-income country you know well. Was its development path similar to that of any of the case studies? Did it pass labor, environmental, educational, and other regulations

before, during, or after rapid economic growth? Talk about two to three specific major programs or pieces of legislation in your answer. For instance, in the case of the United States, consider pieces of legislation such as the Wagner Act, New Deal, Clean Air Act, and so on.

6. Do current middle-income countries face the same sorts of development challenges that industrialized nations such as England, Japan, and the United States did in the last century? What has changed?

FURTHER READING

Wallich, P. (1995). Mystery inside a riddle inside an enigma. *Scientific American*, March, 37.

REFERENCES

Acemoglu, D., & Johnson, S. (2006). *Disease and development: The effect of life expectancy on economic growth*. Cambridge, MA: National Bureau of Economic Research.

BBC World Service. (2008, August 11). *Beijing pollution: Facts and figures*. Available online at http://news.bbc.co.uk/2/hi/asia-pacific/7498198.stm

Collier, S., & Sater, W. F. (1996). *A history of Chile, 1808–1994* (Vol. 82). Cambridge, UK: Cambridge University Press.

Collier, S., & Sater, W. F. (2004). *A history of Chile, 1808–2002* (Vol. 82). Cambridge, UK: Cambridge University Press.

Drèze, J., & Sen, A. K. (1989). *Hunger and public action*. New York: Oxford University Press.

Economist. (2012, November 3). Bangladesh and development: The path through the fields. Available online at www.economist.com/news/briefing/21565617 -bangladesh-has-dysfunctional-politics-and-stunted-private-sector-yet-it-has-been -surprisingly

Ensalaco, M. (2000). *Chile under Pinochet: Recovering the truth*. Philadelphia: University of Pennsylvania Press.

Epel, E. S., Blackburn, E. H., Lin, J., Dhabhar, F. S., Adler, N. E., Morrow, J. D., & Cawthon, R. M. (2004). Accelerated telomere shortening in response to life stress. *Proceedings of the National Academy of Science of the United States of America*, *101*(49), 17312–17315.

Evans, P. (2006). Population health and development: An institutional-cultural approach to capability expansion. *Successful societies*. Washington, DC: World Bank.

Friedman, M. (1982). *Capitalism and freedom*. Chicago: University of Chicago Press.

Heller, P. (2012). Democracy, participatory politics and development: Some comparative lessons from Brazil, India and South Africa. *Polity, 44*(4), 643–665.

Kawachi, I., Subramanian, S. V., & Kim, D. (2010). *Social capital and health*. New York: Springer.

Kim, D., Subramanian, S. V., & Kawachi, I. (2006). Bonding versus bridging social capital and their associations with self-rated health: A multilevel analysis of 40 US communities. *Journal of Epidemiology and Community Health, 60*(2), 116–122.

Muennig, P. (2009). The social costs of childhood lead exposure in the post-lead regulation era. *Archives of Pediatrics and Adolescent Medicine, 163*(9), 844–849. doi: 163/9/844 [pii]10.1001/archpediatrics.2009.128.

Muennig, P., Cohen, A. K., Palmer, A., & Zhu, W. (February 2013). The relationship between five different measures of structural social capital, medical examination outcomes, and mortality. *Social Science & Medicine, 85*.

Neidell, M. J. (2004). Air pollution, health, and socio-economic status: The effect of outdoor air quality on childhood asthma. *Journal of Health Economics, 23*(6), 1209–1236.

Oeppen, J., & Vaupel, J. W. (2002). Broken limits to life expectancy. *Science, 296*(5570), 1029.

Orloff, A. S., & Skocpol, T. (1984). Why not equal protection? Explaining the politics of public social spending in Britain, 1900–1911, and the United States, 1880s–1920. *American Sociological Review, 49*(6), 726–750.

Parayil, G. (1996). The "Kerala model" of development: Development and sustainability in the third world. *Third World Quarterly, 17*(5), 941–957.

Pernet, C. A. (2000). Chilean feminists, the international women's movement, and suffrage, 1915–1950. *Pacific Historical Review, 69*(4), 663–688.

Preston, S. H. (1976). *Mortality patterns in national populations: With special reference to recorded causes of death*. New York: Academic Press.

Putnam, R. D. (1995). Tuning in, tuning out: The strange disappearance of social capital in America. *Political Science and Politics, 28*, 664–683.

Ratcliffe, J. (1978). Social justice and the demographic transition: Lessons from India's Kerala State. *International Journal Health Services, 8*(1), 123–144.

Schwartz, J. (1994). Low-level lead exposure and children's IQ: A meta-analysis and search for a threshold. *Environmental Research, 65*(1), 42–55. doi: S0013–9351(84)71020–6 [pii]10.1006/enrs.1994.1020.

Sen, A. (1999). *Development as freedom*. New York: Knopf.

Singh, G. K., & Miller, B. A. (2004). Health, life expectancy, and mortality patterns among immigrant populations in the United States. *Canadian Journal of Public Health, 95*, 114–121.

Skocpol, T. (1979). *States and social revolutions: Comparative analysis of France, Russia, and China*. Cambridge, UK: Cambridge University Press.

Veron, R. (2001). The "new" Kerala model: Lessons for sustainable development. *World Development, 29*(4), 601–617.

WECD. (1987). *Our common future*. New York: Oxford University Press.

Weir, M., Orloff, A. S., & Skocpol, T. (1988). *The politics of social policy in the United States*. Princeton, NJ: Princeton University Press.

Xu, X., Gao, J., & Chen, Y. (1994). Air pollution and daily mortality in residential areas of Beijing, China. *Archives of Environmental Health: An International Journal, 49*(4), 216–222. doi: 10.1080/00039896.1994.9937470.

PART TWO

Global Health and the Art of Policy Making

CHAPTER 3

The Global Burden of Disease

KEY IDEAS

- The global health community needs to shift our focus from how many people get sick to why they get sick and what we can do about it.

- Burden of disease analysis tells us how much suffering and death there is among a given group or in a given place on earth.

- Cost-effectiveness analysis tells us how many lives we can save with a particular amount of money.

Burden of disease refers to how much disease and death are present in a given place (e.g., Zambia) or among a group of people (e.g., poor rural farmers). Once we know which health problems are present and where, we can start to do something about them. Maybe.

But just how do we figure out how to make public health investments? One approach is to look at where people are dying at much higher rates than in other places. But how do we think about what it is about the characteristics of such places that make people sick? Is it the poorest nations that need our attention? Focusing on such nations might lead us to invest in places such as Cuba, where people only earn a dollar a day. But although this might generally be a good approach, people in Cuba live longer than in many rich nations, so universal investments in the poorest nations do not make complete sense. Another way of thinking about this is by geography. Some parts of the world are sicker than others (thus the *global north* and *global south* designations) but that logic does not consistently work either. Even if we hone our criteria down to focus on regions such as Latin America, Asia, and Africa, we ignore that some nations are doing well in terms of health and others not so well. It is also a problem that neither geography nor wealth really tells us much about what we should be doing to improve people's health. Another way of thinking about health is in terms of which policies are needed and where. Burden of disease analysis can help inform these kinds of policy actions and investments.

In this chapter, we will explore the major causes of disease among adults and children. Some of these can be addressed with very simple, tried-and-true public health interventions: vitamin A supplementation for malnourished people, clean water, vaccination, and healthy meal preparation in the face of food scarcity. These are a few essential steps that will be discussed throughout this book that can be used to address leading causes of disease in low-income countries. For middle- and high-income countries, the solutions are more complicated but can also probably be addressed if only there were enough funding. Let us begin by asking where diseases are located.

WHO DIES WHERE?

The leading causes of death worldwide can be found in table 3.1. These numbers are not perfect. It is very difficult to tell how many people there are in many poor nations, let alone whether they are alive or dead. And if we know whether they are alive or dead, we still have to figure out what they died from. With this in mind, take a look at table 3.1.

We see that the leading causes of death are heart disease, stroke, pneumonia, and chronic obstructive pulmonary disease (COPD), that is, most people worldwide go because either their heart or their lungs give out on them. But as we have mentioned before, the biggest threats to human health vary

Table 3.1. Counting Deaths Worldwide, by Disease

	Number of deaths (in millions)	Percentage of all deaths
Heart disease	7.25	12.8
Stroke	6.15	10.8
Pneumonia	3.46	6.1
COPD	3.28	5.8
Diarrhea	2.46	4.3
HIV/AIDS	1.78	3.1
Tuberculosis	1.34	2.4

Source: WHO. (2011). *The top 10 causes of death.* Fact sheet no. 310. Available online at http://who.int/mediacentre/factsheets/fs310/en/.

Note: COPD is the acronym for chronic obstructive pulmonary disease.

greatly from country to country, so knowing the overall burden of disease of stroke might be interesting to some people, but it does not help us set up policies that will make people any healthier because policies to reduce stroke are usually applied at the local level.

The World Bank argues that it is possible to understand these threats according to a nation's level of economic development. The WHO argues that global region is also important (Murray & Lopez, 1996). (The WHO does look at these problems in many different ways.) In reality, prevalent diseases and other causes of mortality and morbidity vary even *within* countries. At the time of writing, 30 percent of China's population was still living on US$2 per day. (This, in a nation that has put humans into outer space.)

One way to think about the global burden of disease is to explore deaths by level of development. In figure 3.1, we see the relative number of deaths due to infectious and noninfectious causes by level of economic development. Here, we see that noncommunicable diseases dominate in wealthier nations and infectious diseases dominate in poorer nations. (Note that these traditional distinctions will probably one day soon be replaced because we are learning that many noncommunicable diseases, such as obesity, may actually be spread from person to person [Christakis & Fowler, 2007]). At any rate, behaviors such

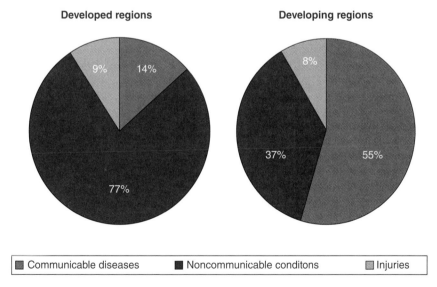

Figure 3.1. Death by broad cause group.

Source: UC Atlas of Global Inequality. Available online from http://ucatlas.ucsc.edu/cause.php.

as smoking are almost certainly transmitted from person to person via social circles (Christakis & Fowler, 2008).

This "big picture" graph hides all of the details. When we look a little deeper, we might consider what the breakdown looks like for specific causes of death for less-developed nations, middle-income countries, and the wealthiest nations (see table 3.2).

If we think in these terms, we see that middle-income countries and high-income countries generally face the same problems. We can get some rough sense of what the policies underlying these causes of death might be. For example, chronic obstructive pulmonary disease (COPD, a condition resulting from damaged lung tissue) and lower respiratory infections (almost all of this is pneumonia) are caused mostly by smoking and air pollution. Those that have lived through smoking and air pollution are more likely to die of lung cancer in their old age. So, we see that middle-income countries have more of an active challenge in confronting smoking and air pollution (because they are facing shorter-term respiratory problems such as pneumonia) and that wealthier countries are confronting the aftermath of these problems (because there are high rates of longer-term problems, such as lung cancer).

But we also see something curious. Stomach cancer is a bigger problem in middle-income countries than in high-income countries. It turns out that stomach cancer is a regional or cultural issue related to diet, and it is a much larger problem in Asia than elsewhere. This may be an argument for thinking in terms of regions, as the WHO does. Figure 3.2 shows what happens when we look at nations by region. This is a graph of child mortality rates. Even here, high-income countries clump together because the problems tend to be similar. When we take this perspective, we see that perinatal conditions are big problems in Africa. (Perinatal conditions—conditions that occur right before, during, and after birth—are highly responsive to quality health care. One definition of perinatal is the period three months prior to birth through one month after birth.)

Sarah Palin, a former candidate for vice president of the United States, was accused of thinking that Africa was a nation and not knowing that Africa was a continent. Whether or not this is true, the WHO is just as guilty—some nations in Africa actually do pretty well with respect to child mortality rates. For example, even with a high rate of HIV/AIDS, child mortality rates in Botswana were 25.9 per 1,000 children, similar to those in the Dominican Republic, Ecuador, and Egypt (UN, 2012).

Simple regional analyses might be useful in helping us decide where, more generally, aid dollars should be going and for what. But that is a pretty crude tool: if we use these guidelines, we should be sending aid to "Europe," given its much higher rate of perinatal conditions than other "high-income" countries. (Of course, high-income countries are not actually included in those

Table 3.2. Leading Causes of Death for the World Overall and by Level of Economic Development

Disease or injury	Deaths (in millions)	Percent of total deaths	Disease or injury	Deaths (in millions)	Percent of total deaths
World			*Low-income countries*		
Ischemic heart disease	7.25	12.8	Lower respiratory infections	1.05	11.3
Stroke and other cerebrovascular disease	6.15	10.8	Diarrheal diseases	0.76	8.2
Lower respiratory infections	3.46	6.1	HIV/AIDS	0.72	7.8
COPD	3.28	5.8	Ischemic heart disease	0.57	6.1
Diarrheal diseases	2.46	4.3	Malaria	0.48	5.2
HIV/AIDS	1.78	3.1	Stroke and other cerebrovascular disease	0.45	4.9
Trachea, bronchus, lung cancers	1.39	2.4	Tuberculosis	0.40	4.3
Tuberculosis	1.34	2.4	Prematurity and low birth weight	0.30	3.2
Diabetes mellitus	1.26	2.2	Birth asphyxia and birth trauma	0.27	2.9
Road traffic accidents	1.21	2.1	Neonatal infections	0.24	2.6
Middle-income countries			*High-income countries*		
Ischemic heart disease	5.27	13.7	Ischemic heart disease	1.42	15.6
Stroke and other cerebrovascular disease	4.91	12.8	Stroke and other cerebrovascular disease	0.79	8.7
COPD	2.79	7.2	Trachea, bronchus, lung cancers	0.54	5.9
Lower respiratory infections	2.07	5.4	Alzheimer and other dementias	0.37	4.1
Diarrheal diseases	1.68	4.4	Lower respiratory infections	0.35	3.8
HIV/AIDS	1.03	2.7	COPD	0.32	3.5
Road traffic accidents	0.94	2.4	Colon and rectum cancers	0.30	3.3
Tuberculosis	0.93	2.4	Diabetes mellitus	0.24	2.6
Diabetes mellitus	0.87	2.3	Hypertensive heart disease	0.21	2.3
Hypertensive heart disease	0.83	2.2	Breast cancer	0.17	1.9

Source: WHO. (2011). *The top 10 causes of death*. Fact sheet no. 310. Available online at http://who.int/mediacentre/factsheets/fs310/en/.

Note: COPD is the acronym for chronic obstructive pulmonary disease.

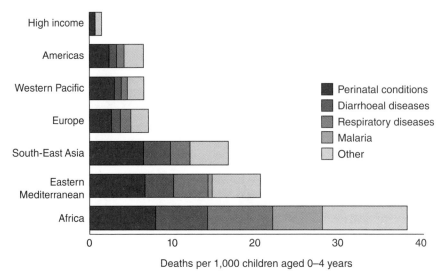

Figure 3.2. Child mortality rates by cause and region.

Source: WHO. (2004). *The global burden of disease: Part 2.* Available online at www
.who.int/healthinfo/global_burden_disease/GBD_report_2004update_part2.pdf.

statistics; it is poor former Soviet nations that are driving the higher rates of
child mortality in these European nations.)

As noted in chapter 2, Kerala has achieved health statistics on par with
the most economically developed nations. Cuba, one of the poorest nations
in the world, is in tough competition with the United States, one of the wealthiest, for the best infant mortality rates and longevity statistics. In either of these
"least-developed" states, we would be hard pressed to find the raging childhood diarrheal illness that the World Bank predicts based on economic indicators or those that the WHO predicts based on geographic location. Within the
United States, Hawaii boasts of a life expectancy of eighty-two years (similar
to Sweden or Japan), whereas Mississippi and the District of Columbia residents live to be an average of seventy-three or seventy-four years (lower than
the impoverished state of Kerala in India) (Burd-Sharps, Lewis, & Martins,
2008).

One last point about figure 3.2 is that perinatal conditions are highly sensitive to access to quality health care, diarrheal illness is highly dependent on
clean water, and respiratory disease is highly dependent on clean air. Therefore,
we would need to effectively invest in these three areas if we are to reduce
childhood mortality in areas where it is high. In fact, too often overlooked in

Table 3.3. Counting Deaths Worldwide by Disease and the Most Relevant Policy for Addressing the Disease

	Number of deaths (in millions)	Percentage of all deaths	Most relevant policies
Heart disease	7.25	12.8	Nutrition, transit, green cities
Stroke	6.15	10.8	Nutrition, transit, green cities
Pneumonia	3.46	6.1	Transit, green cities
COPD	3.28	5.8	Transit, green cities
Diarrhea	2.46	4.3	Sewage, sanitation, nutrition
HIV/AIDS	1.78	3.1	Preventive practices
Tuberculosis	1.34	2.4	Nutrition, medical care, housing

Source: WHO. (2011). *The top 10 causes of death.* Fact sheet no. 310. Available online at http://who.int/mediacentre/factsheets/fs310/en/.

Note: COPD is the acronym for chronic obstructive pulmonary disease.

discussions about the global burden of disease is what one actually does about these problems. Therefore, we have added a category, "most relevant policies," that helps sort out problems by their solution to table 3.1 (see table 3.3.)

COUNTING GLOBAL DEATHS (WITH AN EYE TOWARD SAVING LIVES)

We could also analyze which countries or localities have adopted pro-health policies and which have not. Those that have generally conquered infectious disease have done so via improved sanitation, clean water, and vaccination practices. Safe transit policies also seem to be important (Birn, 2009; Epp, 1986). Looking at the global burden of disease in this way gets around the problem of using geographical or income categories. Not only does this allow us to pinpoint communities in need of policy action, but it also helps us think more about the solutions we need to emphasize rather than the problems we have. Of course, no approach is perfect. Hong Kong, a world leader in life expectancy, has not adopted many of the pro-health policies we discuss. And cultural and historical factors, ones that are not always reflected in social policy, probably matter a lot. It also creates a demand for still more data from areas where data is most difficult to come by. Still, a policy perspective's demand for specificity forces us to measure those things that we should have been measuring all along; rather than just counting bodies of dead children, it forces us to count those things that are killing them in the first place.

INDOOR POLLUTANTS AND THE GLOBAL BURDEN OF DISEASE

When we think of heart disease and stroke, the image of a smoker should immediately come to mind. But many people in low-income countries cook with wood or coal indoors (see figure 3.3). This effectively creates an entire family of smokers. Many organizations are now focusing on combating indoor air pollution as one concrete means to lower chronic disease in low- and middle-income countries.

We might therefore think of one category of nations as those that have succeeded in implementing basic public health policies, heart disease, cancer, stroke, and accidents are the leading killers. Life expectancy in these countries

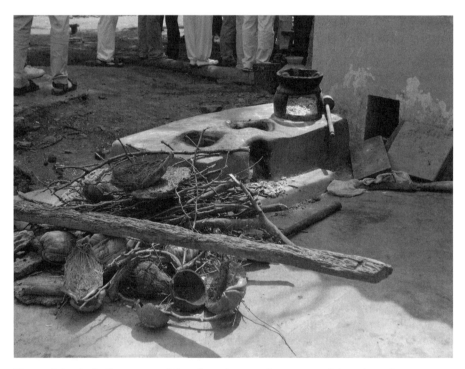

Figure 3.3. A chulla, or a traditional outdoor cook stove used in India. This particular chulla is going to be lit using branches, scrap wood, dried dung cakes, and coconut shells.

Source: McKay Savage. Available online at www.flickr.com/photos/mckaysavage/ 3976613716/.

tends to be more than seventy years. Many believe that the leading causes of death in wealthier nations—a second category of countries that might be added to this list—may be better tackled with improved health systems, education, public transit, and safety net programs.

A third category of countries might also be added. This includes countries that provide comprehensive social services. Similar to the countries in the second category, heart disease, cancer, and stroke predominate but at much lower levels. Accidents and homicides are rare causes of death (Ohsfeldt & Schneider, 2006). These countries tend to have life expectancies more than eighty years. Using this policy approach, Qatar, one of the wealthiest nations on earth, might fall into the same category as Cuba, one of the poorest. Both have similar life expectancies.

Still, a final category might be added. These include the highly socially regulated societies of Asia, including Singapore and Japan. It is too early to convincingly add or categorize these nations as a distinct entity, but they are

SO, WHY DON'T WE JUST PUT IT IN PLACE?

Many experts believe that simple latrines would go a long way toward bumping up the world's life expectancy. At this point, you might be asking yourself: "If poor countries really need latrines the most, and they are so cheap to put in place, why are so many people doing their business on the bare earth?" Imagine that a major aid agency, such as the United States Agency for International Development (USAID), gives a nation such as the Democratic Republic of the Congo a large grant. With poorly developed financial institutions, how do we make sure that the money is deposited and then safely distributed to public health agencies? Without a fully functioning ministry of transportation, how do we get workers and equipment out to rural areas where latrines are needed most? Without a functioning criminal justice system, how do we ensure that things are not stolen along the way? If people believed in these institutions, they would work. But people in the Democratic Republic of the Congo have good reason not to believe in such institutions—they have had their goods stolen from them and seen corruption in action for years. Why would things today be any different? Well, one reason is that this nation began an experiment with democracy in the first part of the twenty-first century that is slowly taking hold. There is hope that these institutions will get strong enough that we actually can one day get those latrines built.

Table 3.4. Counting Deaths Worldwide by Preventive Policy Needed

Potential policy and remedy	Number of deaths averted (in millions)	Percentage of all deaths
Nutrition, transit, green cities	20.0	35.5
Sewage, sanitation, nutrition	2.5	4.3
Preventive practices	1.8	3.1
Nutrition, medical care, housing	1.3	2.4

worth mentioning. In this book, we will mostly focus on the first three categories.

The rank importance of disease by policy can be found in table 3.4. This table rearranges the leading causes of death by the policies that underlie them. Here, the term *green cities* is shorthand for improved reliance on public transit, lower citywide use of fossil fuels and nonrenewable energy resources, industrial pollution control, and opportunities for exercise in the community. Transit is separated out to call attention to the need for transit regulation outside of cities as well. Nutrition interventions can be conceptualized as opportunities to purchase healthy food via improved earnings and enhanced agricultural practices.

Again, these categories are far from perfect. In the poorest countries, fertilizer, seeds, and jobs may be needed for nutritional enhancements. In the wealthiest countries, a decreased reliance on prepared frozen dinner meals may be more appropriate. The point here is to provide a sense of alternative, helpful ways to think about disease causation. A measure that focuses on saving lives, rather than categorizing deaths, is likely to be a big improvement.

RELATED DISEASES, SAME ROOT CAUSES

A policy-oriented approach informs us about what we need to do better than simple mortality statistics. Another benefit to the policy-oriented approach is that we do not have to worry as much about misclassified diseases. If someone dies of a heart attack in a low-income country, it is not usually known whether the heart disease was due to high blood pressure, diabetes, or another underlying cause. In fact, this is also true in some developed countries. For instance, in the United States, medical residents are usually the people filling out death certificates in the hospital in the middle of the night, and they often do not know how to fill out the form or even know the person who died. In practice, this does not necessarily matter. Policies that prevent high blood pressure usually also prevent diabetes. Said more bluntly, it is easier to say that someone died from a disease of the heart than it is to say that they died of congestive heart failure, ischemic heart disease, and so forth. The vast majority of preventable diseases of the heart have the same policy remedy: reduce tobacco consumption, improve the food supply, increase exercise via active living communities, and reduce reliance on the automobile. The vast majority of diseases of the lung, accidents, or most other large categories of mortality also have distinct sets of policy remedies. So, there is no need to worry about what the resident writes on the death certificate at 3 AM.

DEAD CHILDREN MAKE FOR BAD STATISTICS

So we see that there are a number of different ways of thinking about how to lump causes of death into categories, and each has its pluses and minuses. But how do we think about death itself? Is it better to die of a heart attack than cancer? Does a death at age three mean the same thing as a death at age eighty?

As you can see from these questions, *death* is not a very useful or nuanced indicator. Lives taken from an easily preventable disease early in life feel more tragic than deaths due to a lifetime of smoking, which is not only more difficult to prevent but is also more likely to come after a mostly fully enjoyed life.

Fortunately, there are other ways of thinking about and measuring sickness and death than death by cause. One is to consider how many years of one's potential life are needlessly lost by a given condition or risk factor. Figure 3.2 lists causes of death among children by cause and region. We mentioned previously that perinatal conditions are best addressed with health care. That is because it is quite common for problems to arise during childbirth. Health professionals with modest training and facilities can save the mother and child from common problems that occur during birth.

Now, pretend that smoking cessation and maternal and child health care cost the same amount of money and save an equal number of lives. If a baby saved at birth would have lived to be seventy were such a health professional present, then we can say that seventy years of life were lost due to the absence of that professional. However, if a thirty-five-year-old male quits smoking, he will live ten months longer on average than if he continued to smoke for the rest of his life (Wright & Weinstein, 1998). If we merely look at deaths rather than years of life lost, it is possible that smoking cessation and maternal health care workers will come out about equal. But if we think in terms of years of life, if both investments were just as effective, maternal care workers will save a lot more life in absolute terms than will smoking cessation.

And all of this talk of latrines to improve life expectancy? Well, we also see from figure 3.2 that diarrheal illness among children is a major public health problem. When a child dies at age three, it has a much greater impact on a nation's life expectancy than a smoker who dies at age seventy. Why? Because life expectancy is essentially a way of averaging the number of years of life people live within a given area. A death at a young age tends to pull down that average.

So, if we switch to years of life lost or average life expectancy as a way of measuring burden of disease, we are much better off than if we measure numbers of deaths alone. But what about the heart disease versus cancer question? We have a way of dealing with that question as well, using a single measure—a combination of one's years of life lost and quality of life lived with a disease.

THE HEALTH EFFECTS OF EVIL GENIES

Regardless of the category of disease one examines, life expectancy is a fairly lousy measure of a nation's health. For instance, depression saps millions of people's productivity and happiness and interferes with their social relationships. Nevertheless, depression is not captured very well in international mortality statistics. Neither are migraine headaches. In fact, conditions that hurt a lot but kill you slowly or not at all will always take a backseat to those that take lives if we use life expectancy or years of life lost as our only measure of burden of disease.

Public health researchers and policy analysts need more nuanced ways of understanding how specific programs can affect the health of their constituents and target populations. For them, a much better measure would be the **quality-adjusted life year** (QALY). The QALY accounts for morbidity and mortality in a single measure. One QALY is a year of life lived in perfect health.

How does the QALY work? It combines health states ranging from missing limbs to psychosis into a single number between zero and one. Imagine that you have a friend who has faced quite a few health hardships. He lost his hand in a work accident so they fired him. He became very depressed and started drinking, only to develop liver cirrhosis. His wife left him with only their dog, and now he has trouble supporting even the dog. He does not commit suicide in part because he loves his dog so much and fears that no one will care for it.

Macabre as it may be to quantify such grief, imagine that your friend says that every year of life lived is only worth half of what it would be if he were happy and had his hand back. One way of measuring the impact that this has on his life is to just cut his remaining number of years in half—that, after all, is what he thinks that they are worth.

So, let us give him a score of 0.5. Every year lived in his current life is equivalent to half a year of life of someone who is in perfect physical and mental health. If your friend lives for ten years, he will have lived $0.5 \times 10 = 5$ QALYs. This is 10 QALYs − 5 QALYs = 5 QALYs less than someone in perfect health.

Fine, you might say, but where does this 0.5 ratio come from? You cannot just ask people to give a number for how much each year of life is worth to them. Imagine that you were missing a hand like your friend and an evil genie appeared. Imagine that the evil genie offered you a bargain. In a creepy voice, the genie said, "I will give you your hand back. But you must take a risk. We will flip a coin. Heads, you get your hand back; tails, I get to kill you." (The expected outcome here is 0.5 because you have a 50 percent chance of living in perfect health and a 50 percent chance of dying.) You respectfully decline and you start to feel better about your missing hand. But then the genie says, "Okay, 40 percent chance of death." You decline again, until the genie is down to 25 percent. Then, you are ready to bargain. You ask for 20 percent, and the genie counter offers with 22.5 percent. You accept. Your score is 100 percent − 22.5 percent = 77.5 percent or 0.775. This can be used to better value your lost life. It is not perfect but it is something.

Scientists and researchers are in the unenviable position of asking thousands of real-life people how to rate their health using a similar method to the evil genie. These values can be translated into surveys asking respondents to rate different states of ill health according to criteria such as their mobility, self-care, typical activities such as work and study, pain, and anxiety and depression. These surveys are mathematically designed to provide a number between zero and one that can be used to calculate QALYs.

Another important consideration is that lives saved today, similar to money, may be worth more to people than lives saved in the future. Given the choice between US$100 now and US$110 a year from now, most people choose instant gratification, even if a 10 percent interest rate is a great financial deal. In other words, we tend to discount the future. Cost-effectiveness analyses try to incorporate a **discount rate** to account for this, but experts cannot agree on what a realistic discount rate looks like. This is especially controversial when time horizons are long. People tend to leave messes for future generations to clean up, so what is the appropriate discount rate for an intervention that provides cheap food now but will deplete potable water supplies in just two generations?

The problems extend far beyond that. A much bigger problem is that QALY valuations vary from culture to culture, and they are extremely expensive to capture for an entire nation. A cure for a condition such as deafness, for instance, will be associated with many more QALYs in a population in which deaf people are assumed to be "deaf and dumb," stigma persists, and there are few opportunities for deaf people to become educated, communicate via sign language or alternate means, and contribute to society. In a population in which deaf people thrive with their own culture, lead full and active work and social lives, and express high levels of happiness, a cure for deafness will be associated with a low QALY score. In fact, many deaf people do not view deafness as a disability at all but as a different sort of human experience (Ladd, 2003).

Enter the **disability-adjusted life year** (DALY). The DALY represents a gigantic compromise. Refined by the World Bank, Harvard University, and the WHO, the DALY is obtained by asking health experts to value disease states. Of course, health experts are a subculture all their own; therefore, their disease state valuations do not vary much from country to country. Not too many people would want health professionals deciding their fate, but this is the best that these three elite organizations could come up with.

Similar to the QALY, the DALY is scaled from zero to one. In this case, one represents death and zero represents perfect health. (This is the opposite of the QALY and has to do with differences in the math used to estimate the burden of disease.) In its simplest form, the DALY for females is calculated as follows:

Years of life lived + Years lived with disability

The number of DALYs lost to disease is simply:

82.5 DALYs − Years of life lived + Years lived with disability

The 82.5 comes from the idea that Japan is the world's best example of a healthy nation (a notion from the 1990s), and female life expectancy there should be considered the ideal standard for all nations to achieve. It was assumed that the maximum potential for healthy human life expectancy is 80 for males and 82.5 years for females (WHO, 2013). Unfortunately, the DALY is derived from methods that do not validate well with respect to actually capturing the value of health lost relative to the value of life lost (Gold & Muennig, 2002).

Table 3.5. Burden of Disease Worldwide in DALYs

World	DALYs	Percentage of all DALYs
Pneumonia and bronchitis	94.5	6.2
Diarrhea	72.8	4.8
Depression	65.5	4.3
Heart disease	62.6	4.1
HIV/AIDS	58.5	3.8
Stroke	46.6	3.1
Premature birth*	44.3	2.9

*We wish to call attention to a significant categorical oversight here. The premature birth category should really fall under a broader category of prenatal conditions. Once we do this, the category rises to first place, with 126 DALYs worldwide.

Source: WHO. (2004). *The global burden of disease: Part 2.* Available online at www.who.int/healthinfo/global_burden_disease/GBD_report_2004update_full.pdf.

QUANTIFYING THE GLOBAL BURDEN OF DISEASE

Table 3.5 presents the global burden of disease for the world and by the conventions we use in this book in DALYs. Notably, depression pops up on the list of leading diseases. That is because, although it does not kill, it is common and causes a lot of suffering. The DALY has done its job in giving us a better sense of what is important from a public health standpoint. Notice, too, that diarrhea is way up on the list again. This is the DALY in action, too. The number of years of life lost to diarrhea is much greater than heart disease, even though heart disease is more common.

So we see that from the perspective of the DALY, infectious diseases are much more important than chronic diseases. This is true even as the world is rapidly conquering these diseases, primarily by decreasing abject poverty and increasing rates of sanitation, clean water, and vaccination. (See figure 3.4 for current worldwide distributions of sanitation resources. Figure 3.5 demonstrates how many people in low-income countries access clean drinking water.)

From table 3.6, it should become obvious that the poorest countries need better infectious disease control. Middle-income and high-income countries need healthier, greener cities, pollution controls, transit regulations, and anti-smoking interventions, such as cigarette taxation. Occupational health, particularly hearing protection, is needed in wealthy countries.

Of course, such seemingly simple analyses are not that simple. For example, it turns out that hearing loss is a result of poor occupational health standards in the past, more than in the present, in wealthy countries. Hearing

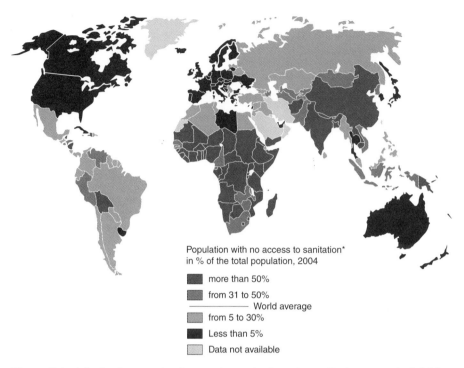

Population with no access to sanitation*
in % of the total population, 2004

■ more than 50%
▨ from 31 to 50%
──────────── World average
▨ from 5 to 30%
■ Less than 5%
□ Data not available

Figure 3.4. A lack of access to clean water and adequate sanitation severely inhibits many countries, especially those in sub-Saharan Africa. This problem inhibits their ability to accelerate their development.

Note: *According to the definition of the WHO and UNICEF: a population having no access to a wastewater or solid waste treatment infrastructure, well-maintained toilets, or a septic tank.

Source: WHO and UNICEF. (2006). *Meeting the NDG drinking water and sanitation target.* Geneva: WHO and New York: UNICEF. Available online at www.grida.no/graphicslib/detail/total-population-access-to-sanitation_136d.

loss mostly occurs among elderly populations in wealthy countries (Davila et al., 2009). When these folks were younger in the 1950s and 1960s, they were not given much in the way of hearing protection. That has changed in wealthy countries, with strong regulations on workplace noise put in place, but such regulations are either not in place or not enforced in many middle-income countries.

As will become painfully evident when you progress through these chapters, policy solutions can be either long term or short term. Smoking can be greatly curtailed in the short term with simple remedies, such as increasing taxes and banning smoking in public spaces, but such solutions can only go so far.

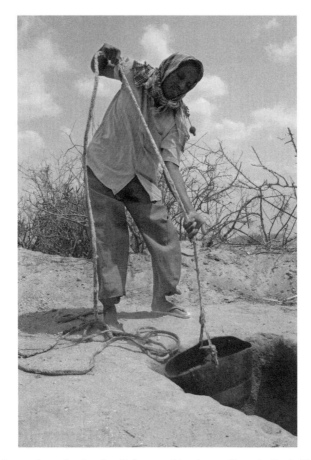

Figure 3.5. A member of a local relief committee in a village in East Africa builds a latrine. This particular village has chosen to use aid provided by the organization Oxfam to build latrines.

Source: Available online at www.flickr.com/photos/46434833@N05/5932332971.

Table 3.6. DALYs Ranked by Country Categories

Poorest	Middle income	Wealthy
Pneumonia	Depression	Depression
Diarrhea	Heart disease	Heart disease
HIV/AIDS	Stroke	Stroke
Malaria	Accidents	Alzheimer's
Premature birth*	Pneumonia	Alcohol abuse
Depression	Emphysema	Hearing loss

*This is the leading cause of DAYLs lost in the poorest nations when all forms of birth complications are combined.

MEASURING THE IMPACT OF POTENTIAL POLICY SOLUTIONS

Genetic studies show that some people are price sensitive to cigarette taxes and others just aren't because they are so addicted (Fletcher, 2012). That is, some people might mortgage their house to buy one last cigarette. Cigarette taxes have therefore essentially changed the characteristics of those who smoke. Prior to initiating high cigarette taxes in wealthy nations, some smokers enjoyed smoking but were able to quit with the right incentives and some could not. Now, increasing taxation on cigarettes will be unlikely to produce further reductions in smoking rates. These folks might benefit from the use of antismoking medications, but this is not yet fully established. If not, policy makers may be left with giving up on trying to treat current smokers, and money may be better spent on preventing young people from smoking in the first place. This can be done through advertising to change the social desirability of smoking, banning images of people smoking in the movies, and increasing investments in schooling. (More educated people are much less likely to smoke, but no one knows for sure whether this is cause or correlation.)

So far, we have talked about how it is important to understand where disease is located geographically, to understand which groups of nations (or people within nations) suffer the most, and to understand how disease is best addressed. We also mentioned that cause of death is a lousy measure of the global burden of disease because it does not account for how long someone lives or how much they suffer with disease. Measuring years of life lost is superior to measuring deaths, but better still is to use a measure such as the QALY or DALY, which provides information on the quality and quantity of life one lives with a given disease.

The point of all of this is to figure out where we should be focusing our precious public health resources to make the world a healthier place. But there is still one piece missing: cost. We know that heart and lung diseases are among the leading killers worldwide, so should we be spending all our money on heart and lung transplants? Or should we be preventing heart and lung disease through active living, improving the food supply, and reducing reliance on polluting automobiles or dirty power sources? The answers to such questions might seem intuitive but not all are.

For example, if we have US$1 million to spend in a given poor nation, are we better off spending it on sanitation or vaccinations? How many lives would we save if we spent it all on one or the other? **Cost-effectiveness analysis** tells us how to maximize the number of lives saved within a given budget. It is a tool that tells us how to appropriately use the resources that are available to us, a concept called **appropriate technology use.**

COST-EFFECTIVENESS ANALYSIS

Cost-effectiveness analyses in health compare the relative costs (money spent, time spent away from work for patients, etc.) to the outcomes (measured in QALYs and DALYs) of different interventions. They differ from **cost-benefit analyses** in that they do not place a monetary value on outcomes. Cost-benefit analysis is much more straightforward in that it tells you if what you are investing in will be a good investment or a bad one. That is, a cost-benefit analysis tells you that the total social value of what you are doing is better than not doing it at all. (This is measured as a value greater than US$0, indicating savings, or a ratio of costs to benefits of less than US$0, indicating that the benefits outweigh the costs.)

If it is so straightforward to report, why not use cost-benefit analysis for everything? It turns out that a cost-benefit analysis has to place a dollar value on everything, even human suffering and the value of a human life. This is not easy to do, and many researchers believe that it is impossible and even unethical. For most health investments, we could make them cost beneficial by simply increasing the value of a human life or suffering until we get the value we want. Or we could kill it by making the value of a human life worth very little (Muennig, 2007).

This is why most health experts choose cost-effectiveness analysis instead. In a cost-effectiveness analysis, programs or items with a monetary value, such as the cost of medical care or lost wages, are left as costs. But unquantifiable goods and states of being, such as suffering and longevity, are measured as QALYs.

So, imagine that we have US$1 million to spend on sanitation or vaccination, as in the previous example. If we know that sanitation costs US$1 to save a life and vaccination costs US$10 to save a life, then we know our US$1 million investment will save one million lives if we put it in sanitation and one hundred thousand lives if we spend it on vaccinations.

Of course, for all the reasons we discussed, we want to use QALYs as our outcome measure rather than lives. That is because QALYs tell us how many years of life we are saving and how much we are reducing morbidity and mortality. These decisions are sometimes made using a **league table**. That is,

Table 3.7. A Hypothetical Cost-Effectiveness League Table

Heath intervention	Cost/QALY
Sanitation	US$1.00
Vaccination	US$10.00
Maternal health	US$100.00
Antibiotics	US$200.00
Medical clinic	US$1,000.00

if we know that we have US$1 million to spend on health, and we have a sense of the cost-effectiveness of the things that we want to spend it on, then we can just run down the table until we have saved the most lives (see table 3.7).

Here, we can see that we can spend our money on sanitation until everyone is covered, then we move on to vaccination until everyone is covered, and then we move on to maternal health. Whenever we run out of money, we run out of money. But one thing is clear. If we spend it all on a medical clinic, we will only save a tiny fraction of the lives than if we spend it all on options that cost less per QALY saved.

TRANSLATING REAL-LIFE QUESTIONS INTO RESEARCH STUDIES IN PUBLIC HEALTH

All of this talk about the burden of disease and cost-effectiveness raises a question that some readers might not be familiar with: how do we know what we know? The answer to this question is, sadly, we do not know a lot because public health is not a "hard" science like physics. In physics, we can come up with a hypothesis about how fast something will fall out of the sky and then actually drop it from the sky. In public health, we ethically cannot design lab experiments to see what happens when we infect people with disease or deny them education. Even if we were to perform such tests, there is a lot of variability in individual circumstances, culture, local conditions, and the way that we run the experiment. In public health, researchers attempt to achieve **internal validity** in their study designs, questioning whether a given study is really measuring the causal interference between two variables and doing that well—making sure that the supposed effect temporally comes after the cause—and that there are no other obvious explanations for the effects left unaccounted for by the study. One example would be a study that randomly assigns mosquito nets to homes in a village in Malawi, carefully following families that did and did not get the nets to make sure that they are using them, and checking whether the families develop malaria.

Another concept is that of **external validity**—that is, can the findings from one study be applied to another? In the example of the randomized trial of mosquito nets, we do not know whether the practices in the village we are studying will be similar to those of other villages. We also do not know what would have happened if we did not have researchers there to check in to make sure that the villagers were using the nets. Maybe without the researchers' check-ins, some families would have made them into wedding veils. To get a better sense of external validity, we might look at patterns of malaria among villages that tend to use mosquito nets and those that do not across sub-Saharan Africa. Why is this approach not necessarily better? Well, those villages that use nets might be in areas with really high rates of infection. If so, we might find that the use of mosquito nets is associated with a higher rate of malaria! Or they might be richer and more proactive about their health, in which case we might conclude that mosquito nets help, when in fact they actually are just used more in villages that happen to also get treated more frequently for malaria.

SUMMARY

The global burden of disease is too often thought of in terms of "what is out there" with respect to the leading causes of death. One improvement on this approach is not just to think in terms of lives lost but rather the number of years of life lost. This allows us to better take into account the total impact of disease over the life course. This way, policy makers can better prioritize diseases that affect children over those that affect adults. (Because life expectancy is an average, preventing childhood deaths also has a greater impact on life expectancy than preventing adult deaths.) Another improvement on this model has been the disability-adjusted life year, which includes not just years of life lost but also makes some attempt to estimate morbidity. This way, diseases such as depression can get the attention they deserve as leading health problems even if they do not increase mortality by much. But perhaps a better way of thinking about diseases still is to consider the policies that produce or prevent them. When we think this way, we can have a good deal more clarity surrounding not just "what is out there" but also "what should we do about it?"

KEY TERMS

appropriate technology use

burden of disease

cost-benefit analyses

cost-effectiveness analysis

disability-adjusted life year (DALY)

discount rate

league table

quality-adjusted life year (QALY)

DISCUSSION QUESTIONS

1. How do global health researchers tend to measure how big a health issue is, that is, its global burden?

2. What are some of the key assumptions of cost-effectiveness analysis? In what sorts of situations is this type of analysis most useful?

3. Why do public health researchers tend to use cost-effectiveness and not cost-benefit analysis?

4. How are cost-effectiveness analyses ideally used in policy making? What are some of the trends in how they are usually used in real-life policy making?

FURTHER READING

Hans Rosling: States that reshape your worldview. (2006, February). TEDTalks. Available online at www.ted.com/talks/hans_rosling_shows_the_best_stats_you_ve_ever_seen.html

REFERENCES

Birn, A. (2009). Making it politic(al): Closing the gap in a generation: Health equity through action on the social determinants of health. *Social Medicine, 4*(3), 166.

Burd-Sharps, S., Lewis, K., & Martins, E. (2008). *The measure of America. American human development report, 2008–2009*. New York: Columbia University Press.

Christakis, N. A., & Fowler, J. H. (2007). The spread of obesity in a large social network over 32 years. *New England Journal of Medicine, 357*(4), 370–379.

Christakis, N. A., & Fowler, J. H. (2008). The collective dynamics of smoking in a large social network. *New England Journal of Medicine*, *358*(21), 2249–2258.

Davila, E. P., Caban-Martinez, A. J., Muennig, P., Lee, D. J., Flemming, L. E., Ferraro, K. F., LeBlanc, W. G., Larn, B. L., Arheart, K. L., McCollister, K. E., Zheng, D., & Christ, S. L. (2009). Sensory impairment among older US workers. *American Journal of Public Health*, *99*(8), 1378–1385.

Epp, J. (1986). Achieving health for all: A framework for health promotion. *Health Promotion International*, *1*(4), 419.

Fletcher, J. M. (2012). Why have tobacco control policies stalled? Using genetic moderation to examine policy impacts. *PloS One*, *7*(12), e50576.

Gold, M., & Muennig, P. (2002). Measure dependent variations in burden of disease estimates: Implications for policy. *Medical Care*, *40*(3), 260–266.

Ladd, P. (2003). *Understanding deaf culture: In search of deafhood*. Clevedon, England: Multilingual Matters.

Muennig, P. (2007). *Cost-effectiveness analysis in health: A practical approach*. San Francisco: Jossey-Bass.

Murray, C.J.L., & Lopez, A. D. (1996). *The global burden of disease: A comprehensive assessment of mortality and disability from diseases, injuries, and risk factors in 1990 and projected to 2020*. Cambridge, MA: Harvard School of Public Health, the World Health Organization, and the World Bank.

Ohsfeldt, R. L., & Schneider, J. E. (2006). *The business of health*. Washington, DC: AEI Press.

UN. (2012). *Millennium development goal indicators*. Available online at http://mdgs.un.org/unsd/mdg/SeriesDetail.aspx?srid=561

WHO. (2013). *Metrics: Disability adjusted life year*. Available online at http://www.who.int/healthinfo/global_burden_disease/metrics_daly/en/

Wright, J. C., & Weinstein, M. C. (1998). Gains in life expectancy from medical interventions—standardizing data on outcomes. *New England Journal of Medicine*, *339*(6), 380–386.

CHAPTER 4

Aid

KEY IDEAS

- Experts differ on whether development aid for health actually improves the health of people in poor nations. Specifically, some pundits argue that aid is harmful and others argue that there is not enough or it is misused.

- Aid comes in different forms, such as humanitarian assistance (aid delivered directly to people), bilateral aid (aid delivered between governments), and multilateral aid (aid delivered from wealthy countries to poorer countries).

- Especially contentious are donors' use of conditionalities and tensions between aid to governments and nongovernmental organizations.

Assumptions. It's part of human nature. We assume things and act without proper due diligence (see figure 4.1). We assume that building more roads will lead to fewer traffic jams, that replacing our diminishing hormones as we age is good for us, and that low-tar cigarettes are less detrimental to our health than high-tar cigarettes. As it turns out, in most situations, these things are not true. Unless tailored to women with very specific risk profiles, hormone replacement can increase a woman's risk of mortality. Low-tar cigarettes will cause most people to smoke more, increasing, rather than reducing, their risk of disease. So, what about giving aid to low-income countries? Some experts have come to question whether aid helps or hurts low-income countries. As with most things human, though, we become so enmeshed in the question that we lose sight of the basic questions: for whom, where,

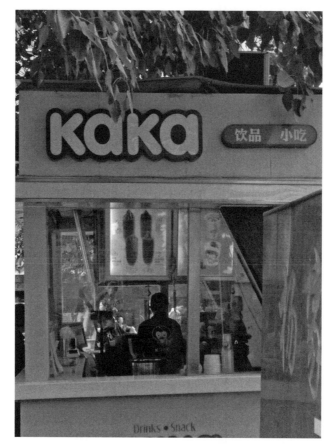

Figure 4.1. Many in international development make the same mistake that this food shop in Chongqing, China, makes. It is important to have a grasp of local and international knowledge before implementation (in this case, a sign suggesting that the snack shack is selling feces).

under what circumstances, and when? In this chapter, we break this debate down to try to better understand the complex reality underlying the relationship between aid and health.

DIFFERENT TYPES OF AID

As we mentioned in chapter 1, the Cold War rivalries between the United States and the USSR, the oil crises in the 1970s, decolonization, and the welfare retrenchment and structural adjustment programs of the Reagan and Thatcher eras all had huge effects on the health and economic development of low-income countries. This history probably shapes not only how well countries are doing today but also how capable they are of effectively using aid that is given to them.

It also influences the kinds of aid that a country receives. Former colonial powers are more likely to favor their former colonies, for instance. So, what is aid and what forms does it take? **International aid** refers to the transfer of funds from one entity or government to another across borders. For instance, it may take the form of a US citizen or foundation writing a check to Doctors Without Borders or the Red Cross. One form of such international aid is **humanitarian aid,** which supports programs to alleviate immediate human suffering. International aid may also take the form of a government transferring cash aid or goods, such as food or even helicopters, to another government. This is often called **bilateral aid** because it goes from one governmental party to another. Aid can also go through an intergovernmental organization, such as the World Bank, providing funding for a project in a specific locale, such as Rwanda. This form is often called **multilateral aid** because organizations such as the World Bank are funded by many different nations. Some forms of multilateral aid, such as those administered by various UN agencies, come from every imaginable source: governments, companies, and even private donors. In fact, Ted Turner, a US media mogul, once wrote a billion-dollar check to the UN. Finally, many scholars consider **remittances** as a form of large-scale, informal, international aid (Maimbo & Ratha, 2005). This chapter will discuss only formal aid. Remittances are payments made by overseas workers to their families. This can amount to substantial portions of a nation's economy.

Bilateral aid and multilateral aid are often called **official direct assistance** (ODA). As the name suggests, it is called this because it comes from official sources and goes directly to the country of interest. Usually, aid takes the form of a grant, but it can also take the form of a loan or smaller shipments of in-kind goods, such as tents and nonperishable foods in a disaster situation.

The United States is the largest donor overall, but this is because it is the world's largest economy. As a percentage of its GNP, the United States ranks toward the bottom of the industrialized nations with respect to ODA, providing about 0.2 percent of GNP (UN, 2006). This is well below the official target set by the United Nations of 0.7 percent of GNP. The only nations that actually meet this goal are Sweden, Luxembourg, Norway, and the Netherlands, which tend to donate between 0.8 and 1 percent of their GNP. However, if aid provided directly by US citizens is added to the overall figure, the United States rises to the top of the list. This is partly because the US government offers tax incentives for its citizens to contribute to charities under the belief that NGOs are a more effective way to deliver aid, particularly humanitarian aid, than are government agencies. (Of course, the US government

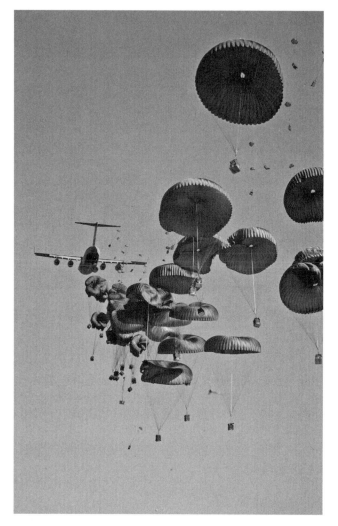

Figure 4.2. Aid is delivered to Port Au Prince, Haiti, following the magnitude 7 earthquake that hit the city in 2010.

Source: Available online at www.flickr.com/photos/walkadog/4317655660/.

itself does not have a history of small, intimate aid delivery as illustrated in figure 4.2.)

In fact, the government agencies that actually deliver this aid tend to be quite specific about the things that they fund, so it is likely that a lot of smaller project work would not get done without the help of NGOs. That these agencies are sometimes bureaucratic and inflexible is underscored by their long and sometimes ironic acronyms. Take the Swedish International Development

Cooperation Agency (SIDA), which happens to have the same acronym as HIV/AIDS in Spanish.

THE AID CONTROVERSY

There is some debate about the effectiveness of this aid, though—not just the aid delivered by large government agencies but also that delivered by small NGOs with very targeted and effective missions. Some prominent researchers and policy makers believe that aid is, in some cases, harmful for the health and economic well-being of people living in low-income nations (Easterly, 2006; Moyo, 2009). These critics see aid as fostering dependency, complacency, and corruption. After all, since the end of World War II, rich nations have spent more than two-and-a-half trillion dollars on aid to poor countries, and many of those have little to show for it. Maybe, some experts argue, if these countries had been left alone, they would be much better off. For example, the Democratic Republic of the Congo has been a recipient of aid for many decades but its development indicators remain abysmally low.

The experts who argue for international aid to be abolished are certainly in the minority. And the two-and-a-half trillion-dollar figure is less impressive when you think about the number of people that it covered over that time span. Moreover, as mentioned in chapter 1, there is strong global convergence—that is, life expectancy is increasing, economies are developing, people are getting more education, poverty rates are declining, and infant mortality is dropping in most nations on earth. This leaves these critics in the position of arguing that aid simply isn't working fast enough.

Still, even those who believe in aid have reservations. The majority of international policy makers, researchers, and other experts also have gripes with the way that aid is being delivered. Most people involved in international aid, whether on the ground in Kenya or sitting in air-conditioned office cubicles in Geneva, would argue that aid to poor countries is poorly used. They are right to think this way. Some official aid is diverted for nefarious uses or wasted and much is probably not effective or efficient (Doucouliagos & Paldam, 2009). But the money is difficult to follow, so it is exceptionally difficult to know how much is in fact useful or wasted (Bourguignon & Sundberg, 2007). There is also evidence that aid for health merely displaces government spending on health services, leaving health services vulnerable to fluctuation in global giving (Lu et al., 2010).

There are also researchers who argue that conditions in low-income nations would improve dramatically if they just received more aid (Sachs, 2006). These folks point to times when it has worked in the past as part of aid promised to alleviate suffering in poor nations. South Korea is now one of the world's wealthiest nations, and its economy was largely built on aid. In this chapter, we will take a look at the key arguments and bodies of evidence for each of these schools of thought.

MODELS OF GLOBAL AID FOR PUBLIC HEALTH

Development and public health experts have forwarded several ways of thinking about how global aid should *ideally* improve global health. One model assumes no specific prescriptions for public health. This model is just a way of thinking about decision making. The model argues that policy decisions (to allocate global aid in ways that will maximize public health) are best made via the **ex ante approach** (Harsanyi, 1953). In this approach, one is asked to imagine that he or she is making decisions prior to being born into the world, for example, without knowing whether you will become a hungry villager in rural Malawi or a well-fed venture capitalist in Silicon Valley.

Now, imagine that you are in this state, that you have not yet been born into a body on earth. Imagine further that you are asked to allocate US$30 billion in aid on earth. US$30 billion is not enough to solve the world's problems, but it could make a significant dent in suffering—if used properly. One way of using it is via cost-effectiveness, which we discussed in chapter 3. Remember the league table? Imagine we had the following league table:

1. Sanitation projects: US$0.50/QALY gained
2. School projects: US$0.75/QALY gained
3. Vaccination projects: US$1/QALY gained
4. Bed nets: US$3/QALY gained
5. Primary medical care: US$15/QALY gained
6. HIV/AIDS testing and treatment: US$300/QALY gained

We could invest our US$30 billion in the poorest areas without clean water, schooling, or vaccinations and save well over thirty billion lives. Alternatively, if we focused the same funding on HIV/AIDS treatment, we might save just one hundred million lives. One other thing we did not mention is that we could ignore the list altogether and invest in dams in Myanmar, nuclear power plant construction in South Africa, or a transnational superhighway through Southeast Asia. These projects could save or could take lives over the long run, but it is relatively safe to assume that they would not be ideal investments if our objective is to maximize the health of low-income people over the short run. Yet, those large-scale, infrastructural megaprojects were exactly where most foreign aid money went for most of the twentieth century. When investments from China are included, a high percentage of aid money still goes to infrastructure rather than health and education. Worse, when aid is spent on health, the reality is that aid money is more likely to be spent on these priorities in reverse, with significantly more money going to HIV/AIDS than to sanitation projects.

Certainly, some of these "suboptimal" investments may actually be ideal for certain countries or localities. For instance, a country that has achieved reasonable vaccination rates and has invested in schools may need roads and power plants. Likewise, a locality with very high rates of tuberculosis and HIV/AIDS will maybe benefit more from medical clinics than an area that is afflicted with diseases that can be prevented with public health measures, such as diarrhea and malaria. Context is the most important factor in international aid.

Other reasons for ignoring this list of priorities include overriding political priorities, ethical concerns, or lack of clear information (on the part of the donor, the recipient requesting the funding, or both).

Political concerns often top the list. The World Bank was once the world's largest funder of dams internationally. Now it is China. In both cases, the money was, and still is, often donated or lent for political reasons. The Chinese government has become one of the major sources of aid in Southeast Asia and Africa alike, largely in the hopes of acquiring rights to timber, oil, or minerals. The World Bank continues to fund large infrastructure projects despite also funding studies showing that dollars invested in schools would be a preferred investment.

Ethical concerns also play a large role. For instance, the anthropologist Paul Farmer argues that the "reigning ideologies" of public health favor "efficiency over equity" (Farmer, 2004, p. 18). Although not denying that cost-effectiveness is an important life-saving tool, Farmer argues that it is wrong for a treatment to be seen as "cost effective in New York, but not in Siberia" (Farmer, 2004, p. 131). Applying this example to an ex ante perspective, Farmer essentially argues that we should refuse the US$30 billion dollars and instead demand that all resources be distributed with preferential treatment for the poor who need it most. Of course, he doesn't say this outright because it would make him look naive. After all, although a lot of people in rich countries would choose to live less extravagantly if they knew that doing so would save lives elsewhere, it is not clear how to actually effectively redistribute their resources. But the larger question of whether we should help someone who is dying in front of us, no matter how expensive and inefficient, is real. This is especially true if we believe that the money might not actually benefit the unseen thousands of people whose lives could have been saved with that same money that could save one.

Finally, a lack of information often plays a role in funding decisions. Small NGOs too often invest in hospitals to treat diseases such as cholera when latrines are needed instead (Dichter, 2003). Few NGOs and donors prioritize appropriate technology use.

Some development experts argue that aid agencies have conducted enough ex ante exercises and analyses. It is clear enough, they say, that human development is best achieved via heavy investments in schooling and agriculture (Strauss & Thomas, 1998). The idea is that education and nutrition build human capital, the platform needed for economic development. Schooling also confers important survival skills—humans adapt to a harsh ecological niche via cognition. Investments in schools and agriculture may be one important reason why so many Asian nations have undergone rapid human development. It is difficult, however, to parse out the relative contributions of investments in schools and the agricultural reforms (or green revolutions) that occurred at the same time.

A second model, forwarded by the economist Jeffrey Sachs (2006), proposes that aid projects be pooled in such a way that they synergize. For instance, in addition to a full stomach, learning is best achieved if students have a safe home environment, are healthy, have employment, and have a means of transport to the school. This model differs from the one described previously in that it does not isolate or prioritize specific programs and projects. This approach is typified by the Bolivar Health Center in the 1960s or the recent Millennium Villages Project (Geiger, 2002).

In the Bolivar Health Center model and the Sachs model, the emphasis is on nonmedical determinants of health. Both recognize that health cannot be created within fundamentally unhealthy environments. Thus, both strive to accomplish sanitation, vaccination education, jobs, roads, and agriculture programs as a means to improving health. The Bolivar county example primarily involved building a farming cooperative and food distribution center that also included education and other programs. When this program was investigated for using federal dollars earmarked for health care on food, the program director, Jack Geiger, famously informed Congress, "The last time I checked in a medical textbook, the treatment for starvation is food" (Geiger, personal communication).

This model has been derided by William Easterly as "utopian social engineering." He argues that outsider meddling in others' practices is doomed to failure, equating it with "IMF/World Bank-sponsored comprehensive reforms called structural adjustment" (Easterly, 2006, p. 13). He argues that Professor Sachs has forwarded 449 interventions, but in trying to get any one accomplished, "[p]lanners are distracted by doing the other 448 interventions" (Easterly, 2006, p. 6).

A final dominant model uses an institutional approach to policy making, to emphasize not the specific public health programs to be implemented but the ways in which local knowledge, incentives, and reform can be brought together for effective service delivery. For instance, one project in a poor county in Brazil managed to break through entrenched bureaucracy and cronyism to dramatically increase vaccination rates and public health service provision (Tendler, 1997). It did so by creating competition between local governments on measures of efficacy and paying workers high wages for what was seen as important work, among other reforms. However, this sort of nuanced approach is difficult to implement in different contexts.

ARGUMENT: AID IS HARMFUL

A number of researchers and aid officials have come to believe that aid is harmful. This line of reasoning gained prominence in the 1960s with Milton Friedman and Peter Bauer. For instance, Friedman has argued that foreign aid "strengthened governments that were already too powerful." By this, he meant that aid was encouraging public investment rather than private, thereby limiting free trade and economic growth. Although ODA is the primary target of most critics, humanitarian aid provided by NGOs has also come into question (Carapico, 2000; Gugerty, Kremer, Center, & Floor, 2000).

Humanitarian Assistance

One common argument regarding humanitarian assistance is that aid abdicates governments from their rightful responsibilities (Rahman, 2006). If enough organizations are providing vaccinations, schooling, and primary health care, then the recipient government comes to believe that it no longer needs to provide these services. If true, this is problematic for a number of reasons. First, NGOs, which tend to be smaller in size and capacity, do not have the broad reach or regulatory powers of governments. Therefore, many poor areas will be left without service or serviced by a now-neglected ministry of education. Second, NGOs tend not to coordinate with one another. Thus, when many NGOs are providing schooling, there is no way of ensuring that school staff members are trained in a consistent manner or that they meet a minimum standard. Local curricula are replicated from scratch for each NGO, resulting in the proverbial "reinvented wheels" and highly variable quality of service delivery and wasted resources. Third, different NGOs have very different missions, with many having religious backing. This can turn parents away when, for instance, a Christian organization sets up a school in a predominantly Muslim area. Finally, humanitarian aid is highly dependent on charitable trends in developed nations and foreign economic fluctuations. Given that donors do not have their own children in these schools, there is sometimes little incentive to make sure that they remain viable.

Responding to such concerns, some NGOs have moved to work more closely with recipient governments. For instance, a health NGO might work through the ministry of health to improve coordination and service delivery. However, when delivered this way, such aid essentially becomes ODA, which has also been deemed harmful by some, especially in contexts with little governmental democratic accountability.

Official Direct Assistance

As with funding from smaller organizations, ODA can foster dependency, corruption, and poor governance. For instance, Dambisa Moyo argues that the responsibility for development be handed back to governments so that they can take charge of their own destiny (Moyo, 2009). Moyo's objective is to restate and update the ideas of Bauer and Easterly. For instance, she provides more details of hypothetical links between ODA and corruption. She argues that the solution is market reform and autonomy so that poor countries can naturally undergo economic development. Moyo sees debt forgiveness as a major source of this harm (because it provides the temptation to apply for loans and steal the proceeds) and sees stipulations attached to loans as problematic because "conditionalities carry little punch" (Moyo, 2009, p. 52). Conditionalities are the restrictive conditions, or "strings attached," to international loans and development aid. They are usually spelled out by the funding organizations and countries and might, for example, dictate that the loaned funds be used only for capital projects and not for health or education services.

The idea that ODA is harmful also has been forwarded by activists, who argue that financial interventions from the IMF and the World Bank have done more harm than good (Klein, 2001). They point out that during the 1997 Asian financial crisis, China, the one country that ignored the advice of the World Bank and the IMF, emerged from the crisis unscathed; the rest of the countries languished in recession for many years. Likewise, they place the blame for the Argentinean financial crisis of 1999 on the IMF. However, unlike Moyo, activists generally see the imposition of free market reforms (e.g., via the Washington Consensus) as the fundamental problem rather than the solution. For instance, they argue that free market reforms are only superficially neutral, if at all. Moreover, they argue that reforms are often structured in ways that protect subsidies in the United States and Europe, even as they require that poor nations rid themselves of similar subsidies. In contrast to Moyo, many activists argue that the solution is to forgive debt, terminate the use of donor-oriented and time-limited projects, allow for flexible budgets, and invite participatory decision making.

Aside from this anecdotal evidence that aid produces harm, there is a body of research to support the claims of naysayers. For example, it may be that the more aid a nation receives, the less it saves (Hadjimichael, 1995). Generally, such researchers argue that free-market and trade-oriented reforms will foster economic development in contrast to human development–oriented approaches that emphasize schools and public health projects (such as latrines and water purification projects). These studies, however, are based largely on weak ecological data. Although the biggest aid recipients in sub-Saharan Africa have a dismal record of economic growth and human development, it is difficult to know whether aid recipients do poorly because they were weakly governed to begin with (and thus in the need for aid) or whether they experienced continued decline precisely because they received aid. Some organizations, such as Oxfam, have argued that "trade not aid" approaches will fail until wealthy countries open their markets to poor ones and as long as poor countries lack the infrastructure or markets needed to take advantage of trade opportunities (Watkins, 2002).

ARGUMENT: AID IS POORLY MANAGED

Other development and health experts argue that global aid is not inherently harmful; rather, the essential challenge lies in allocating aid in helpful, context-appropriate ways. Although there are few comprehensive studies, development projects are often criticized for mismanagement and for introducing disruptions and wage disparities to the local economy (Gasper, 2000). Here, we provide one anecdote of the challenges faced in the field. One mid-sized aid project in the Sudan sought a new Kenyan hire to conduct fieldwork and to help with administrative tasks. The organization, funded by the USAID, sought to hire a local worker. Because there were no skilled locals available, the NGO settled for an African national, a Kenyan.

The organization pays Western wages, a king's fortune to a Kenyan. This worker already owned a large business bought with past aid jobs and was busy with the task of running it. Therefore, despite the fact that the foreign workers were putting in eighty-hour weeks, the new hire demanded a nine-to-five job and a light workload and got it. Of course, the ideal situation for many NGOs would be to have a highly trained and motivated local workforce who knew the landscape and culture and worked for local wages. That way, more aid can be delivered more effectively. The reality is too often the exact opposite of this ideal.

Management at all levels is a major challenge. The world's most highly trained managers tend not to want to work in poor nations for low wages. It is therefore difficult to recruit good managers for aid work. This does not stop many aid agencies from hiring expensive consultants who are often unfamiliar with the local context and who dole out advice that the aid agency has little capacity to incorporate.

Since the end of the Cold War, NGOs have amassed great power in shaping global health policy. This is partly because many funders wanted to funnel aid outside of inefficient or corrupt governments, and they hoped that NGOs would be more efficient. However, this explosive growth of NGOs has also led to serious critiques that NGO aid is misguided or poorly managed.

For instance, Doctors Without Borders is a private, nonprofit organization that works in many countries to deliver emergency medical and public health services. It operates in many different nations at the same time, performing services that those nations are not able to provide because they are too poor or too poorly governed to do so. One can imagine that Doctors Without Borders has a lot of company in providing medical services. After the 2010 Haiti earthquake, for example, groups as varied as the Church of Scientology and the Red Cross descended on the island to help victims, but most did not have expertise in the Haitian institutional and public health context; more important, many also did not necessarily know whom to ask or how to establish networks and connections with locals on the ground.

Some of these organizations do the exact same thing in the exact same place. Others are scattered randomly around the world. It is quite rare that these organizations work together to plan and coordinate service delivery. When disaster strikes, some do more harm than good by interfering with the logistics of the bigger operations. For example, they can clog runways or ports and confuse the people they are trying to help. Some are so poorly prepared that their own workers just become additional victims at the disaster site, consuming critically needed food and water.

Still, the net effect of NGOs is probably positive. According to the WHO, NGOs affect global health by bolstering existing resources; acting as liaisons among large governmental agencies, foundations, and intergovernmental institutions; and helping to implement health initiatives of many sorts. For example, they can promote public health campaigns such as the eradication of polio, reach out in emergencies such as tackling guinea worm in Sudan, enhance local capacity by providing technical assistance, mobilize volunteers to build toilets in Indian slums, and produce "best-selling" training modules for midwives (Barboza, 2002).

WHAT DO NGOs DO?

Actual NGO activities can be generally categorized into (1) internal organizing or services, (2) lobbying or advocacy, and (3) fundraising. Internal organizing includes leadership development, education, documentation, speechwriting, research, and outreach for the NGO. NGOs do everything from on-the-ground health education programs (such as teaching mothers to use special **oral rehydration solutions** so that their children do not die when they develop diarrhea) to advocating for better human rights policies. An NGO working for safety standards in textile factories, for example, may work on teaching factory workers about their rights, documenting violations of such rights, coaching and encouraging workers to speak out on their own and on behalf of the organization, compiling and publishing materials supporting their agenda, and coordinating demonstrations or meetings about their policy goals. Service activities include health, nutrition, education, legal, or other assistance. For instance, the International Rescue Committee is an NGO that helps to set up emergency schools, psychological counseling, and health services for refugees and asylum seekers around the world. In public health, NGOs do play a pivotal role in providing nutrition, health education, education, deworming, vector control, basic medical care, specialized surgical procedures, and other life-saving services.

Lobbying or advocacy activities include networking, participation and presentations in conferences, protest, and dissemination of case histories, policy goals, and work via media. Although use of media is often crucial in obtaining popular support, executing outreach, publicizing and threatening protest, and fundraising, participation in conferences helps NGOs to gain institutional legitimacy and entrée into the academic, foundation, and policy-making worlds. Fundraising is not always a discrete activity but one enmeshed in advocacy and organizing overall. Nevertheless, most NGOs have at least one staff member solely dedicated to fundraising, primarily through foundation grants or public relations and individual contributions.

Given the diversity of NGOs, it is quite difficult to draw general conclusions about shared benefits and weaknesses. Nevertheless, a review of common points of praise and criticism highlights the theme of grassroots relevance, legitimacy, and scalability as key points of debate.

ARGUMENT: AID IS MISUSED

Too often, one-size-fits-all policies are applied with disastrous results by ODA and humanitarian organizations. On the ODA side, structural adjustment is one commonly cited example of the application of theory that might work for a rich nation but when administered to poor nations that the decision makers had, in many cases, never even visited, these structural adjustment policies proved disastrous. Another example, documented by the anthropologist Paul Farmer, is the WHO's use of a standard package of tuberculosis drugs. These drugs, which often carry side effects, were repeatedly used to treat tuberculosis in regions that had a high degree of drug resistance. Such trends have led some practitioners to argue for sets of "good" practices rather than oft-donor-dictated "best" ones (Feek, 2007).

Although the list of misadventures goes on, a persistent problem today is the use of inappropriate technology. In 2009, the WHO, among others, initiated a drive for universal primary health care in poor nations. Although it is true that many nations can and should invest in primary health care, the poorest nations do not yet have the public health infrastructure in place. As a result, funding for primary health care systems will largely be spent treating illnesses that would have never happened if clean water, sanitation, vector control, and vaccination programs were in place.

WHAT IS A VECTOR FOR DISEASE?

In global health, we usually talk about vectors for disease as insects or other critters that carry a disease and can transmit it to humans. One very common form of aid is directed at vector control, which generally means trying to get rid of such critters. A central part of malaria control involves spraying stagnant water so that the mosquito larvae are killed. This reduces the number of mosquitoes that ultimately spawn and go on to bite people and animals that, in turn, themselves carry malaria. Removing stagnant water is even more effective but much more difficult. When the Panama Canal was built, for instance, international workers were protected in part by very aggressively draining and preventing stagnant sources of water, even removing people's flower pots and old automobile tires that might collect water inside. Once you get the total number of infected mosquitoes down to a critical number and treat people with the disease, the disease tends to drop off and becomes quite uncommon.

Other diseases, however, are not quite easily contained by spraying. For instance, aggressive spraying programs have not rid New York City of the West Nile virus, a disease also carried by mosquitoes. Tsetse flies and snails are other common carriers of parasitic disease.

ARGUMENT: "AID" FURTHER CONSOLIDATES POWER FOR THE POWERFUL

Another critique of global aid, one primarily aimed at NGOs rather than ODA, is that NGOs sometimes forward the missions of governmental and private business interests under the guise of civil society. (The critique that foreign aid further consolidates power for the powerful, or that "the revolution will not be funded," applies to ODA as well, but its bite is sharpest when applied to NGOs because NGOs often profess to hold global north and global south governments accountable.) As with business, just what renders an NGO independent from government is debatable. At the very least, NGOs must prove to be nonprofit in order to avoid private sector taxation. Still, in some countries, NGOs may undergo such stringent evaluations that NGO activities are greatly censored and only those that support governmental policies are accredited. Indeed, in countries with more restrictive NGO accreditation laws, many NGOs are actually government or donor organized. Thus, there exists the acronym GONGO for the rather counterintuitive term *government-organized-NGO.*

Even in less-restrictive countries, some NGOs, especially those that provide services to the poor, receive some funding from governments. Government-NGO relations are especially contentious when NGOs receive some funding from governmental development agencies. Recently, then, NGOs such as Mercy Corps have begun to refuse money from governments if they feel that contracts come with clauses limiting their public relations or activities. NGOs that focus on human rights issues or review of government actions, such as Human Rights Watch, tend to have policies prohibiting financial aid from any government.

STUDYING AID

In chapter 3, we briefly reviewed the importance of internal validity and external validity in public health research. The ideal situation is to have a mix of studies that make trade-offs between these two concepts. For instance, we might have a randomized trial of aid but also study the effects of aid across different nations. One of the reasons that it is so difficult to know whether aid is working or not is that it is broadly considered unethical to give out aid randomly to some countries but not others. So, we are stuck with looking at patterns of aid use. Unfortunately, countries that need more aid often get it. This makes aid look bad because relative to countries that do not need aid, countries that do tend to have poor governance and weak institutions.

ARGUMENT: ALL IS WELL, JUST SEND MORE

In the three decades following the Korean War, the United States provided more aid to South Korea than just about any other country that has received aid in the history of international aid. South Korea is now one of the most powerful nations on earth, economically and in terms of its human capital. Some argue that nations in sub-Saharan Africa could join South Korea's ranks if only the aid packages were large enough. Such critics assert that donor governments have consistently failed to meet the 0.7 percent of GDP giving targets established at the UN General Assembly in 1970 (Hirvonen, 2005).

Although there are staunch camps, each with their strong beliefs about aid, the reality is that they are probably all partly correct. There are likely some countries that cannot absorb aid, there are leaders who would steal it, and others who would put it to good use. This highlights one of the most enduring problems associated with aid: the human tendency to overgeneralize a valuable hypothesis.

ARGUMENT: WE ARE MAKING PROGRESS, BUT THE HURDLES ARE HIGH

Even among aid projects that accomplish targeted, short-term goals, three challenges remain: (1) they must balance services provision with working toward larger social goals and missions, (2) they must attend to questions of sustainability and length of stay, and (3) they must try to achieve goals on a large scale.

First, NGOs and aid projects often shape global health not just by providing services but also by advocating for change, changing, or shifting the policy goals and priorities of governing bodies (Allison & Macinko, 1993). For example, they may emphasize human rights (such as preventing violence against women and empowering the disabled to shape public policy), attempting to balance private sector interests (developing guidelines for drug donations) or changing rules governing foods, drugs, and health care services (Barboza, 2002). Another prominent role of NGOs in global health lies in raising awareness and funding for certain diseases.

Because of their focus on policy or social change, NGOs are sometimes compared to **social movements.** Social movements are conscious and sustained efforts by organized groups of people trying to achieve social goals (Polletta & Jasper, 2001). NGOs and social movements are assumed to work toward some form of social change via extra-institutional means or outside official political parties. Whereas social movements capture the popular imagination in demonstrations and marches, the speeches, preparation, and agenda are often outlined by relatively formalized collectives or NGOs. For example, the global movement to address HIV/AIDS is certainly greater than the American NGO Act Up!, the South African NGO Treatment Action Campaign, and the Product RED campaign and its spokesperson Bono (of the band U2). Health-related aid projects and NGOs often benefit from social movements but they also work on more immediate issues and programs.

Second, there are questions of sustainability and just how long aid projects can remain effective or helpful. How long should they stay? Will locals be able to continue the work when the project ends or the NGO leaves? In the short term, NGOs and aid projects can raise awareness of humanitarian crises, such as famines or postearthquake injuries. In the medium term, NGOs can draw attention to pressing policy issues that governments are not sufficiently addressing, such as endemic malaria or tuberculosis in certain populations. In these cases, NGOs are an important component of civil society that help to hold governments accountable. In the long term, even if governments do not bristle at most NGO activities, ongoing activities raise the risk that governments will come to rely on NGOs to pay for and provide services that would have otherwise been their responsibility. In such cases, NGOs help governments to abdicate public responsibilities.

Finally, there are questions of scale. At what level should aid projects be implemented? In what forms? How big should they be? Many aid projects end up addressing this question via division of labor within the organization, but this can be perilous. An NGO focusing on women's reproductive rights may operate support groups and health services in a neighborhood or village, lobby for family planning legislation at the national level, and participate in the promotion for multilateral funding or resolutions at UN conferences and other venues. Because there is so much going on within the organization at so many different levels, it sometimes happens that NGO participants at the international level may not be aware of activities at the local level, and vice versa.

CAN CIVIL SOCIETY CURE CORRUPTION?

As with the word *freedom*, it is difficult for global citizens to argue against *civil society*—after all, it has become one of the great buzzwords of public policy and international development. But it is also a phrase that has different meanings to different people. Officially, it refers to things that bring people together that are not related to one's family or the state. So, civil society can be an NGO, a community organization, or even just a club.

Current uses of the term *civil society* became more popular in the 1980s, when organized groups such as Solidarno in Poland used civil resistance tactics to promote workers' rights, protest authoritarian communist regimes, and build a social movement for democratic change. In that context, civil society held the state politically accountable for its policies.

By the turn of the new millennium, amid growing protests over structural adjustment programs overall, policy makers no longer trumpeted civil society as a cure-all remedy. Its allure, however, remains. And although a robust civil society—one with active and informed citizens—is certainly essential to healthy democracy, it also comes with dangers. Many robust civil society movements exclude less-powerful groups. The growing anticorruption movements in India, for example, tend to be funded by the right-wing Hindu nationalist groups. It is important, then, to remember that civil societies are not monolithic and that no one group represents all of civil society. Indeed, a robust civil society is inherently pluralistic. Otherwise, civil society groups are likely to simply trade one network of corruption for another.

SUMMARY

There is little question that aid can be better used, but the solutions are not easy to come by. There is not yet a clear cure for corruption, even in democratic nations. Moreover, ODA is still largely driven by political agendas, and humanitarian aid is driven by pet projects. Ideology even plays a role in the very existence of NGOs; NGOs probably would not have grown so much or become so important if institutions such as the IMF had not so emphasized privatization and the devolution of the state as remedies to governmental corruption and inefficiency.

NGO and aid projects are probably most beneficial when they fill service, advocacy, or assistance gaps left by governmental and intergovernmental bodies. The wide diversity of these overlapping NGOs and government agencies has also led to criticisms of their apparent lack of coordination and waste of funds. Critics assert that NGOs and funded development projects sometimes duplicate work rather than reach those who are most in need of help (Gugerty et al., 2000). Ideally, if NGOs and aid projects are governed well and give local residents the sort of training, skills, and decision-making opportunities necessary to participate meaningfully in planning, then they are empowering communities not just to follow instructions, supervise safer childbirths, or fix potable water pumps, but also to ask questions and participate in governance (Morgan & Rau, 1993).

International aid for health and economic development comes in many forms. It arrives officially from governments and unofficially through private sources. One government might give directly to another government or it might choose to pool funds with other governments (e.g., through the World Bank). However it comes, there is serious controversy over how best to administer it or coordinate it. There are so many different entities giving out aid that it is difficult to figure out who is doing what, let alone how to target it to where it is needed most.

Aid has long been assumed to improve the health and economic conditions of people in poor countries. However, a minority of development experts have questioned this assumption and regard aid as potentially expensive and harmful.

KEY TERMS

bilateral aid

civil society

ex ante approach

humanitarian aid

international aid

multilateral aid

official direct assistance

oral rehydration solutions

remittances

social movements

DISCUSSION QUESTIONS

1. What are some of the key arguments for increased aid funding to low-income countries? What are some debates on what this aid should look like?

2. What are some of the key arguments against increasing aid funding to low-income countries? Or for more restrictive aid?

3. Is it possible to generalize across contexts? Should Sierra Leone receive the same sorts of aid as Bangladesh or Ecuador? Should they face similar conditionalities?

4. What are the key debates on what the role of high-income countries and intergovernmental institutions (such as the World Bank) should be? Why do so few countries meet the UN goal of providing 0.7 percent of one's GNP in aid?

5. Does the ex ante approach change your opinion on what aid should look like in, say, Paraguay?

6. What are some of the key recommendations you would have to make sure of so that aid is used well? Who should be in the room? What

should the role of national policy makers, civil society groups, NGOs, business groups, diplomats, bankers, and policy analysts be, if any?

FURTHER READING

Bearak, B. (2003, July 13). Why people still starve. *New York Times*.

REFERENCES

Allison, A., & Macinko, J. A. (1993). *PVOs and NGOs: Promotion of democracy and health*. Cambridge, MA: Harvard University Data for Decision Making Project.

Barboza, G. (2002). *WHO and civil society: Linking for better health*. Geneva: World Health Organization Civil Society Initiative.

Bourguignon, F., & Sundberg, M. (2007). Aid effectiveness: Opening the black box. *The American Economic Review*, *97*(2), 316–321.

Carapico, S. (2000). NGOs, INGOs, GO-NGOs, and DO-NGOs: Making sense of non-governmental organizations. *Middle East Report*, Spring (214), 12–15.

Dichter, T. W. (2003). *Despite good intentions: Why development assistance to the third world has failed*. Amherst: University of Massachusetts Press.

Doucouliagos, H., & Paldam, M. (2009). The aid effectiveness literature: The sad results of 40 years of research. *Journal of Economic Surveys*, *23*(3), 433–461.

Easterly, W. R. (2006). *The white man's burden: Why the West's efforts to aid the rest have done so much ill and so little good*. New York: Penguin Press.

Farmer, P. (2004). *Pathologies of power: Health, human rights, and the new war on the poor*. Berkeley: University of California Press.

Feek, W. (2007). Best of practices? *Development in Practice*, *17*(4), 653–655.

Gasper, D. (2000). Anecdotes, situations, histories-varieties and uses of cases in thinking about ethics and development practice. *Development and Change*, *31*(5), 1055–1083.

Geiger, H. J. (2002). Community-oriented primary care: A path to community development. *American Journal of Public Health*, *92*(11), 1713–1716.

Gugerty, M. K., Kremer, M., Center, L., & Floor, T. (2000). Outside funding of community organizations: Benefiting or displacing the poor? *NBER Working Paper w7896*.

Hadjimichael, M. T. (1995). *Sub-Saharan Africa: Growth, savings, and investment, 1986–93* (Vol. 118). Washington, DC: International Monetary Fund.

Harsanyi, J. C. (1953). Cardinal utility in welfare economics and in the theory of risk-taking. *The Journal of Political Economy*, *61*(5), 434.

Hirvonen, P. (2005). *Stingy Samaritans: Why recent increases in development aid fail to help the poor*. Global Policy Forum. Available online at www.globalpolicy.org/component/content/article/240/45056.html

Klein, N. (2001). Reclaiming the commons. *New Left Review*, 9, 81–89.

Lu, C., Schneider, M. T., Gubbins, P., Leach-Kemon, K., Jamison, D., & Murray, C.J.L. (2010). Public financing of health in developing countries: A cross-national systematic analysis. *Lancet*, *375*(9723), 1375–1387.

Maimbo, S. M., & Ratha, D. (2005). *Remittances: Development impact and future prospects*. Washington DC: World Bank Publications.

Morgan, R., & Rau, B. (1993). *Global learning for health*. Washington, DC: National Council for International Health.

Moyo, D. (2009). *Dead aid*. New York: Farrar, Straus and Giroux.

Polletta, F., & Jasper, J. M. (August 2001. Collective identity and social movements. *Annual Review of Sociology*, *27*, 283–305. DOI: 10.1146/annurev.soc.27.1.283.

Rahman, S. (2006). Development, democracy and the NGO sector: Theory and evidence from Bangladesh. *Journal of Developing Societies*, *22*(4), 451.

Sachs, J. D. (2006). *The end of poverty: Economic possibilities for our time*. New York: Penguin.

Strauss, J., & Thomas, D. (1998). Health, nutrition, and economic development. *Journal of Economic Literature*, *36*(2), 766–817.

Tendler, J. (1997). *Good government in the tropics*. Baltimore, MD: Johns Hopkins University Press.

UN. (2006). *Official development assistance, 2005*. United Nations Millennium Project. Available online at www.unmillenniumproject.org/press/07.htm

Watkins, K. (2002). Last chance in Monterrey: Meeting the challenge of poverty reduction. *Oxfam Briefing Paper.*

CHAPTER 5

Health Systems

KEY IDEAS

- Health systems focus on ways to improve population health by preventing disease. Activities range from delivering clean water to protecting worker safety.

- Health care *delivery* systems tend to focus on medical services and tend to focus on curative rather than preventive care. These vary according to whether they are universal or have good accessibility, their level of comprehensiveness, and their comprehensiveness in financing.

- Health care systems in high-income countries focus most on chronic diseases and issues of cost control, whereas health care systems in low- and middle-income countries tend to focus more on selective primary health care, especially for early childhood, disease-specific strategies, and good governance.

- As countries develop more, the amount of money spent on health care decreases in importance; rather, researchers worry about the distribution of capabilities-enhancing resources.

Health systems can be thought of as the collections of organizations, people, and policies that work to improve population health. Many of the factors that influence health, but are outside of the traditional roles of medicine and public health, are not always thought of as part of a health system. For example, education and public transit might play a bigger role in population health than medical care delivery (Muennig, Fiscella, Tancredi, & Franks, 2010). But this is changing now, particularly at the local level, as cities ramp up investments in bike lanes, parks, and even schools or welfare programs in the name of health (City and County of San Francisco, 2013; Srinivasan, O'Fallon, & Dearry, 2003).

They were right to do so. When one thinks of health policy aimed at improving population health, it is important to think outside the health system box and to think of the broader, **nonmedical determinants of health,** which encompass anything that improves health but falls outside of the purview of traditional medical care. For instance, environmental protection regulations can reduce people's exposure to potentially harmful chemical compounds (Muennig, 2009; Perera et al., 2003; Schwartz, 1994). Some investments in nonmedical determinants of health, such as environmental regulations, may slow down an economy in the short run while improving health. For instance, it may be better for one's health to reside within a developed nation that lumbers along with thirty-five-hour work weeks and lots of environmental and occupational regulations than it is to reside within a rapidly expanding but poorly checked economy such as China's.

Health systems are distinct from other entities that improve population health in that health betterment is the explicit, primary purpose of such systems. A health system is quite different from a **health care delivery system**. Health care delivery *is* part of a health system, and similar to other parts of a health system, it can improve health (or adversely affect health if too little or too much health care is delivered). Consider, for instance, a system rife with medical errors, overtesting, and unnecessary procedures. Such a system may, in net, improve health but it may do so at the expense of some lives. Some have argued that such problems explain why the United States does so poorly relative to other nations with respect to life expectancy (Muennig, Sampat, Tilipman, Brown, & Glied, 2011).

Some might also narrow the definition of a health system to the set of institutions that are explicitly responsible for health. This would, of course, include health care delivery systems but would also include national efforts to provide clean water, sanitation, vaccination, parasite control, and the like. When thought of this way, the United States suddenly becomes a world leader with respect to health systems. In the United States, for example, the Centers for Disease Control and Prevention tend to do an exceptional job of limiting exposure to infectious diseases, and the National Institutes of Health have successfully invested hundreds of billions of dollars into understanding and combating noncommunicable diseases, such as cancer. By these standards, we can state that the United States does a better job than any other nation in the world with respect to battling disease with technology. The benefits that US institutions realize in tackling disease are public property, so they are enjoyed not just by US citizens but also by everyone in the world.

In this chapter, we will focus primarily on health care delivery systems. However, we will also touch on some aspects of research and development in the public and private sectors that constitute part of health systems.

PREVENTION OR PLASTERS?

Literacy is increasing, poverty is declining, and nutrition is improving in most parts of the world. As a result, rates of infectious diseases are declining and people are living longer lives. Longer lives mean that countries that used to worry about diarrhea and malaria are now forced to grapple with hypertension, obesity, diabetes, heart disease, and cancer. For many, this means medications to lower blood pressure, blood sugar, and cholesterol. Because these conditions are typically diagnosed by health providers and treated with medications, many global experts are pushing for health care delivery systems in every nation.

But does this mean that health care delivery systems are the future of public health in low-income nations? Every nation needs a health care delivery system, but scarce funding for chronic diseases can also be diverted to preventing them in the first place. **Primary prevention** refers to preventing disease before it appears. Primary prevention is usually accomplished via public health measures such as taxing cigarettes to prevent people from smoking. **Secondary prevention** refers to detecting and addressing a disease before it has had a chance to take a toll on the body. Secondary prevention is usually managed by clinicians who provide screening tests, such as cholesterol screening or colonoscopies. In these cases, the person already has a lifetime of a sedentary lifestyle behind her and has elevated cholesterol or has already developed cancer but it is addressed and managed early. **Tertiary prevention** is also performed by clinicians and refers to reducing the harms of a disease once it has taken hold, such as chronic pain management programs. It is possible that many more lives could be saved by redirecting scarce resources to primary prevention interventions, such reducing tobacco use, reducing air pollution, and building communities that promote healthy lifestyles. This way, it becomes possible to prevent the diseases before they happen for the entire population, not just medicating individuals after the disease is already there and taking a toll.

HEALTH CARE DELIVERY SYSTEMS

Health care delivery systems tend to focus on curative services, such as those provided in clinics, hospitals, and doctors' offices. Most health care systems research has focused on issues most present in high-income countries. This includes different types of health care delivery systems, insurance markets, private for-profit versus nonprofit hospitals, and the taxation systems necessary to fund doctors, hospitals, and pharmaceutical companies. But lower- and middle-income countries are interesting start-ups, and they need information on how to actually deliver services most effectively and efficiently. Fortunately, a good deal of recent attention has been given to how to deliver care in low- and middle-income countries (Yip & Mahal, 2008).

Although a nation's per capita GDP income is not the only way to think about health system needs (we would be hypocrites if we said so), the amount a nation has to spend on health care versus other health-producing services is one indicator of how fancy a nation's health system might be. Recall that the terms *primary, secondary,* and *tertiary prevention* refer to at what stage in the disease process we intervene to prevent harms. A similar scheme is used to describe levels of medical care. The ideal deluxe health care delivery system would offer **primary care** (the first point of contact a patient has with a provider, often a generalist), **secondary care** (the care provided by medical specialists, such as cardiologists), and **tertiary care** (the care provided by high-level medical centers that have highly specialized equipment for diagnosis and treatment of complex diseases). However, it does not make a lot of sense for a very poor nation to invest in tertiary care because, after spending money on heart transplants, no money would be left over for basic, life-saving treatments for the masses, such as antibiotics.

Another important consideration is how broadly the health care delivery system reaches into the population. **Universal health care** refers to a nation's ability to cover nearly everyone in the population (a core concept called **universality**). Many poor nations offer some form of health care assistance to their poorest citizens but leave care of others up to the free market. This strategy, providing **targeted services**, saves money by providing care to those who need it most. But it also means that better-off citizens usually lend less political and public support to the public health care system and that they might even fight it or leave it languishing. Such systems tend to have little by way of funding and tend to be poorly managed so that the lack of trust and buy-in prompts a self-fulfilling prophecy and vicious cycle—the public health programs are not funded well, so they are not very good, so politicians refuse to fund them, so their quality worsens further, and so on. For this reason, some believe that universal primary health care is important for poor nations; the more people use the system, the more voters a nation has to improve the system.

Without universality, it is difficult to make sure that all citizens—urban or rural, rich or poor, sick or healthy—have the same access to quality care (a concept sometimes referred to as **accessibility**). It is also important to make sure that no one has to pay very much out of his or her own pocket for health care (a concept known as **comprehensiveness**). Finally, a health care delivery system may also want to have a means of paying for care when citizens are outside of their local area, such as when a rural worker travels to a big city in search of work (a concept known as **portability**).

In addition, all patients would ideally have some form of **electronic medical record** (EMR). An EMR provides a means of entering information about the patient into a computer. This has a number of important advantages. One is that the patient's medical information can be called up and care paid for using a simple card or via a secure networked computer system. By increasing the efficiency of a system, the EMR would allow for all people (universality) to receive the same high-quality care (accessibility) wherever they are (portability) without paying too much for it (comprehensiveness). Another advantage of an EMR is that the computer can provide feedback to the provider. For instance, if the provider orders a medication that the patient is allergic to, the system will alert the provider. Some systems can even help guide the provider to a better diagnosis and treatment plan (see figure 5.1).

But, as mentioned previously, such a system would not necessarily be appropriate in a nation that can barely afford vaccines. Very poor nations would ideally invest in those things that saved the most lives and ignore costly, high-tech treatments, even if they alleviate suffering. This concept, appropriate technology use, was mentioned in chapters 3 and 4. Recall that it is coupled with the notion of cost-effectiveness analysis, which within a given budget provides policy makers with information on which technologies they might invest in to maximize the number of lives saved. Until now, we have primarily discussed cost-effectiveness among individual public health programs. Cost-effectiveness analysis can also be applied within health care delivery systems. When used this way, we can determine which sorts of medical treatments (e.g., paying for medications for high blood pressure or paying for more expensive surgeries) a government should invest in, given its health care delivery budget.

Then, there are practices or programs that virtually all nations can afford to implement but few actually practice. One of these is the concept of **transparency and accountability** in health care delivery and administration. That is, the system should be well managed and its budget, objectives, and outcomes should be widely available to the public for feedback and comment. There should also be a mechanism for remedying problems with specific, trained staff members or departments to hold accountable. A system that is simple to administer and easy to use is possible under most budgets. Nevertheless, most systems end up as quite complex to access for the providers, patients, and administrators anyway.

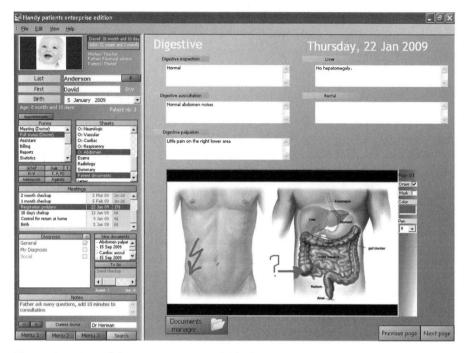

Figure 5.1. One of the many EMRs available from commercial vendors. Nations that are now converting to EMR systems face the challenge of either navigating the many systems that were in place prior to implementing a mandate for providers to use such records or forcing providers to drop their existing systems in favor of a universal system.

Source: Wikimedia Commons/Handylife.

HEALTH CARE PAYMENTS

Nations vary greatly in the way that they pay for health care delivery services. In Canada, funding comes from the federal and provincial governments, and it is derived from payroll taxes, corporate taxes, and a wide array of other schemes (including premiums, the lottery, and sales taxes). In the United States, a very large number of public and private entities pay for health care services, using general tax revenue, employer risk pools, and private insurance. However health care delivery is initially financed, getting the money to doctors and hospitals can be a tricky business.

In Thailand, payments are made from the central government to local health authorities in a **capitated** form. This payment structure provides a lump sum of cash for each patient who is covered. Some patients will not show up for care at all, and the provider can pocket the money. Others will be quite sick and consume much more care in a single shot than the provider would ever receive for the patient. This mechanism has the advantage of forcing providers to be very careful with their expenditures. If providers spend too much, they lose money. The disadvantage is that this often compels providers to be stingy with their care. Capitation payments provide a strong incentive for providers to dump sick patients or to withhold tests and treatments that may be beneficial. A large number of countries use capitation in some form, but few use it as the only way of paying for care.

The capitated payment system is not too different from just paying physicians a salary. In both of these systems, the provider knows how much money he or she will be getting up front. The difference between these systems and capitated payment systems is that salary systems do not usually include the cost of tests or procedures that the providers do in the payment.

In the Medicare system in the United States and elsewhere, hospitals are paid using the **diagnosis-related group** (DRG) system. This system pays according to the overall product (such as a hernia repair) that a provider, usually a hospital, would deliver. Thus, all of the necessary lab tests, surgical procedures, and so forth are all lumped together in a single payment. The advantage of this system is that it strongly encourages providers to stay within the limits of appropriate care (with respect to laboratory tests and nothing fancy on the side). The disadvantage is that it is not very precise. So, a provider with very sick patients who need additional care could potentially lose money. To compensate for this shortcoming, they are sometimes repackaged for routine versus more severe cases.

Fee-for-service (FFS) payments are undoubtedly the most common form of payments made to providers. In this scheme, the provider bills for the medical visit, laboratory tests, and so forth on a per-item basis. This is very common in part because, whether payments are made in livestock or cash, many people pay for care out of their pockets. This payment mechanism has the disadvantage of greatly inflating medical costs—providers are incentivized to provide more care than is necessary. Its effects are often exacerbated by **information asymmetries** between consumer and provider. Just as a taxi driver might take advantage of a tourist by taking the long way between the airport and the hotel, the doctor can order tests and perform procedures that might not line up with optimal practice. Just as the tourist does not know the town he or she is visiting, the patient often has little idea of what constitutes the best medical treatment.

Out-of-pocket (OOP) payments are components of a lot of systems. In France, otherwise healthy and wealthy patients must pay 15 to 30 percent of their medical bills as a copayment. Because this can get expensive, many choose to buy supplemental private insurance to cover the gap (Rodwin & Le Pen, 2004). Many other systems also require copayments for services, including

Medicare in the United States. Some health care delivery systems are mostly free market (e.g., Somalia), leaving citizens exposed to their entire health bill. This can get quite expensive when catastrophic illness strikes, bankrupting friends and family members of the unfortunate patient.

Most countries cover care using some mixture of payments. For instance, in Denmark and the Netherlands, some services are covered under capitated payments but others are covered under FFS. In the United States, some insurance policies pay salaries, others pay FFS, and still others pay capitated rates. Even the government itself uses many different methods of payment. In general, systems that pay up front are thought to deliver less care (and sometimes inferior care) than systems that do not but they also are much better at containing costs. Systems that use FFS can provide *too much* care, ordering tests and procedures that can lead to false positive results. When this happens, perfectly healthy people can suffer from complications, such as infection or bleeding, from procedures that they never needed in the first place.

HEALTH CARE MARKETS

The challenges associated with FFS treatment highlight one of the central problems with market-based solutions to health care delivery: health care is not a perfect market. When we think of a market, we think of grocery shopping. There are many grocers, and we can comparison shop for the best-looking tomatoes at the lowest prices. In health markets, though, we have little idea what we are shopping for. It is very difficult to comparison shop between different recommended treatments or between different doctors, and it is very difficult to know what constitutes good service.

Partly for this reason, medical care costs tend to inflate very rapidly. Imagine you have to get an MRI and that you are paying for it with your hard-earned money. If we all know that, when shopping for an MRI, you should look for a half-Tesla magnet machine and that Siemens is better than GE, you might think to ask these questions before comparison shopping. You might be willing to pay $200 for a GE scan and $250 for a Siemens scan, but if you found a place with high ratings and a radiologist who trained at Harvard that offered a Siemens scan for $235, you would probably go for that. This would put downward pressure on other places that offered scans, and they would try to remain competitive by offering a lower price or a higher quality. But, of course, none of this is actually the case in the real world. Few people have to pay for their own scans, and those who do have a difficult time comparison shopping. Without the downward pressure on prices, prices will rise for a given level of quality. After all, if no one knows how much something is worth, why not just keep charging more and more for it? (You may have experienced this phenomenon in markets within low-income countries, where bargaining starts at 50 percent of the requested price.)

As time goes on, providers, pharmaceutical companies, and device manufacturers become increasingly sophisticated at exploiting imperfections in the health care marketplace. Pharmaceutical companies looking to introduce a new drug into the market for people with moderate hypertension can formulate a half-dose antihypertensive medication and charge more than they did for the full-strength version. No one is the wiser. As a result, medical inflation tends to greatly outstrip consumer price inflation unless strict governmental controls on price increases are put into place. This is one of the reasons why governments do a much better job than private entities when it comes to holding down prices and maintaining quality. Commonly, governments do not come close to working as well as private entities within efficient markets. But in inefficient markets, governments generally do a much better job than companies with a profit incentive.

WHAT DOES *PRIVATE* MEAN, ANYWAY?

Public health and health care delivery services can be delivered by private entities and governments alike. But within the "private sector," some intend to make a profit and others do not. The ones that do not are called *not-for-profit* entities. This profit motive is a critical distinction, but it is nevertheless sometimes misleading. A not-for-profit entity can be an NGO that relies entirely on donations to survive and does not pay any of its workers (this is still "private" because it is not run by a government). But it can also be a large, aggressive hospital chain or health insurance company that is reinvesting its profits back into its operations and is not traded on a stock exchange. Such not-for-profit entities can pay executives millions of dollars a year and adopt delivery practices we usually associate with the for-profit private sector.

HEALTH CARE DELIVERY SYSTEMS IN HIGH-INCOME COUNTRIES

The US system is often used as a convenient counterfactual (comparator) for understanding other national health delivery systems, so we will jump in line and follow that trend here. After all, it represents many different kinds of health systems within a single nation.

Within the industrialized world, the United States is the only country without universal health insurance. Approximately forty-seven million Americans live without health insurance and many more are underinsured—living with some health insurance but not enough to cover most basic expenses.

More than 50 percent of the people declaring bankruptcies in the United States have unpaid medical bills (Himmelstein, Thorne, Warren, & Woolhandler, 2009). This suggests that medical care is a major contributor to bankruptcy in the United States. President Obama's 2010 reforms—the Patient Protection and Affordable Care Act—will help an estimated thirty-two million Americans become insured. Nevertheless, the reform is akin to a new, big patch in a larger patchwork quilt health care system that, in essence, remains unchanged and does not provide blanket coverage.

The basic statistics are alarming. The United States spends twice as much on health care as the next most expensive country, Switzerland, but it ranks thirty-eighth in life expectancy, despite a per capita income that is the third highest in the world, at US$46,716. It is, however, zooming ahead of other nations with respect to health care costs, even as it steadily falls behind other nations with respect to life expectancy (Muennig & Glied, 2010). In fact, as costs are soaring, health is declining in the United States (Salomon, Nordhagen, Oza, & Murray, 2009). Life expectancy may soon follow because it has already started to decline in some counties (Ezzati, Friedman, Kulkarni, & Murray, 2008). In figure 5.2, we see that forty-five-year-old females have made great progress between 1975 and 2005 with respect to the chance that they will survive to their sixtieth birthday. However, in 2005, US forty-five-year-old females had still not passed Switzerland's fifteen-year survival in 1975 (figure 5.2).

Health costs are also eating into Americans' disposable income. In figure 5.3, we see that Americans began to feel less healthy around 1993, reversing a general trend of improving health (after accounting for age and a host of other factors). We also see that medical costs were eating into the after-tax income of the median household, resulting in a decline in purchasing power. This all means that Americans are experiencing a dramatic decline in health and economic well-being and that the health system might be contributing to some of this malaise.

On the upside, waiting times for care in the United States are shorter and Americans have more access to expensive medical technology than anywhere else in the world. In the United States, a patient's treatment is primarily based on her insurance status and ability to pay. An insured patient can receive the latest cutting-edge diagnostics and treatments. The United States is also the leader in innovative medical technology, and this innovation is probably at least partly being driven by its largely free-market health system. These trends are reflected in the fact that approximately one-third of all US medical

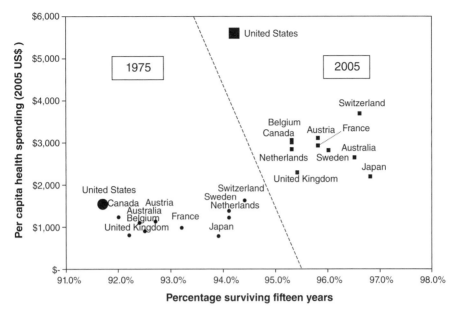

Figure 5.2. The chances that a forty-five-year-old woman will survive to her sixtieth birthday (fifteen-year survival) in twelve nations in 1975 (left half) and 2005 (right half). These fifteen-year survival estimates are plotted against health expenditures (*y*-axis).

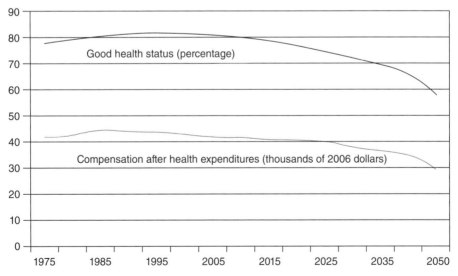

Figure 5.3. Trends in self-reported health status and total household income after accounting for medical expenditures (from the *General Social Survey, 1972–2008*, provided by the author).

care costs are spent on end-of-life care, the last six months before a patient passes away. Such end-of-life care is much more likely to consist of very expensive, technology- and innovation-driven attempts to keep someone alive for a bit longer; this contrasts with more preventative, cheaper care that more dramatically prolongs life expectancy earlier in life.

In other industrialized countries, treatments are based primarily on need, but care can be limited in some cases. Many national plans come with waiting times, for instance. This is true even in wealthy nations with national health programs. But when everyone has health care, more diseases tend to be caught and treated early, reducing the need for tertiary care later on. So, one way of thinking about the state of wealthy health systems is that the average citizen is better off with a rare or very serious disease in the United States than anywhere else, provided one has insurance. On average, though, the average citizen would be better served in France, Germany, Sweden, Norway, or the United Kingdom.

So we see that the extent to which one has access to all of the basic elements of a health plan—universality, comprehensiveness, access, portability, transparency, and appropriate technology use—varies greatly from one nation to the next. In addition, many nations allow their national health insurance plans to run alongside private plans. This way, those who can afford to purchase insurance can ensure that they also get deluxe health care benefits when they want them (though this does not apply to Canada).

THE CANADIAN HEALTH SYSTEM

The Canadian health system is often described as a *single-payer* system, meaning that there is one source of funds to pay for all medical costs. This is not exactly true because each province within Canada has its own system, with some payments coming from the province and some from the federal government. Although the system is financed by tax dollars, care is delivered by private physicians, with payments negotiated between the state and provider groups. All citizens receive a card that entitles them to free physician visits or hospital care anywhere in Canada, and coverage is close to 100 percent (though some provinces do not offer dental or visual care). Canada is a bit different from other nations with national health care in that private insurers are technically not allowed to provide the same services as the government. In theory, this prevents wealthy people from "jumping the queue" to get priority access to elective care, such as a knee replacement. (In some countries, wealthier citizens are allowed to "top up" national health insurance with private care that allows them to receive premium services.) Of course, none of this matters in an emergency; everyone receives timely and comprehensive care, if needed, in virtually every wealthy nation. Recently, waiting times for elective services in Canada have fallen, and the vast majority of Canadians are pleased with their health system.

All wealthy nations other than the United States tend to direct their financing toward preventative care, and many emphasize cost-effectiveness. For instance, if two drugs are of equal effectiveness and have the similar side-effect profile, such nations will favor the cheaper drug. (In the United States and China, the more expensive drug is often favored, possibly because it is prescribed by physicians who indirectly or directly will benefit from prescribing the drug.) Cheaper drugs also tend to be older and to have undergone more extensive testing, so they may also be safer.

Most wealthy nations also tend to streamline administrative channels. For instance, in nations where the government pays for care, only one medical billing system is needed. (Though this does not always mean that just one is actually used, it does mean that in virtually all cases, *fewer* systems are used in nations with government-financed care.) In the United States, where many different insurance companies have many different bureaucracies, medical offices need a large front office staff. Insurance companies also duplicate a lot of services, billing systems, websites, and so on. There are, in fact, so many redundant people in the United States working in medical billing and support that streamlining the system overnight could produce great short-term harm for the US economy by increasing unemployment.

However, the increased efficiency of government-driven health care does not mean that such systems are impervious to inflation. Medical inflation is a natural by-product of increasingly high-tech care and an aging world. All wealthy nations are therefore struggling with high health care delivery costs, and they tend to pass these costs directly on to taxpayers or create deficit spending.

A TALE OF MANY NATIONS

Any health care tourist or traveler with an injury abroad can tell you that no two systems in industrialized countries look exactly the same. For example, veteran *Washington Post* foreign correspondent T. R. Reid traveled to ten countries in attempts to treat his chronic shoulder pain, the result of an injury in the Navy years before. In the book *The Healing of America* (Penguin Press, 2009), he focuses on five countries that, similar to the United States, have industrialized, market economies—Canada, France, Great Britain, Germany, and Japan.

Although analyzing entire health care systems via the lens of a patient with shoulder pain is a bit gimmicky, the focus ensures that Reid engages readers in a systematic analysis rather than a hodgepodge of convenient anecdotes. Along the way, we learn that, indeed, the UK government will not cover his shoulder surgery (arthroplasty, or joint repair), which would have cost US$40,000 in the United States. (He was free to go purchase the procedure himself, though, for a lot less than it would have cost in the United States.) His doctor in France thought that Reid's shoulder pain was occasional enough, and his injury different enough, that he would not be a good candidate for shoulder arthroplasty. The doctor then admitted that because Reid could go to another orthopedist in France, he could eventually find one to agree to the arthroplasty for him. If he did that, the surgery and five-day hospital stay would cost around 5,000 euros, or US$7,000, but his sickness funds would pay for them. In Japan, Reid's prestigious doctor offered him a wide assortment of treatments to choose from, from injections to acupuncture to surgery. The price control system ensured that the total shoulder arthroplasty, also including five nights at a hospital, would cost US$10,000. Scheduling it for "[t]omorrow might be a little difficult," he was told. But the "next week would probably work."

In the United States, Reid's treatment was based primarily on his insurance status and ability to pay. In the other countries he visited, his choice of treatments was based primarily on need and choices were more likely to be affordable. Some came with waiting times, but it turns out that when everyone has health care, one is more likely to plan ahead for surgeries. Someone whose shoulder is beginning to wear out, then, will probably be placed on a waiting list long before the surgery is actually needed.

Nations with strong, centrally controlled plans have historically done a better job of holding down health care costs. For instance, Canada's expenditures as a percentage of their GDP have not changed much since the 1980s. Here are some of the ways in which most wealthy nations maintain a high-quality, low-cost health system:

- In many countries, doctors get bonuses for patient satisfaction, payments for patients even if they don't get sick (thus placing value on the patient's wellness rather than sickness and overuse of care), and for preventative measures such as flu vaccines. Certainly few doctors intend to keep their patients sick, but in the United States, there are perverse incentives to keep patients sick in parts of the health care delivery system. That is, sick patients mean more business.

- There are no columns or piles of paper charts, no repeated lab tests, no inaccessible records, no coterie of receptionists and staff members asking about the patients' latest insurance plans, haggling with insurers, or checking formularies in the offices. Even excluding insurance industry personnel, administration may account for 31 percent of US health care costs (Woolhandler, Campbell, & Himmelstein, 2003).

- Cost-effectiveness league tables can be used to hold down costs. That is, policy makers can use state-of-the art economic research to decide how to maximize the number of lives they save under their health budget by approving some treatments and prohibiting others. This practice is highly contentious in the United States because many people believe that those who can afford it should get care regardless of how much it costs (or whether it actually works). This practice creates openings for drug companies to sometimes market drugs that are more expensive and less effective (or have worse side effects) than available generics. Physicians tend to respond to this marketing, so these drugs receive priority over others.

Not all universal health care delivery systems have centralized, government-financed payment delivery systems. On one end of the spectrum, doctors in the UK's National Health Service are paid with government money. Toward the middle, Canadian, South Korean, and Taiwanese patients use government-run insurance to attend private doctors and hospitals. On the other end of the spectrum, in Japan, Switzerland, and the Netherlands, private insurers use payroll deductions to finance private health care providers. These private insurers are heavily regulated so that they cannot arbitrarily drop patients from their rolls or create redundant costs. Japanese doctors are entrepreneurial enough to blanket Tokyo public transit with posters advertising cures for sweaty palms and balding hair.

In most of these health care systems, even socialized ones such as the United Kingdom's or Norway's, patients with financial means are free to buy supplemental or private health insurance so that they can always get private hospital rooms, for instance. Relatively few opt to do so.

In "corporatist" welfare states such as Germany and Japan, patients choose between plans based on the occupation and union, and the government pays for the unemployed. (We provide a full definition of "corporatist" welfare states when we delve into the subject of political economies in chapter 6.) Further, around eighty million Americans are already covered by "socialized" systems such as Veterans' Affairs, Medicare, Medicaid, and the Department of Indian Affairs. Indeed, these programs regularly score higher patient satisfaction marks than "regular" health insurance.

In the rest of the industrialized nations, doctors do tend to make quite a bit less than they do in the United States, but they seem to still be able to afford comfortable lifestyles. This is partly because medical training is free or nearly free and malpractice insurance fees are negligible. Practicing medicine has just as much prestige as in the United States.

HEALTH CARE DELIVERY SYSTEMS IN LOW- AND MIDDLE-INCOME COUNTRIES

Priorities for donor agencies and intergovernmental entities, such as the World Bank, tend to follow trends that seem to come and go in waves. For several decades after World War II, the WHO and major governmental agencies focused on health issues by disease (see chapter 3). Major antimalarial and antismallpox campaigns in the 1960s and 1970s, for instance, were carried out by agencies dedicated to those specific causes without much effort directed at building on-the-ground health care delivery systems.

In the 1980s, UNICEF shifted away from this disease-specific approach and toward a focus on selective primary health care, especially for early childhood. Thus, growth charts and the "three F's" (female education, feeding programs, and family planning) rose in prominence at donor agencies.

However, many low-income countries were unable to implement even this selective primary health care approach. They simply did not have the money for other priorities, such as building schools. Worse, the timing of this approach followed cuts in public spending associated with structural adjustment programs. Many low- and middle-income governments were not equipped to balance quality and quantity in their health care services. Some of the issues discussed in chapter 4, such as corruption, also kept some countries from building primary health care delivery systems.

Since the 1990s, policy makers have been infatuated with the concept of **good governance** when planning reforms for health care systems around the world. Good governance is just a broad term used to mean what it sounds like—improving the way that government works. This can mean increasing transparency, giving decision-making authority to local governments (a process called **decentralization**), and getting employees to perform better by giving them incentives.

But even when management is outstanding, money is still needed. Already, almost 10 percent of the world's economy is devoted to health care, but much of that money is spent in rich countries. In 2002, the WHO's Commission on Macroeconomics and Health concluded that roughly $30 per capita per year is needed to provide basic health care to everyone, but most low-income countries only manage to spend roughly US$5 per capita (Lindstrand, Bergstrom, Stenson, Tylleskar, & Rosling, 2006) (see table 5.1).

The delivery systems that most commonly exist in low-income countries tend to be private FFS systems. Even states such as Kerala, with strong cultural and political histories of solidarity over the past few decades, face growing health care costs because they have a large private sector. Because the poor cannot afford private sector health care, even middle-income countries or states with well-developed health policies now see growing inequalities in morbidity and mortality.

HEALTH BEHAVIORS, POLLUTION, AND HEALTH EXPENDITURES IN MIDDLE-INCOME COUNTRIES

Middle-income countries, even more than wealthy countries, are grappling with populations that smoke, eat poorly, and do not exercise. This has led to a higher incidence of heart disease in middle-income nations than in high-income nations. But not all nations are the same. China—the largest middle-income country—probably suffers more from air pollution than diet and lack of exercise (though smoking is a serious problem). India—the second largest—probably suffers more from problems due to diet and lack of exercise (though air pollution is horrendous in some cities in India, too). These risky health behaviors increase health care delivery costs, making it difficult to establish a stable health care delivery system.

Traditionally, risky health behaviors have been addressed through advertising campaigns that have the goal of changing the way that people think about their health. These campaigns can be quite innovative—such as those delivered through popular soap operas or, in big corporations, workplace incentive programs to improve health. But current conventional wisdom is that these campaigns must be delivered in combination with programs that force us into a more active lifestyle. Population health can be improved directly by addressing air pollution, but it is easier to exercise in a clean air environment. Public transit can be beneficial because it forces people to walk more and also contributes to improved air quality. Buildings are now being designed to encourage dwellers to take stairs rather than elevators, and urban planners are designing neighborhoods to make more efficient use of space. This allows for shopping by foot and for more cost-effective transit systems.

At roughly US$300 per person in annual expenditures, Thailand has implemented health reforms commonly known as the "30 baht plan" (Hughes & Leethongdee, 2007; Towse, Mills, & Tangcharoensathien, 2004). This plan derives its name from the 30 baht (roughly US$1 at the time of printing) payment for every visit or service on the part of the patient. In exchange, patients can receive basic primary care services, with referral for secondary care when needed. It is a universal plan that every citizen is eligible for. As in many wealthy countries, beneficiaries receive a card that is presented to the patient's provider for payment. The system is a bit more restrictive than that found in wealthier countries—patients have to stick with their provider and providers are paid under capitated payments—but it is remarkable for having achieved universal coverage in a country that falls on the low end of middle-income nations with respect to per capita GDP.

Mexico, Turkey, and the Philippines are other examples of lower- and middle-income countries that have made great progress toward national health care. Although relatively wealthy, South Korea implemented its nearly universal health care system long before it became the modern economy that it is today (Kwon, 2009). Two of our case study locales, China and Kerala, serve to illustrate divergent policy paths that some nations take.

In figure 5.4, we see yet another illustration of how complex the relationship between money and health outcomes (as measured by life expectancy) can be. More money does not necessarily lead to proportionally more doctors' visits or to higher life expectancy. Yet, even in this complicated picture, the United States stands out in the amount of money spent on health care as well as the relatively few doctors' visits (on average) and the low health outcomes we get in return (see figure 5.4).

Table 5.1. Health Care Spending in 2009, per Person, in US Dollars

Country	Government spending	Private spending	Private prepaid plan spending	Private OOP spending	Other private spending, including donor spending	Total spending	Life expectancy
Zimbabwe	US$9	US$11	US$3	US$5	US$3	US$20	44
India	US$29	US$81	US$6	US$73	US$2	US$109	65
Kerala	US$38			US$111			
China	US$104	US$129	US$9	US$119	US$1	US$233	73
Chile	US$507	US$356	US$167	US$190	US$0	US$863	79
Sweden	US$2,716	US$607	US$7	US$529	US$72	US$3,323	81
United States	US$3,317	US$3,967	US$2,519	US$896	US$553	US$7,285	78

Sources: WHO National Health Accounts for all spending figures, www.who.int/nha/country/world_tables/en; United Nations for life expectancy figures, World population prospects (2006). Available online at www.un.org/esa/population/publications/wpp2006/WPP2006_Highlights_rev.pdf; Kerala figures, Ashokan and Ibrahim (2008), Dilip (2010), Ekbal (2006).

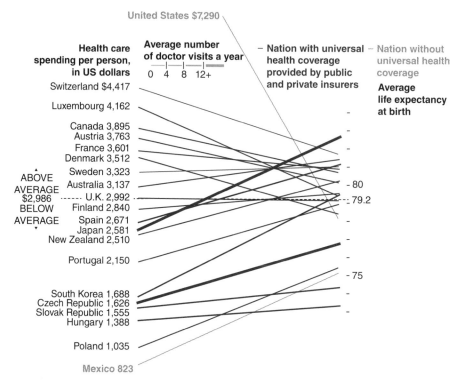

Figure 5.4. Global health expenditures, average number of doctor visits per year, and life expectancy.

Source: Uberti, Oliver. (2011). "The Cost of Care" [Information graphic] in *National Geographic* using OECD Health Data 2009, which draws on data gathered in 2007.

Health Care Delivery in China

Each of the three case study locales in this textbook—China, Chile, and Kerala—has been struggling to tackle the issue of distribution of health care to their populations. Doing this involves using the right mix of private and public health care providers. It is also important to use the right organizational structures for financing while maintaining balance of quality and affordability.

In China, dramatic policy changes since the 1980s have transformed the health care system from one of low level—but widely distributed—primary and preventive care to one of immense inequalities but with technological advances. The main challenges for China's health care system now lie in cost control, expansion of health insurance, ensuring greater access to high-quality health care for its massive population, and greater attention to chronic diseases such as hepatitis and cancer (Hesketh & Wei, 1997; Ramesh & Wu, 2009).

After the Communist Revolution in 1949, China focused its health resources on a three-tiered system that emphasized preventive rather than curative care. Most health campaigns, for instance, focused on public infrastructure such as sanitation, or getting rid of the "four scourges"—rats, sparrows (perhaps perceived like the much-maligned pigeons in New York City), flies, and mosquitoes. These mass campaigns helped to stem infectious diseases such as cholera.

Recall that for most minor ailments, most Chinese citizens saw barefoot doctors who usually completed secondary school and received an additional six months' worth of training in first aid, vaccination, a mixture of traditional Chinese and Western medicine, and other basic care. At the next level, patients could see lower-level doctors in the outpatient township health centers. If an illness or ailment was more serious, patients could go see senior doctors at the county hospital. In addition, many industry factories and state enterprises had their own "company" doctors and health care facilities. This tiered system used few cutting-edge technologies, but it probably covered many of the most prevalent and life-threatening conditions with basic treatments.

When cooperatives could no longer sustain barefoot doctors at the beginning of the 1980s, many of the former barefoot doctors took exams in order to become village doctors, who charged patients money and earned their incomes that way. As a result, medical practices overall also shifted from preventive practices to treatments of chronic conditions.

Affordability and a doctor shortage remain pressing issues. There are three main public systems in China today: the Urban Employee Basic Medical Insurance (UEBMI), the Urban Resident Basic Medical Insurance (URBMI), and the New Rural Cooperative Medical Insurance (NRCMI) (The World Bank, 2010). The first two cover people in urban areas. UEBMI covers employees and URBMI covers lower-income people without jobs (mostly the elderly and children). Although UEBMI was set up in the 1990s, its sister for unemployed elderly and children was not set up until 2007. China introduced the New Rural Cooperative Medical Care System in 2003 to help the rural poor bear the burden of medical costs, but the country still doesn't have a national primary health care system, and these three systems are still poorly integrated and deliver low-level care with expensive copayments. Doctors, especially ones trained in Western medicine, are concentrated in wealthy urban areas, earning relatively low wages but receiving most of their income from prescription medications and other additional medical services.

Health Care Delivery in Kerala

As compared to other Indian states, Kerala boasts of a much more developed health care system, with a large number of public and private hospitals and clinics as well as a supply of well-trained doctors. Kerala is somewhat known as a medical tourist destination for low-cost, high-quality Western medicine and for Ayurvedic medicine. Ayurvedic medicine is a traditional Indian form of medicine that emphasizes maintaining equilibrium in the body by following certain dietary, lifestyle, and religious practices (see figure 5.5).

Even before the arrival of European medicine, Kerala had an organized system of Ayurvedic practitioners. Thus, Keralans were used to having caregivers rather than treating themselves for medical ailments. When colonial powers, especially the British Empire, took over the area, a royal proclamation in 1879 mandated vaccination for civil servants, prisoners, and students (Kutty, 2000). Throughout the twentieth century, local governments engaged in preventive health (such as controlling the parasites hookworm and filariasis), health care (such as in the construction of general hospitals), and other public health and social services (such as safe drinking water and girls' education).

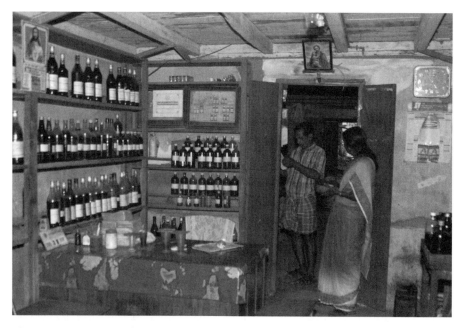

Figure 5.5. An Ayurvedic medicine shop in India.

Source: Brian Snelson. Available online at www.flickr.com/photos/exfordy/ 365079488/.

From the official formation of the Kerala state in 1956 until the early 1980s, the government greatly expanded health care facilities, with expenditures growing at an annual, non-inflation-adjusted rate of 13 percent, exceeding government expenditures overall and the state domestic product growth rate of 9.8 percent (Kutty, 2000). For instance, the number of hospital beds for non-Ayurvedic care grew from around thirteen thousand in the early 1960s to around thirty-six thousand in the mid-1980s. By contrast, only two thousand additional beds were constructed between 1980 and 1996.

In Kerala, the economy has been fair or poor for some time. This is partly because organized labor unions and government employees demanded high salaries, and the state government paid for workers' wages instead of paying for further medical infrastructure.

The availability of medicines, technologies, range of services, and quality of services in governmental hospitals and clinics suffered as a result of cuts to health care spending. But people in Kerala became used to easy access and availability of health care overall. Kerala's "glorious tradition of public health," as the Kerala minister of health's website describes it, helped to lay down medical infrastructure and led people to demand high-quality health care (Ashokan & Ibrahim, 2008; Dilip, 2010).

NECESSARY CARE?

One way of thinking about unnecessary medical care is to consider Caesarean section rates. These are operations that women receive when certain complications arise in childbirth and they cannot give birth vaginally. *C-sections*, as they are commonly called, potentially place the mother in jeopardy for future birth complications, but many women want them because the baby comes out through an incision in the abdomen rather than through the vagina (which tends to be very painful). Mothers also request C-sections because they like to induce labor before a due date for reasons of convenience and they are often unaware of the risks. Because C-sections are not often needed, their use is a good indicator of excessive medical care. They also cost twice as much as vaginal births.

Caesarean rates in urban areas of Kerala hit 34 percent, exceeding US rates of C-sections (which itself exceeds the rates of other industrialized nations) (Menacker & Hamilton, 2010). This all suggests that the government has relatively less control over ideal health practices than it might seem from the outside.

In Kerala, private sector growth in health care far exceeds that of the public sector, and there are serious signs of trouble with government health centers. For instance, only 30 to 40 percent of low-income people currently seek state medical care, including care at primary care health centers. This suggests that even free care isn't seen as a good value by many. Only 10 to 15 percent of Keralans currently receive free medical care, poor people now spend 40 percent of their income on health care, and high-income households spend 2.4 percent of their income on health care (Kunhikannan & Aravindan, 2000; Varatharajan, Thankappan, & Jayapalan, 2004).

PHARMACEUTICAL SPENDING

In the industrialized world, *big pharma* is big business. New drugs receive patents that give the patent-owning companies exclusive rights to sell these drugs, and thus command high prices and high profits for a limited period of time—usually, twenty years. This patenting system allows pharmaceutical companies to invest heavily in **research and development** (R&D), with the hopes that they can recoup the money spent to develop a drug by charging higher prices for it.

However, Marcia Angell, a former *New England Journal of Medicine* editor-in-chief and professor at Harvard Medical School, disagrees (Angell, 2004). According to Angell, the National Institutes of Health, universities, private-public ventures, and the governmental agencies of other industrialized nations around the world pay much of the research conducted in the development of new drugs. Pharmaceutical companies, she argues, thus pay for a smaller percentage of R&D costs than one might think (or pharma might claim). More-over, some policy analysts suggest that marketing costs account for a large percentage of drug company costs, but most of these data are not publicly available. One fact that is certain is that pharmaceutical companies tend to have much higher profit margins than most Fortune 500 companies.

The companies counter that it costs upwards of a billion dollars to develop a new drug. Although the studies tabulating these costs were conducted by recognized scientists, they were funded by the drug industry, raising serious questions about the validity of the research (DiMasi, Hansen, & Grabowski, 2003). Some research suggests that this cost is closer to US$55 million (Light & Warburton, 2011).

Regardless of who funds the R&D, policy makers and researchers also debate the extent to which the current system leads to true innovation in drug making. Of seventy-eight drugs approved by the FDA in 2002, for instance, only seventeen used new active ingredients, and only a handful were considered improvements over existing drugs (Angell, 2004). The bulk of drugs are sometimes called "me-too" drugs, ones that technically bear different molecular formulae from older drugs (that are either generic and widely manufactured or hold patents that are about to expire) but that use the same active ingredients and essentially work the same way.

In their searches for "blockbuster" drugs (that yield high profits), pharmaceutical companies often focus on certain diseases more than others. For example, drugs abound for common allergies, depression and anxiety, high cholesterol, and the side effects of menopause. But effective medicines for tropical diseases, particularly new vaccines, remain scarce (Trouiller et al., 2002).

More money is spent treating parasitic diseases among US pets, such as canine heartworm (Wise, Heathcott, & Shepherd, 2003), than is spent on similar conditions among humans in the poorest nations. Thus, such diseases tend to receive greater private R&D for animals in wealthy nations than for lower-income humans in low-income nations (Makinen et al., 2000). This is for one simple reason. Poor people have no money and little access to health care, so they would not be able to pay high prices for them if they were on the market. In fact, the cost of one pill or injection of some of the newer drugs far exceeds the entire annual per capita health budget in most nations (Martin, Pater, & Singer, 2001).

Bill Gates cited these patterns in R&D when he and his wife founded the Bill & Melinda Gates Foundation and their Global Health Program. One of their ideas is to guarantee that there is a market for these drugs by funding their development and paying for them (creating a market for them) after they are developed.

Although the costs of prescription drugs have risen so considerably that they are now controversial even in high-income countries, they move to the forefront of health economics debates in lower-income countries. Although the World Trade Organization (WTO) states that low-income countries can appeal to obtain drugs by importing cheaper versions, some critics state that the process is prohibitively difficult. Some middle-income countries, such as Brazil, South Africa, and India, have sought to produce cheaper, generic versions of AIDS drugs themselves. When pharmaceutical companies attempted to end these government-led practices, public outcry was severe enough that the drug companies dropped several lawsuits. They quickly changed the new arrangements to charity gifts instead.

In addition to political issues regarding drug manufacturing, there are safety concerns stemming from the lack of oversight and protection of intellectual property rights in low- and middle-income countries. These countries tend to focus on generic medicines. Especially troublesome are tainted drugs or those with lower-than-stated doses of active ingredients. Such drugs may not only kill people with the disease they are meant to treat but they may also lead to greater drug resistance.

WHAT MAKES US HEALTHY?

In 1998, Amartya Sen won the Nobel Prize in economics in part for his idea (developed with Martha Nussbaum) that a nation's development should be measured on much broader terms than by economic growth alone. The alternative development measures he discusses include the measures we humans tend to say we value most: a democracy, education, a longer and healthier life, and thicker wallets.

Policy makers mostly emphasize economic growth in development, especially in terms of improvements in the GNP. People in cities in rich nations are inundated with stock market quotes scrolling across the bottom of their television screens. Indexes like the Dow Jones Industrial Average are presented in real time and serve as a great moment-by-moment measure of economic progress.

Within the field of welfare economics, Sen and Nussbaum forged alternative ways to measure the quality of a country's development, such as its literacy or health, in what they call the **capability approach**.

Although Sen is wary of prescribing to different countries what *their* core sets of capabilities should look like, Nussbaum is a bit more forward in asserting a universal set of important capabilities for any society (Nussbaum, 2001). The functional capability we are most concerned with in this book—living long and healthy lives—appears to be nonnegotiable. As Deborah Stone has written, health is a prerequisite to everything else in life (Stone, 2005). More bluntly, "the dead cannot do so much" (quoted in Kawachi & Kennedy, 2002, p. 42).

Individuals might not always do what is best for them, but they should have the *practical* choice of good options for their health and well-being if they choose them. The role of the state is to set up the figurative playing field so that citizens are able to do so. Policies should help individual citizens to better and fully participate in their social, economic, and political worlds.

The capability approach also might help us think more clearly about our existing priorities. For instance, if we really want to ratchet up life expectancy, improvements in health care delivery will help. However, improvements in our schools, transit system, food supply (and consumption), and changes in our behavioral risk factors (smoking, drinking alcohol, using illicit drugs, poor diet, and lack of exercise) might matter more.

Following the Money

One of the lessons that we can draw from the US and Brazilian experience alike in health care delivery is that it is not enough to spend money on social programs. The money must also be spent well. For instance, Hsieh and Pugh (1993) conducted a meta-analysis on the literature exploring the effect of income inequality on crime. Most of these studies are based on simple international comparisons so they have potential flaws. That kept in mind, they find that social safety net programs that redistribute wealth from wealthier people to the poor probably help to significantly reduce crime (Hsieh & Pugh, 1993). Some public programs may actually increase crime. For instance, US public housing construction was thought to concentrate poverty in dense institutional living environments, worsening the social problems it was meant to fix. Well-meaning policies are important, and how thoughtfully and carefully they are applied also significantly shapes their effects.

Review: Elements of a Health System

Imagine that you are a citizen of the world, a butterfly, but are looking for a place to land. You are solidly middle class. One thing that you want in a country is a great health care system. But what do you look for? Here is a brief shopping list:

1. How is it financed?
   a. General taxes, payroll, or out of pocket. Systems that are financed by general tax revenues carry huge advantages not only because it makes things simple, but also because it gives the government a good deal of leverage when trying to push through reforms. Still, systems financed by employer and employee contributions can also work well. France's system was ranked best in the world at the turn of the millennium, and it is financed by deductions from employee's paychecks. OOP financing plays a role in many countries, but few use OOP as a primary financing mechanism. Of course, countries with tax-based systems can have high income taxes, but a lot of that is paid by wealthier citizens.
   b. Granted versus mandated versus voluntary enrollment. In some countries, particularly those with tax-financed national health systems, people who are citizens are covered from birth or at the time of legal residence or citizenship. Others are required to purchase health insurance by law. Still others have voluntary enrollment (as was the case in the United States until 2014). Still others, such as Germany, allow certain citizens (e.g., those who are well off and self-employed) to either buy into government plans or to use private plans.
   c. Is the system means tested? Some systems, such as Norway's, provide the same insurance to everyone. Others only offer government-financed care to those with lower incomes.

d. How many payers? As is the case with tax-financed systems, those systems with single-payer models benefit from administrative efficiency and control. They can also be more equitable because poorer regions or populations are not left with poorly financed plans or high medical costs. However, single-payer models can lack local input or controls and can be more bureaucratic than smaller, simpler plans. Many single-payer plans tend to exist within very sparsely populated nations. (If the entire population of Norway were fit into Shanghai's suburban city, Suzhou, it would be half empty.)

e. What is the mix of public versus private? Although governments rarely manage to run anything well, free market failures in health care mean that health care cannot be effectively delivered in unregulated capitalistic markets. In theory, systems that have fewer privately financed components to them will be more efficient and therefore less expensive. In practice, highly regulated insurance markets (e.g., those in the Netherlands, Japan, and Switzerland) perform quite well on most measures.

f. What cost controls are in place?

   i. Deductibles? These are amounts of money that must be paid before the insurer takes over. Thus, a deductible of $1,000 on a medical bill of $10,000 means that the user pays $1,000 and the insurer pays $9,000. Not bad, unless the medical bill comes out to $1,001 dollars. (The insurer only covers $1 in that case.)

   ii. Copayments? These are fixed amounts or percentages that the user must pay. For instance, one might pay $30 for every medical office visit.

   iii. Administrative efficiency? Is the system automated? Are there uniform and known amounts paid for a given service? Are insurance companies allowed to refuse a payment (and thereby require two parties to bargain and barter for care)? Highly computerized billing and EMR systems tend to be inexpensive and save more lives.

   iv. Appropriate technology use (cost-effectiveness panels)? Is care only provided in cases when it is deemed "affordable"? The National Health Service in the United Kingdom is infamous for denying some forms of care to the elderly or those in need of very expensive treatments that produce only small benefits. Although rationing saves money and lives under any given budget, it can also add frustrating bureaucracy.

v.   Range of benefits offered (dental, vision)? Not all health plans offer all benefits, even when those benefits are cost-effective (as is the case with preventive dental care or corrective vision assistance).

vi.   Is coinsurance needed? Plans' fixed percentage deductibles can leave users with high medical bills. Although falling at the time of press, deductibles are particularly problematic in China, where costs can reach those of wealthier countries but incomes lag far behind.

vii.   Are price lists used (drug formularies or formal price lists for specific services or diagnoses)? Medical prices can be derived from collective bargaining with physician groups or by central mandate. These can mean that physicians rush through patients (as in Japan, where the volume of care determines their income). This can be expressed by the formula: income = price × volume.

viii.   Medical information systems for records and billing? An electronic billing and medical records system is one of the few administrative measures that is almost uncontroversially beneficial for patients and increases cost savings. Of course, some technophobic providers push back.

ix.   Allow or disallow profits (by providers or insurers)? Although profits and competition provide huge incentives for providing quality products at a low price for most consumer goods, market failures in health care mean that, in most cases, profits just add inefficiency to already inefficient systems.

x.   Average length of stay in hospitals? These can be unnecessarily long (e.g., in Chinese and Japanese hospitals) leading to unnecessary exposure to hospital-acquired infections, sleepless nights among beeping machines, annoying neighbors coughing or vomiting all night, and loneliness or despair. One strength in the US system lies in the very short hospitalizations for many conditions.

xi.   Litigation controls? By reducing payouts for malpractice or injury, there is more money that can be spent on medical care. Of course, litigation can also keep providers on their feet.

g. What forms of payment are used?

i.   Capitated

ii.   Fee for service

      iii. DRGs

      iv. Out of pocket

2. What is the nation's population aging and disease distribution structure like?

    a. Are the numbers of the young increasing (e.g., India or sub-Saharan Africa) or are the proportions of older populations increasing (e.g., Europe, Japan)? Older people consume a disproportionate share of health dollars.

    b. Is the population healthy? What are the risk factor profiles? Most health care budgets are consumed by a minority of the population that is sick. If that minority is large, then costs will be high.

3. What is the nation's political economy (corporatist, market socialist, free market)? Market socialist systems appear to offer outstanding care at lower prices but also tend to exist only in small countries. Were the same patients in larger systems, they might be crushed under a mountain of bureaucracy.

SUMMARY

Health systems aim to increase population health through health care delivery and nonmedical policies, such as occupational, road, and food safety. There is growing recognition that the way that we implement our education policy, design our communities, and build our homes can have large effects on population health as well. Health care delivery systems seek to provide medical care alone and serve as a key part of broader health systems. Some health care delivery systems provide government-controlled universal health care and others leave health care delivery up to the free market (with differing degrees of regulation). One of the biggest problems facing health care delivery systems is cost control. Medical inflation outstrips other forms of inflation in most nations, which means that it increasingly consumes larger portions of government and consumer budgets alike.

KEY TERMS

accessibility

capability approach

capitated

comprehensiveness

decentralization

diagnosis-related groups

electronic medical record

fee-for-service (FFS) payments

good governance

health care delivery system

health systems

information asymmetries

nonmedical determinants of health

*out-of-pocket (OOP)
   payments*
portability
primary care
*primary
   prevention*

*research and
   development*
secondary care
secondary prevention
targeted services
tertiary care

*tertiary
   prevention*
*transparency and
   accountability*
universal health care
universality

DISCUSSION QUESTIONS

1. What are the basic components of health systems? How do they tend to be organized? What are some of the key factors that shape the effectiveness of health care delivery?

2. How do people pay for health care? How is health care financed in different countries?

3. What are some of the key factors that determine the prices and distribution of the medicines we take?

4. What are some of the key challenges that high-income countries currently face in their health systems? Low- and middle-income countries?

5. What are some of the strengths and weaknesses of your health care system? For a wealthy person? A poor person? Does the capability approach—thinking about just what policies enable you to live until at least age eighty-five, let us say—change your evaluation of your health care system? For a wealthy person? A poor person? How so or why not?

FURTHER READING

Aspalter, C., Uchida, Y., & Gould, R. (2012). *Health care systems in Europe and Asia*. New York: Routledge.

Budrys, G. (2012). *Our unsystematic health care system* (3rd ed.). Lanham, MD: Rowman & Littlefield.

REFERENCES

Angell, M. (2004). *The truth about the drug companies: How they deceive us and what to do about it*. New York: Random House.

Ashokan, A., & Ibrahim, P. (2008). Inpatient health care expenditure: Some new evidences from rural Kerala. *Indian Journal of Economics and Business, 7*(2), 297–307.

City and County of San Francisco. (2013). *Program on health, equity and sustainability*. Available online at www.sfphes.org/about

Dilip, T. R. (2010). Utilization of inpatient care from private hospitals: Trends emerging from Kerala, India. *Health Policy Plan*, *25*(5), 437–446. doi: 10.1093/heapol/czq012.

DiMasi, J. A., Hansen, R. W., & Grabowski, H. G. (2003). The price of innovation: New estimates of drug development costs. *Journal of Health Economics*, *22*(2), 151–185. doi: 10.1016/S0167-6296(02)00126-1.

Ekbal, B. (May 2006). Kerala's health sector: Crying for cure. *Kerala Calling*, 37–39.

Ezzati, M., Friedman, A. B., Kulkarni, S. C., & Murray, C.J.L. (2008). The reversal of fortunes: Trends in county mortality and cross-county mortality disparities in the United States. *PLoS Medicine*, *5*(4), e66.

Hesketh, T., & Wei, X. Z. (1997). Health in China: From Mao to market reform. *BMJ*, *314*(7093), 1543–1545.

Himmelstein, D. U., Thorne, D., Warren, E., & Woolhandler, S. (2009). Medical bankruptcy in the United States, 2007: Results of a national study. *The American Journal of Medicine*, *122*(8), 741–746. doi: 10.1016/j.amjmed.2009.04.012.

Hsieh, C. C., & Pugh, M. D. (1993). Poverty, income inequality, and violent crime: A meta-analysis of recent aggregate data studies. *Criminal Justice Review*, *18*, 182–202.

Hughes, D., & Leethongdee, S. (2007). Universal coverage in the land of smiles: Lessons from Thailand's 30 baht health reforms. *Health Affairs*, *26*(4), 999.

Kawachi, I., & Kennedy, B. P. (2002). *The health of nations*. New York: New Press.

Kunhikannan, T. P., & Aravindan, K. P. (2000). Changes in the health status of Kerala, 1987–1997. *Discussion Paper No. 20*, 26–36. Thiruvananthapuram, Kerala: Centre for Development Studies.

Kutty, V. (2000). Historical analysis of the development of health care facilities in Kerala State, India. *Health Policy Plan*, *15*(1), 103.

Kwon, S. (2009). Thirty years of national health insurance in South Korea: Lessons for achieving universal health care coverage. *Health Policy Plan*, *24*(1), 63–71. doi: 10.1093/heapol/czn037.

Light, D. W., & Warburton, R. (2011). Demythologizing the high costs of pharmaceutical research. *BioSocieties*, *6*(1), 34–50.

Lindstrand, A., Bergstrom, S., Stenson, B., Tylleskar, T., & Rosling, H. (2006). *Global health: An introductory textbook*. Copenhagen, Denmark: Studentlitteratur.

Makinen, M., Waters, H., Rauch, M., Almagambetova, N., Bitran, R., Gilson, L., et al. (2000). Inequalities in health care use and expenditures: Empirical data from eight developing countries and countries in transition. *Bulletin of the World Health Organization*, *78*(1), 55–65.

Martin, D. K., Pater, J. L., & Singer, P. A. (2001). Priority-setting decisions for new cancer drugs: A qualitative case study. *Lancet*, *358*(9294), 1676–1680.

Menacker, F., & Hamilton, B. E. (2010). *Recent trends in cesarean delivery in the United States*. Washington, DC: Department of Health and Human Services.

Muennig, P. (2009). The social costs of childhood lead exposure in the post-lead regulation era. *Archives of Pediatric and Adolescent Medicine, 163*(9), 844–849. doi: 163/9/844 [pii]10.1001/archpediatrics.2009.128.

Muennig, P., Fiscella, K., Tancredi, D., & Franks, P. (2010). The relative health burden of selected social and behavioral risk factors in the United States: Implications for policy. *American Journal of Public Health, 100*(9), 1758–1764. doi: AJPH.2009.165019 [pii]10.2105/AJPH.2009.165019.

Muennig, P., & Glied, S. A. (2010). What changes in survival rates tell us about US health care. *Health Affairs, 29*(11), 2105–2113. doi: hlthaff.2010.0073 [pii]10.1377/hlthaff.2010.0073.

Muennig, P., Sampat, B., Tilipman, N., Brown, L. D., & Glied, S. A. (2011). We all want it, but we don't know what it is: Toward a standard of affordability for health insurance premiums. *Journal of Health Politics, Policy and Law.* doi: 10.1215/03616878-1407640.

Nussbaum, M. C. (2001). *Women and human development: The capabilities approach.* New York: Cambridge University Press.

Perera, F. P., Rauh, V., Tsai, W. Y., Kinney, P., Camann, D., Barr, D., et al. (2003). Effects of transplacental exposure to environmental pollutants on birth outcomes in a multiethnic population. *Environmental Health Perspective, 111*(2), 201–205.

Ramesh, M., & Wu, X. (2009). Health policy reform in China: Lessons from Asia. *Social Science & Medicine, 68*(12), 2256–2262. doi: 10.1016/j.socscimed.2009.03.038.

Reid, T. R. (2009). *The Healing of America.* New York: Penguin Press.

Rodwin, V. G., & Le Pen, C. (2004). Health care reform in France—the birth of state-led managed care. *New England Journal of Medicine, 351*(22), 2259–2262. doi: 10.1056/NEJMp048210.

Salomon, J. A., Nordhagen, S., Oza, S., & Murray, C. J. (2009). Are Americans feeling less healthy? The puzzle of trends in self-rated health. *American Journal of Epidemiology, 170*(3), 343–351. doi: 10.1093/aje/kwp144.

Schwartz, J. (1994). Societal benefits of reducing lead exposure. *Environmental Progress, 66*(1), 105–124.

Srinivasan, S., O'Fallon, L. R., & Dearry, A. (2003). Creating healthy communities, healthy homes, healthy people: Initiating a research agenda on the built environment and public health. *American Journal of Public Health, 93*(9), 1446.

Stone, D. (2005). How market ideology guarantees racial inequality. In J. Morone & L. Jacobs (Eds.), *Healthy, wealthy, & fair: Health care and the good society* (pp. 65–89). New York: Oxford University Press.

Towse, A., Mills, A., & Tangcharoensathien, V. (2004). Learning from Thailand's health reforms. *BMJ, 328*(7431), 103.

Trouiller, P., Olliaro, P., Torreele, E., Orbinski, J., Laing, R., & Ford, N. (2002). Drug development for neglected diseases: A deficient market and a public-health policy failure. *Lancet, 359*(9324), 2188–2194.

Varatharajan, D., Thankappan, R., & Jayapalan, S. (2004). Assessing the performance of primary health centres under decentralized government in Kerala, India. *Health Policy Plan*, *19*(1), 41–51.

Wise, J. K., Heathcott, B. L., & Shepherd, A. J. (2003). Results of the 2002 AVMA survey of US pet-owning households regarding use of veterinary services and expenditures. *Journal of the American Veterinary Medical Association*, *222*(11), 1524–1525.

Woolhandler, S., Campbell, T., & Himmelstein, D. U. (2003). Costs of health care administration in the United States and Canada. *The New England Journal of Medicine*, *349*(8), 768–775. doi: 10.1056/NEJMsa022033.

The World Bank. (2010). *The path to integrated health systems in China*. Available online at www.worldbank.org/research/2010/06/13240422/path-integrated -insurance-system-china-vol-2-2-main-report

Yip, W., & Mahal, A. (2008). The health care systems of China and India: Performance and future challenges. *Health Affairs*, *27*(4), 921–932. doi: 10.1377/ hlthaff.27.4.921.

CHAPTER 6

Social Policy and Global Health

KEY IDEAS

- A nation's political and economic structures help to shape the way that social services, such as health care, are delivered or whether they are delivered at all.

- Nations are commonly grouped according to the way that they pay for social services. For instance, "market socialist" countries are those that tend to finance and deliver services solely using tax dollars and government employees.

- Democracy plays an important role in health. However, the role that it plays is not always clear-cut, and some authoritarian governments do a good job of maintaining the health of their people.

Government regulations have saved thousands of lives by mandating seat belt use, banning tobacco advertising to children, mandating worker safety rules (such as noise protection, safety goggles, safety harnesses, protection from toxic exposures, and safeguarding against the loss of limbs), and taking away other unsafe choices from people in order to protect them from themselves. Governments take money from people and corporations to build safer roads, schools, and airports. They also use tax dollars to build health care infrastructure. But getting all of these rules implemented and programs funded is not a simple task. In democracies, people resist being told what to do and generally do not like governments taking money out of their pockets. In autocratic and totalitarian governments, leaders too often would rather pocket money than spend it on social programs.

This chapter explores the relationship between health and a government's provision of social services, such as health care, income-redistribution programs, and pension programs. We start off by discussing how social policies are made. We then visit low-income and middle-income countries, where colonial legacies have been blamed for weak governance. This weak governance has, in some cases, led to the provision of services to only relatively elite, urban citizens. We then move on to high-income countries. In these nations, policies tend to be more generalized to everyone. Regardless of the context, politics matters, so we discuss how different types of political systems affect health through social policies.

HOW POLICIES ARE MADE

Ideally, policy makers have the insight, clarity, and authority to make decisions based on cost-effectiveness analyses as well as the capacity to implement the interventions they choose. Should policy makers subsidize condoms for distribution in restaurant restrooms to reduce transmission of sexually transmitted diseases? Should they mandate new safety brakes in cars? Should they regulate car emissions to lower air pollution and reduce respiratory diseases? Should they stop subsidizing gasoline, even though it will feel like a new tax to drivers?

According to the **traditional policy-making cycle,** (1) problems are presented; (2) policy makers come up with some solution to the problem; (3) these policy proposals are then accepted or rejected; (4) if accepted, these policies are implemented. They are then (5) monitored and modified as needed (Lindblom, 1968). Cost-effectiveness analyses, which were discussed in chapter 3, try to give us a sense of how well "reasonable" alternatives might work, helping policy makers with steps three and four, and everyone moves on.

This does not happen very often in real life. Even when cost-effectiveness analyses are available, they are presented in rather messy larger **policy environments**. A policy environment describes the cultural, legal, and political context in which policies are made. Even well-informed politicians mostly "muddle through" politics to get something passed, and that something is usually suboptimal (Kingdon, 1984). Sometimes, policy makers come up with solutions (e.g., lower taxes, incentives, a new database of information) even before they articulate a policy problem. Other times, a **window of opportunity** opens up so that the public need for immediate attention to existing problems and solutions makes the policy possible. For example, policy makers and public health advocates had been asking for regulations or fines on text messaging while driving for years, but several states in the United States have managed to pass laws regarding this only in the one week or so after major accidents, such as a train accident in Los Angeles that occurred because the conductor had been texting on the job.

THE ADVANTAGE OF AUTHORITARIANISM?

In 2008, the United States and China were undergoing major health reform proposals. China's health reform was implemented deliberately, with policy makers carefully looking at the international evidence and data coming back from homegrown experiments before acting. In China, health reform has come at a snail's pace, with urban workers' programs complemented by rural programs, complemented in turn by urban programs for nonworkers. This has led to a highly fragmented system. But fixing the system is seen mostly as a technical issue, and the program is expanded as funds and expertise become available.

In the United States, however, experts have studied how to implement different types of health reform for decades. Optimal plans gave way to politically viable plans. And even these have proven to be scarcely viable at all. Even after the Great Recession in 2009—when all branches of government were ruled by one political party—a great deal of wrangling occurred to get one of the compromises of politically viable plans in place. Then after the Democratic Party lost a majority in Congress, the health care plan was chipped down into something barely resembling a comprehensive plan at all.

As it turns out, policy making in the idealized world is very similar to **program evaluation.** Program evaluation is a systematic way of understanding how a program or policy fares as well as how it might be reformed to work better.

Imagine that you wake up one morning and settle down to read the paper with a nice hot cup of coffee. In the *New York Times*, you read an article about child labor and decide that you are going to start an organization to help children who were sold off to factories. Where do you start? You would ideally follow the same four steps we've discussed, more or less. You would work to understand why children are forced into labor. (Reasons might include being sold by parents to pay off a debt, working for family income while living at home, being orphaned and therefore needing to work, or being kidnapped and trafficked.) You would come up with a set of proposed ways of fixing the problem and settle on one of them (say, monitoring factories and placing orphaned children with families that will send the children to school). You would also want to look at the broader picture, such as the role of women in societies with a lot of child labor. This may provide additional opportunities for intervention and also raises the possibility that you could address two or more problems at once. That is, if you find a strong correlation between low roles of women in society and child labor, you might hypothesize that established forms of women's advocacy could solve your child labor problem because women may be less likely to trade or abandon their children than men, but may not have much say in the matter in some places. You would then want to figure out if what you are doing is working or whether there is a better way of doing it.

Identifying the Problem

Before anything happens in policy making, the problem has to be identified. This is the point of burden of disease analysis that we mentioned in chapter 3. Identifying the problem helps us understand what the health problems are out in the real world. Being too thin is unlikely to be heralded as a problem among supermodels, and being too fat is probably unfathomable to entire populations suffering from famine. For advocates of adolescents in industrialized countries, then, naming eating disorders such as anorexia was an important step in getting their concerns on the public agenda. Likewise, the notion of marital rape was not considered a public health issue until advocates could convince policy makers that a wife has the right to refuse sex to her husband. Once violence against women becomes a public—and public health—issue, and not just a private one, then we begin to worry about it. Of course, the urgency of the problem and the time it spends in the media limelight are also important factors. Another consideration is that places where it is most prominent are also likely to be the most resistant to change (see figure 6.1).

Identification is also a problem for marginalized groups. In the early days of the HIV/AIDS crisis in the United States, groups that had been disproportionately hit by the disease—mostly gay men—had trouble advocating for it to be on the national agenda or getting funding for research toward treatment. A turning point came about when hemophiliacs, who are less politically stigmatized constituents than gay men, joined the so-called "4-H Club," alongside homosexuals, hard-drug users, and Haitians.

Even getting to identifying and understanding the problem can be very hard. How big is the high-risk population of clients who visit HIV-positive sex workers, for example? This population tends to be quite mobile (e.g., truck drivers) and not exactly forthright about their sexual habits. When epidemiologists first approached sex workers asking about the numbers of their clients each night, they severely underestimated vulnerable populations because most

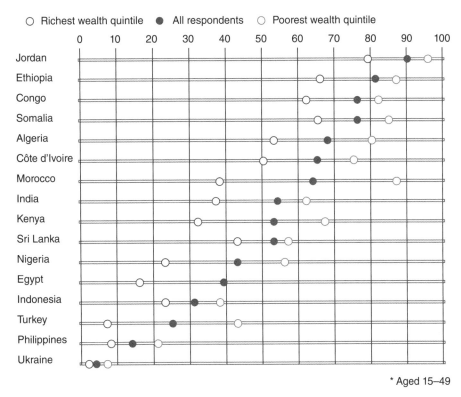

Figure 6.1. The percentage of women who feel that husbands are justified in hitting their wives under certain circumstances by selected nations. The data for each country are broken down by wealth so that we see that poorer women are more likely to favor beatings than wealthier women.

Source: UNICEF.

busy sex workers were, frankly, unavailable to speak with field-workers. They were busy working. Workers talked to the less-busy sex workers and therefore got smaller numbers. This is a problem known as **selection bias.**

THE PROBLEM OF SELECTION BIAS

Selection bias refers to a distortion in statistical data that happens when the people you end up including in a story are not quite representative of the population you think you are studying. This is particularly a problem when you are trying to compare health outcomes for people who do or do not do something that you think might be harmful. For example, perhaps you are conducting a three-month study on maternal health in Quito, Ecuador, and you survey women at vegetable markets and health clinics about the prenatal care they attempt to receive while pregnant. You conclude that poor women in Quito tend to receive care in their first trimester, but their prenatal care visits taper off until it is time to give birth. Then, your boss asks you to use your survey data to develop a community health program. You do so and your thoughtfully developed program turns out to be somewhat successful. You later discover, however, that your program was not designed to reach housewives who neither worked at the market nor had the money to attend clinics— these women had different health care habits, and they got no care in the first or second trimesters. Instead, they only went to clinics in the third trimester if complications arose. Your conclusions about maternal care practices in Quito were somewhat distorted because your survey suffered from selection bias.

There are a few ways of getting around this problem. Usually, researchers try to compare only women that are similar in age, race, income, educational attainment, or other characteristics. (In statistical speak, this is called *holding constant* the variables or factors that might bias the data.) The best way to evaluate a program is to conduct a **randomized controlled trial.** In this kind of study, you take one group of women and randomly give half of them one treatment and the other group another treatment. This is not always easy or possible.

Coming Up with Proposed Solutions

The ideal is to draw **causal** links between the problem at hand and proposed solutions. Causality means that one action (selling children to factory work) causes another (child labor). That link or pathway appears to be straightforward, but can you say that raiding factories causes children to stop working in factories? It could be that most of the children just go on to be sold to a different factory owner and the problem is not solved.

Proving causality is not always easy from either a research standpoint or from a political one. Despite many decades of evidence on the harmful effects of cigarette smoking, cigarette smoking bans are rarely mentioned for cigarettes the way they are for marijuana plants. Higher taxes, banning smoking in restaurants, and regulating advertising to children might have different likelihoods of emerging as the most cost-effective analyses, but they are also given different political priorities.

Evaluating Your Policies or Program

As stated previously, cost-effectiveness analysis helps us identify the policies that will get us the biggest bang for the buck (maximize the total number of lives saved on a fixed budget). In the ideal world, policy makers consider the interests of all of their constituents. In real life, marginalized groups lose out to powerful political constituents. If these groups do not have the ears of policy makers, they might not even get to first base, identifying what needs to be done.

Unlike this example using randomized trials, cost-effectiveness analyses can be tailored to local conditions and can incorporate a good deal of uncertainty. But they are rarely done this well. And most politicians have to strike compromises not mentioned in the cost-effectiveness analysis. For example, a politician might be loath to order evacuations given an uncertain hurricane forecast or nuclear plant meltdown. If so, the politician can bypass articulated choices such as "order evacuation" or "do not order evacuation" by instead dropping hints or suggesting that vulnerable groups, such as young children and the elderly, within a three-kilometer radius evacuate. Cost-effectiveness analysts might use arithmetic to calculate answers, but constituents sometimes have to read between the lines.

WHY IS RISK TRICKY TO CALCULATE IN POLICY MAKING?

Consider this hypothetical scenario: Epidemiologists forecast that a cholera outbreak in Haiti will kill twelve hundred people. In response, nongovernmental organizations can distribute (1) a vaccine that will save three hundred people or (2) another, riskier treatment that has a 25 percent chance of saving everyone and a 75 percent chance of saving no one. In another scenario, (3) an established vaccine will probably kill nine hundred people and (4) another, new treatment will have a 25 percent chance of saving everyone and a 75 percent of killing everyone. Most people would choose option one in the first scenario and option four in the second scenario. They would like a guaranteed saving of lives but might take greater risks if conventional medicines are guaranteed to kill a certain number of people. Yet, according to decision analyses and probability calculations, the expected outcomes are the same for all four vaccines. People tend to be **risk averse** when they think about maintaining the status quo, but they tend to be **risk seeking** in the midst of crisis and when they wish to remedy a situation (Stone, 1997).

Finally, it is difficult to truly calculate the likelihood that a substance abuser will stick to a drug regimen, that an information campaign will prompt mothers to start feeding their infant girls as much as they feed their infant boys, or that subsidies will induce construction companies to build more expensive and safer scaffolding for their low-income workers. Imagine the difficulty of measuring the predicted effects of different public health programs, such as needle exchanges or condoms, among vulnerable groups such as sex workers (Belani & Muennig, 2008).

Nor do governmental agencies act alone. Policy analysts, judges, media pundits, constituents, political aides, business leaders, and others all play roles in decision making. A provincial governor in China might decide that a hospital is not worth the cost because the national government is giving hints that it will open a new model village in the province and a new bullet train route to this village. The governor guesses that the chances of the village and train actually transpiring are 50 percent and is therefore indifferent to the hospital. One can mathematically calculate the likelihood of getting the hospital is thus 0.5, but real life sure feels a lot more complicated. In real life, decisions are not made only by thoughtful consideration but by bargaining, pleading, trading, fulfillment of roles according to hierarchy and differential levels of power, and luck.

These problems were evident when HIV/AIDS first shifted from a spotlight on people in high-income countries in the 1980s to one on the millions more in low- and middle-income countries in sub-Saharan Africa and Asia. In a candid memoir, Elizabeth Pisani talks about her days as a policy analyst for the UN AIDS program in Geneva (Pisani, 2008).

She describes the Kafkaesque labyrinth and absurdity of different agencies (at the UN, for example) that take credit for tackling AIDS. For example, within the UN, the women's agency, the children's agency, the WHO, and the development program all wished to spearhead campaigns. This happened alongside the World Bank and other intergovernmental institutions that were not related to the UN, and few of these efforts were coordinated. To make matters worse, each of these institutions had different rules, hierarchies, water cooler politics, and major funders, making it difficult to coordinate among agencies at the same organization.

As stated previously, all economic and statistical analyses come with assumptions conducted through **sensitivity analyses,** the technical term for outlining the upper and lower boundaries of the different assumed numbers they are using in estimates, which are themselves the results of hundreds of numbers put together. So, Pisani talks about how they would go to the upper or lower boundaries depending on what fit their story.

Pisani's job also consisted of writing in ways that wove a narrative around the numbers, to try to make them sound important, and to try to make people pay attention. Epidemiologists predicted that hundreds of millions of people would die in Asia, Latin America, and Eastern Europe. Better not to mention that many of these people would be drug injectors, gay men, and sex workers. Analysts such as Pisani thus regularly translate life-or-death numbers about politically unpopular groups into stories about money and babies. They might highlight the number of women who had never had sex with anyone but their husbands in rural India, for example, and highlight mother-to-infant transmission in their policy proposals about the HIV/AIDS crisis.

> For the price of a condom or a sterile needle today, you can save yourself several thousand dollars in health systems costs caring for an AIDS patient ten years from now. But . . . as a lobbying tool, the "buy needles now, save on hospital costs later" argument rests on the assumption that politicians give a damn about what happens "later." . . . If you do something cheap but unpopular now, you'll get voted out of office. It is no consolation that some opposition government will save money in the future. (Pisani, 2008, p. 27)

Finally, policy analysts have to walk the fine line between "it just gets worse and worse," emphasizing the need to do something, and "we know how to stop this thing," emphasizing the ability to address the public health issue. Policy analysts must not only use their best abilities for objectivity to present accurate numbers, but also use their best interpretive abilities to help policy makers read between the lines.

A final consideration is that policy makers sometimes see health as secondary to other goals. We mentioned some of the problems with economic policies versus public health policies. For instance, the rise of cancer with economic development is linked to increased longevity (a good thing, in case you were wondering), but it is also linked to increased exposure to the by-products of industrialization and unregulated tobacco markets. Yet, in addressing the rising incidence of cancer in the low-income world, many experts have called for investments in improved screening and treatment rather than primary prevention via smoking campaigns and environmental regulations (Kendler, Neale, Kessler, Heath, & Eaves, 1993). Cancer screening and treatment in the clinical setting is extremely expensive and does extremely little to prolong life. In fact, in many low-resource settings, one would be hard-pressed to find a hospital that can effectively treat most cancers.

POLITICAL ECONOMY AND HEALTH

As in any development context, politics reflect who gets what, where, when, how, and why. Economics reflect the allocation of resources within society.

The term *political economy* describes how political and economic institutions interact in a given environment. In this section, we describe how political economy influences the social policy landscape, and ultimately health, in low-income, middle-income, and high-income nations.

Political Economy and Health in Low-Income Countries

We have talked a lot about how income can be used to predict life expectancy in poor countries and how some poor countries do well in life expectancy. Another way of thinking about this ranking is to look at life expectancy by political economy in low-income nations. For instance, as we have mentioned many times previously, Costa Rica, Kerala, and Cuba have a long history of universal benefit social programs. They also tend to have extraordinarily high life expectancies given their level of development. Chile's dramatic shift from an emphasis on social programs did seem to slow its meteoric rise in life expectancy. This rise returned with the resumption of democratic regimes in the 1990s, even though the new regimes employed many more means-tested programs.

For instance, recall that a market socialist country will tend to provide social services directly through government agencies. A corporatist state will work closely with associations to provide social services. And a market economy will typically leave social service delivery up to private firms. These are all aspects of a nation's political economy in that the local politics and cultural norms drive how services are delivered. By dividing political economies into categories, we can get a better sense of how different approaches might affect health. "Liberal," market-driven political economies tend to provide a better business environment, but they also tend to do worse on delivering services to their people.

WHAT IS A *LIBERAL* ANYWAY?

Our US readers may become confused when reading the international health literature. In the United States, the word *liberal* generally refers to individuals on the political left who believe in civil liberties, social rights, and a stronger welfare state.

In most other countries, however, *liberal* is not supposed to contrast with *conservative,* as in contemporary US parlance; rather, it probably harkens back to the original use of the word as in the Scottish Enlightenment. (The larger European Enlightenment was a cultural movement in the seventeenth and eighteenth centuries, marked by intellectual develop-ments emphasizing secular rationality and scientific methods in fact finding.) In those contexts, *liberal* was used to refer to individuals as drivers of behavior, especially in the marketplace. More contemporary versions of this strand of thinking, called *neoliberalism*, include the idea that policies should be created with as little state interference as possible.

It is difficult for governments in middle- and low-income countries to provide social protections and services to their citizens. Within the urban areas of these nations, large numbers of workers scrape by in the informal sector. Poor peasant farmers populate the countryside. In good times, urban workers garner enough to feed their families and farmers grow more than what they need for their own subsistence. In bad times, they go hungry. Because informal sector workers such as these are not on the books, they do not pay taxes. Without tax revenues, governments cannot fund the social policies and pro-grams that are needed to lift such lower-income citizens out of poverty.

In low-income nations, the usual social protection schemes that residents in rich countries are used to—such as unemployment insurance or social security programs—too often do not exist. If they do exist, they are sometimes provided mostly to help powerful interests, such as the military, civil service workers, and organized labor (Sandbrook, Edelman, Heller, & Teichman, 2007). In short, they are mostly for those with "formal sector" government jobs.

In low-income countries, the provision of social benefits to those in the formal sector has been a problem throughout modern history. For example, in the 1970s, social insurance expenditures accounted for 15 percent of GNP in some Latin American countries, but they only benefited a very small slice of the population (Mesa-Lago, 1978). This situation has since improved somewhat in Latin America with the proliferation of new services (e.g., the conditional cash-transfer programs discussed in chapter 13 of this book). Today, in low-income nations within Africa, where large swaths of the popula-tion live in poverty, only between 1 to 12 percent of people in the labor force actually have access to social insurance programs (Zwanecki, 2001). Even in modern capitalist China, a person with a government job ("the iron rice bowl") is a highly desired mate. On the upside, these groups within government jobs constitute the seeds for a growing middle class, and there is a clear trend toward expanding social services out of the government sector and into the general population.

The Urban-Rural Divide

In sub-Saharan Africa and Latin America, only Mauritius, South Africa, Namibia, and Costa Rica have managed to develop benefit schemes that cover informal sector workers. Mauritius provides pensions for everyone, even those (such as the disabled or subsistence workers) who were unable to make enough money to contribute to a plan (Sandbrook et al., 2007).

Universal social benefits in areas such as health care are relatively rare in most lower-income and middle-income countries because the poor within these nations tend to have little voice. For example, land reforms in India, Peru, El Salvador, and Bangladesh were largely circumvented by landowners who would otherwise have to give up their land deeds to the government (Sandbrook et al., 2007).

This forces governments to primarily raise revenue through a **value-added tax** (VAT), which is a type of sales tax on consumer goods. This VAT taxation system has some drawbacks. First, it is not a form of **progressive taxation**. Progressive tax is so called because the percentage one pays on his or her income becomes progressively higher as income increases. Thus, if someone is working in a low-paying job, she will pay few or no taxes under a progressive system. Someone with middle income might pay 20 percent of his or her income in taxes. Someone with high income might have to pay 30 percent, 40 percent, or more. The wealthy can continue to earn wealth and perhaps become wealthier, but they will help pay for public programs, such as schools, along the way.

There are other problems with VAT-reliant taxation; for instance, it creates an incentive for a black market (informal sector) economy. People will buy goods in countries with relatively low VAT and then smuggle them across the border to countries with higher VAT. This creates a huge disincentive for governments to spend more on health or other social services (because if they do, their citizens will just start to buy things from their neighbors rather from them). Finally, with a VAT, the poor are paying taxes on goods that help them survive, such as food, shelter, transit, and school supplies.

Corruption is another significant problem that keeps governments from implementing programs. If most of the money for a program is lining the pockets of politicians and contractors, the program itself probably won't be adequately funded or work. It is also difficult to get citizens behind government programs when they feel as if they are only paying corrupt officials with their tax dollars. **Clientelism** also often prevents social policies from working. Clientelism describes "a tie between two parties of unequal wealth and influence" that "depends upon the exchange of goods and services" (Powell, 1970, pp. 412–413). One egregious example is buying votes in exchange for governmental construction contracts, but the process is often a bit more subtle. Clientelism can even prompt officials to provide important services, for example when a politician builds a park in a slum neighborhood in exchange for votes. But clientelism usually is not sustainable in the long run. For example, with the next election cycle, who will clean and maintain the park? Even when put to good ends and backed by long-term funding, clientelism makes it difficult for central governments to coordinate and plan. For instance, park space should be built, mapped, and planned for by the central government, not the priorities of local politicians. Clientelism is thought to be more rampant in certain low-income nations, where weak governments seek to win the favor of powerful elites and little transparency exists.

Clientelism and **populism** tend to go hand in hand (Sandbrook et al., 2007). Take, for example, Hugo Chávez, the former president of Venezuela. Chávez seized oil assets to redistribute resources, allocated material rewards to loyal masses, and reasserted governmental regulations in popular economic life. The Chávez administration clamped down on opponents and built on clientelistic ties to maintain power, but it did this in the name of providing social services to the poor. As a result of poor coordination and a lack of transparency, incompetent administrators who supported the administration were sometimes favored over competent ones. Despite expansion, some programs languished because of inefficiency and corruption.

Legacy of Colonialism?

Some people attribute the poor state of social policy in low-income countries to these nations' colonial histories. For at least eight centuries, colonial powers conquered territories around the world and competed for advantages in trade, raw materials, labor, and investment opportunities. In many cases, colonial rule led to nondemocratic regimes that did little to build institutions (Blanton, Mason, & Athow, 2001). In Latin America, Africa, and Asia, leaders educated in wealthier nations sometimes led nationalist alliances for independence. In Latin America, in particular, these governments built democratic institutions. But, as we just mentioned, some of them nevertheless excluded the vast majority of their poor inhabitants. In Asia and Africa, low-income, postcolonial nations were too often nondemocratic (Sandbrook et al., 2007).

Recall, as mentioned in chapter 1, that the 1960s, 1970s, and 1980s were marked by military dictatorships, which took over many democratic governments in Latin America, Africa, and Asia. Many of the dictators were supported or even guided along by either the United States or the USSR during the Cold War. Around one-third of low-income countries were governed by their own military in 1970. By 1983, the number governed by their own military dictatorships doubled to 60 percent (Midgley, 1987).

We mention this here again because the former colonial governments helped set the stage for modern social policies in most of these nations. In Africa and Latin America, for instance, the first social security programs were designed under colonial rule. Sometimes, these programs were originally designed for the Europeans living there or indigenous groups who were willing to help Europeans maintain their power.

COLONIAL POLITICS AND WAR

Many wonder how rich nations could conquer poor nations with much larger armies in foreign territories. One trick was to join forces with rival ethnic groups. These smaller groups, who were often discriminated against by the dominant powers, knew the terrain and provided additional person power on the battlefield. The unfortunate side effect of these policies was to instill deeper religious and ethnic conflicts using more lethal weapons. In the postcolonial period, this sometimes left a legacy of civil war that remains difficult to break.

Democratic Socialist States in Low-Income Countries

The political economies of low- or middle-income countries sometimes change swiftly and dramatically (as Chile's did from Salvador Allende's administration to Augusto Pinochet's administration).

The case of Kerala exemplifies a "social democracy," a democratic form of government that does not adopt the sort of socialism of the Soviet Union or pre-1980s China but does adopt more government-oriented social policies. In China and the Soviet Union, the state claimed that, through revolution, a centrally planned (and worker-owned) production and distribution of goods would make everyone more or less equal. Instead, Kerala operates with a multiparty system in which political parties on both the left and the right of the political spectrum have ruled in the past few decades. In addition, although Keralans use a parliamentary system, they have also implemented a decentralized decision-making system whereby ordinary citizens, rather than elected officials, help shape local budgets and policies. Keralans have, though, brought the communist party to power multiple times in recent history. Kerala's communist party has advocated for strong workers' rights and incomes and generous health, education, pension, and other benefits. The communist party has also, in the past, passed land reform legislation (Heller, 1999; Isaac & Heller, 2003).

On the whole, social policies in Chile and Costa Rica theoretically focus on "good jobs with good wages" (Sandbrook et al., 2007). They emphasize private property and market forces, but they also tend to operate and subsidize basic public services (education, health, national forests and roads, etc.). Costa Rica, for instance, is famous for its ecotourism, protected forests (which especially stand out in contrast to the rapid deforestation of other global south countries rich in natural resources), a highly educated populace, and for not having a national army.

Finally, post-1990 Chile attempted to translate Tony Blair and Bill Clinton's "third way" approach to the low-income context (Blair, 1996). This usually means that market forces are unleashed but social programs are still emphasized (Muntaner, Lynch, & Smith, 2000). They also tend to recognize that good social programs account for common responses to incentives (alongside other social forces). Table 6.1 organizes these different forms of government into named categories.

Authoritarian States in Low-Income Countries

Overall, as we have mentioned throughout the book, democratic states tend to report better health outcomes than autocratic or authoritarian ones. But there are plenty of exceptions.

CHINESE CAPITALISM AND HEALTH

China's experiment with capitalism had lifted four hundred million people out of poverty in a period of just thirty years at the time of press. It has also led to a slightly more open society with somewhat fewer political executions and prisoners (both of which are obviously major public health issues). Although the beneficiaries of capitalism traded barefoot doctors for care in high-tech tertiary care medical centers, others have not fared as well. There are still few worker protections, and widespread lead poisoning in the community and exposure to occupational toxins at work abound. "Cancer villages" sprouted up all over China as a result of industrial waste. Although many have greatly benefited from China's economic rise, others have lost out. The net effect is a modest deceleration in the life expectancy gains that were realized during the communist heyday.

Table 6.1. Three Forms of Social Democracy in Low- and Middle-Income Countries

	Radical social democratic	Classical social democratic	Third way
Main unit of organization in society	Class (workers and peasants are organized into own associations)	Society as a whole, with everyone in it	Mostly individual, sometimes society as a whole
Main social goals	Equity	Solidarity and growth	Market-based growth
Main patterns in social policy	Universal entitlements; redistributive policies	Universal policies, no eligibility requirements	Means-tested benefits, accessible education, poverty reduction
Benefit levels for most policies	Traditionally high, but reduced in recent decades and now varying according to decentralized decisions	Pretty high, same for everyone	Fairly low, but with subsidized support for capacity building
Conception of democracy, ideal decision making	Decentralized, participatory decision making, high-level representation	Representative system, consultations with stakeholder groups	Electoral, representative, competitive system with elites
Example countries	Post-1960s Kerala, 1977–1990s West Bengal	1950–1980 Costa Rica, post-1970s Mauritius	Post-1990 Chile, 1985–2004 Uruguay

Authoritarian states are diverse. Some are nation-states in war, with no predictable patterns in political or economic activity. Some are also dictatorships, such as those in Turkmenistan and North Korea. And of course, there is Cuba, which, until recently, emphasized health care in its social policies, even as its government was known to torture political prisoners. These nations vary in their economic and social policies, but all tend to consolidate power through a combination of populism and political repression. Governance systems similar to the multiparty representative democracy in Russia can be incredibly difficult to categorize (Sakwa, 2010; White, 2010).

China remains an important case study in authoritarian rule. It is a rising superpower (economically and politically, especially because it sits on the UN

Security Council) and the most populous country in the world. It produced improvements in health outcomes for decades despite a lack of democracy and, similar to Cuba, has a number of pro-public health programs. It is currently embarking on a universal health insurance program.

Despite its nominal status as a communist country, most of China's economic policies since 1979 have been anything but. Instead, as briefly described in chapter 2, they not only charged for health care but in some cases also charged for vaccines. There are few worker protections or safety regulations that are actually enforced. By the start of the twenty-first century, health care delivery was on par with some of the poorest nations in the world (WHO, 2000).

According to some Chinese activists who participated in the famous 1989 Tiananmen protests, their rallies were not just about abstract democratic rights such as freedom of speech and assembly. They were also about economic security, social security, and health. Indeed, the 1989 protests probably would not have happened if 1988 had not been the "Year of the Contract," with quickening privatization and closures of state enterprises, precipitously falling incomes for "iron rice bowl" farmers, new configurations in foreign trade departments and finance contracts, and inflation. Many Chinese scholars have struggled to articulate what a new political economy—one that rejects the social and economic tumult of these unregulated market forces but that looks like neither a US-style capitalist democracy nor the brutal repression of the Cultural Revolution—would look like (Hui, 2010).

Although China may be headed on the path toward greater freedoms and better social services, there remains a long way to go. Entrepreneurs and status-hungry conspicuous consumers abound. Protestors, human rights lawyers, and religious practitioners are sometimes tolerated, sometimes not. The state often heeds their complaints to address poor labor conditions in the factories that make Apple's iPhones, for example, but the government does not do so systematically. Finally, crimes against the state continue to be broadly defined, and years at "re-education" labor camps continue to serve as punishments in lieu of explicit prisons, as in traditional twentieth-century communist regimes. All of this has a profound effect on people's health.

This form of "state capitalism" is quite different from prominent state capitalist examples from the twentieth century, that is, operating the state as a giant corporation or as a coordinated alliance between the government and Big Business, especially in the name of the so-called military industrial complex (Bukharin, 1915/1972; Hossein-Zadeh, 2006; Jansson, 2001; Rothbard, 1973). Overall, the Chinese government's social policies have attempted to draw on the country's comparative advantages (low labor costs, large consumer base) for market-based growth, at the expense of social or economic equity, and environmental protection. China's emergence as an economic powerhouse, then, is not the result of a transition to traditional "free market" policies with

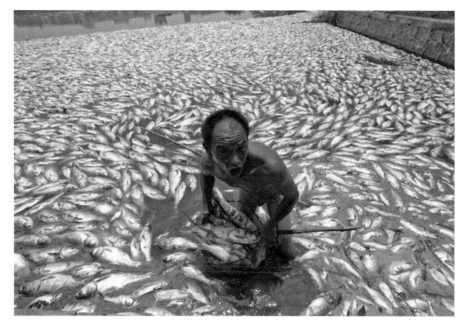

Figure 6.2. A man appears to collect fish for human consumption after extreme river pollution and high temperatures lead to large numbers of fish dying in the river in Wuhan, China.

Source: Copyright © China Daily/Reuters/Corbis.

an "invisible hand," but the result of a set of very visible, heavy-handed policies aimed at coastal economic development, largely at the expense of the rural poor (figure 6.2).

At the same time, the state must maintain high economic and quality-of-life outcomes for a large swath of the population so that mass popular unrest does not transpire. China's governmental leaders see the need to address this, but efforts to do so have been spotty (Evans, 2006). Indeed, comparative politics scholars also rightly argued that we need more research on the widespread expansion of welfare states in low-income countries (Mares & Carnes, 2009). As table 6.2 suggests, low-income countries have a great deal of catching up to do in terms of social insurance policies; Africa, for example, has a whole lot more than four countries. That said, it is remarkable that out of those countries that have developed old age pensions, disability payments, and health insurance schemes, most have been associated with authoritarian regimes. The only such policy that democratic regimes tend to undertake more often is that of unemployment benefits (Mares & Carnes, 2009). Table 6.2 summarizes some traits of two prominent types of nondemocratic mixed political economies in low-income countries.

Table 6.2. Two Types of Nondemocratic Governance

	State-capitalist authoritarian	Populist corporatist
Main unit of organization in society	Mostly individual, sometimes as representative of society as a whole	Interest groups and supporters vis-à-vis leader in office
Main social goals	State-led economic growth	Clientelism
Main patterns in social policy	Both public and private investments; eligibility rules to target specific low-income populations, especially in impoverished rural areas	Popular redistribution and nationalization of resources; no systemic universal policies or safety nets
Benefit levels for most policies	Traditionally low except in capacity-building education and certain priority policies; big shift from post–Cultural Revolution in the 1970s	Varies according to key beneficiaries and constituencies
Conception of democracy	Not democratic; the party makes decisions for the people's benefit	Generally democratic but without strong voter monitoring
Example countries	Post-1978 China	Venezuela

Indeed, prospects for global health in the near future greatly depend on the extent to which countries such as China can remain responsive to emerging health crises without the sorts of democratic accountability that help other countries avert disasters. Indeed, Mao Zedong himself said the following:

> Without democracy, you have no understanding of what is happening down below; the situation will be unclear; you will be unable to collect sufficient opinions from all sides; there can be no communication between top and bottom; top-level organs of leadership will depend on one-sided and incorrect material to decide issues, thus you will find it difficult to avoid being subjectivist; it will be impossible to achieve unity of understanding and unity of action, and impossible to achieve true centralism. (Sen, 1999, p. 182)

The great famines during the Cultural Revolution and the Great Leap Forward, (on a smaller scale), the slow release of information and response to the SARS outbreak, the failure to protect families from melamine-infested infant formula and toothpaste, and the failure to uphold safety standards in the school buildings that fell during the Sichuan province earthquake show the direct ways in which a lack of democracy has affected China's social policies. The government has responded with harsh punishments, including the death penalty, for the heads of companies with tainted infant formula, for example. Still, it has yet to implement the sorts of systemic policies necessary to make sure ordinary citizens are protected from tainted foods and consumer products, corrupt police and governmental officials, and the ravages of poverty in a country that calls itself communist. We will explore episodes such as the Great Leap Forward in greater detail in chapter 7.

POLITICAL ECONOMY IN HIGH-INCOME COUNTRIES

One way of dividing up the world's political economies is to think of them as corporatist capitalist states, social democracies, and liberal capitalist states (Esping-Andersen, 1990). In terms of social policy, liberal capitalist or market economies—a group that includes our case study, Chile, and the Anglo-Saxon ones, such as the United States, Canada, Ireland, Great Britain, and Australia—tend to implement **means-tested policies.** Means-tested policies require that individuals and families qualify for services by showing that they are poor. For example, Medicaid is a government insurance program that is only available to the poorest residents of most states in the United States. By contrast, Medicare is nearly universally available to all persons over the age of sixty-five in the United States; even wealthy elderly Americans collect Medicare benefits. Although Medicare was originally designed as a universal program (for the elderly) under the presumption that most cannot afford to pay for medical care while on an old-age pension, its near-universality has made it much more politically popular than means-tested Medicaid. (In Australia, Medicare is universal but other services tend to be means tested.)

Of course, the lines among market, corporatist, and social democracy nations are blurry. Aside from the United States and Turkey, all of the other OECD countries have universal health insurance. But even in the United States and Turkey, universalist programs (similar to those in social democracies) exist, such as free kindergarten through twelfth grade education and social security. And the United States has various "socialized" health programs, such as the Veteran's Administration. Despite the blurry lines, social, economic, and health inequalities tend to be the highest in market economies of industrialized countries (Navarro & Shi, 2003).

DOES POLITICAL ECONOMY PREDICT HEALTH IN WEALTHY NATIONS?

One distinguishing feature of nations that tend toward market economies is that they often have a lower life expectancy than those of corporatist states or social democratic states. Although some corporatist states, such as Japan, have extraordinarily high life expectancies, the social democracies tend to cluster at the top in this regard. They also fall in similar line with respect to educational performance and income equality. Some researchers have used these statistics to suggest that efficiently run social programs drive up life expectancy (Marmot & Wilkinson, 2006; Wilkinson, Pickett, Trust, & Foundation, 2009). However, it is important to remember that correlation does not mean causation. Correlations could mean that countries that tend toward social democracies tend to be more cohesive and supportive and that this, in turn, explains their better health. Moreover, some of the leading areas with respect to life expectancy—Hong Kong and Singapore—provide very little in terms of social services and are highly unequal. Although this higher life expectancy might be explained by these nations' large immigrant populations, their impressive health statistics cannot be discounted.

In corporatist states, such as Belgium, the Netherlands, Germany, France, Italy, Switzerland, and Japan, individuals tend to rely on their extended families, not on employers or the state, for provision of social services to the elderly, disabled, and children. Accordingly, certain social policies (such as the minimum wage) are often much more generous than in either liberal or social democratic countries so that fathers can earn a "breadwinner wage" and mothers can stay home; others (such as free or subsidized child care) are virtually nonexistent. Some of these corporatist countries have begun to reform their policies; for instance, Germany now boasts of some of the most generous child care policies in the world. Nevertheless, most primary schools still dismiss students by lunchtime, and tax rates tend to be lower for married couples in which one person has a lower income (Bennhold, 2011). The *corporatism* name comes from the fact that these states grant quite a bit of policy-making power to groups—corporations—of different kinds, such as labor unions and other interest groups.

Finally, in social democratic states, policy makers attempt to offset the unequal consequences of the marketplace via social programs. In turn, taxation

Table 6.3. Main Political Economy Types in Industrialized Countries

	Social democratic Scandinavian	Corporatist Christian Democratic	Liberal-residual Anglo-Saxon
Main unit of organization in society	The society as a whole, with everyone in it	The most immediate group (family in welfare and assistance policies, unions in labor policy)	The individual
Main social goals	Solidarity	Communitarianism, a place for everyone and everyone in his or her place	Meritocracy, competition
Main patterns in social policy	Universal policies; no eligibility requirements	Some differences in coverage by gender or age; no eligibility requirements	Means-tested policies; varying eligibility rules to target specific populations
Benefit levels for most policies	High and the same for everyone	Fairly high, but benefit levels vary according to the group the person belongs to	Fairly low, ideally just enough to get the person back into the labor market
Example countries	Sweden, Denmark, Norway	France, Germany, Italy, Netherlands	England, Canada, United States, Australia, Chile

rates are also predictably higher. Policies emphasize full employment and universal entitlements so that a citizen is entitled to all benefits regardless of his or her income, occupation, or marital status. Table 6.3 summarizes some of the key traits of each of these political economies, which are of course idealized here and more nuanced in real life.

LESSONS FOR HEALTH-OPTIMIZING SOCIAL POLICIES

As we mentioned in chapter 5, Amartya Sen argues that participation is an integral capability that should be accorded to all people and that political and economic rights cannot be separated (Sen, 1999). He suggests that economic prosperity is no excuse for the denial of political rights in Singapore. But he also argues that programs for the unemployed in some European countries would be improved if they provided jobs rather than extensive welfare benefits.

No one type of political economy or set of governance structures will work across all countries. Nevertheless, some patterns emerge. For instance, cross-national analyses suggest that education outcomes are one of the most powerful predictors of a nation's life expectancy. Health and other welfare expenditures matter, too, but to a lesser extent. Long-term experiences with democratic practices, especially the freedom of information and freedom to organize, make a difference, even when the governmental administration (such as Pinochet's in Chile) is authoritarian (McGuire, 2010). Here is a list of overarching elements of political economies that, according to comparative research, lead to health-benefiting social policies:

- A state that has the pulse of its populace and knows what it needs
- An organized state with the federalist or multilevel communications and efficiency to carry out social policies
- An organized state with the resources and infrastructure to implement the plans it chooses
- A robust civil society to demand some distribution of new wealth amid market reforms and to keep the state itself in check
- A history of multiparty competition, cross-class compromise, institutional channels of democratic accountability and feedback, and a free press
- A strong political party, possibly with superpower allies, to coordinate efforts and help lead the way

In the following chapter, we delve into how our case studies' political economies have or may have affected health. In the case of China, where tens of millions of people died due to misdirected government policies, the tie between political economy and life expectancy is clear. In other cases, students should be skeptical of the associations that researchers claim.

SUMMARY

This chapter builds on the idea that a nation's political economy and its health are intertwined. We consider whether nations that tend to invest more in social policies really do have better health outcomes than those that do not. The political economies of nations have been loosely grouped into the categories *market, corporatist,* and *market socialism.* In reality, it is very difficult to pigeonhole a nation into one of these categories because most overlap. Nowhere is this more true than in low-income nations. The answer as to whether political economy even matters for health is complicated because such investments are lost to various forms of corruption in nations that otherwise suffer from poor governance. What is clear, though, is that if the very rough analyses currently available are correct, a nation's ability to implement medical and non-medical social policies may be the single most important determinant as to whether citizens lead short or long lives.

KEY TERMS

causal

clientelism

means-tested policies

policy environments

political economy

populism

program evaluation

progressive taxation

randomized controlled

  trial

risk averse

risk seeking

selection bias

sensitivity analyses

traditional policy-

  making cycle

value-added tax

window of opportunity

DISCUSSION QUESTIONS

1. What are some of the main types of political economies of low-income countries?

2. Do you find the typology of political economies in industrialized countries convincing? What do you think the most important characteristics of political economy are in terms of health?

3. Do you think that there are relationships between a nation's political economy and its health outcomes? Through what potential pathways? Why or why not?

FURTHER READING

Acemoglu, D., & Robinson, J. (2012). *Why nations fail: The origins of power, prosperity, and poverty*. New York: Crown.

Economist. (2008, August 28). The bottom 1.4 billion. Available online at www.economist.com/node/12010733

Graeber, D. (2011). *Debt: The first 5,000 years*. New York: Melville House.

REFERENCES

Belani, H. K., & Muennig, P. A. (2008). Cost-effectiveness of needle and syringe exchange for the prevention of HIV in New York City. *Journal of HIV/AIDS & Social Services, 7*(3), 229–240.

Bennhold, K. (2011, June 28). Women nudged out of German workforce. *New York Times.*

Blair, T. (1996). *New Britain.* Boulder, CO: Westview.

Blanton, R., Mason, T. D., & Athow, B. (2001). Colonial style and post-colonial conflict in Africa. *Journal of Peace Research, 38*(4), 473–491.

Bukharin, N. (1915/1972). *Imperialism and world economy.* London: Merlin.

Esping-Andersen, G. (1990). *The three worlds of welfare capitalism.* Princeton, NJ: Princeton University Press.

Evans, P. (2006). *Population health and development: An institutional-cultural approach to capability expansion.* Washington, DC: World Bank.

Heller, P. (1999). *The labor of development: Workers and the transformation of capitalism in Kerala, India.* Ithaca, NY: Cornell University Press.

Hossein-Zadeh, I. (2006). *The political economy of US militarism.* New York: Palgrave Macmillan.

Hui, W. (2010). *The end of the revolution: China and the limits of modernity.* New York: Verso.

Isaac, T. T., & Heller, P. (2003). Democracy and development: Decentralized planning in Kerala. In A. Fung & E. Wright (Eds.), *Deepening democracy: Institutional innovations in empowered participatory governance.* New York: Verso Books.

Jansson, B. S. (2001). *The $16 trillion mistake: How the U.S. bungled its national priorities from the New Deal to the present.* New York: Columbia University Press.

Kendler, K. S., Neale, M. C., Kessler, R. C., Heath, A. C, & Eaves, L. J. (1993). A test of the equal-environment assumption in twin studies of psychiatric illness. *Behavioral Genetics, 23*(1), 21–72.

Kingdon, J. (1984). *Agendas, alternatives, and public policies.* Boston: Little, Brown.

Lindblom, C. E. (1968). *The policy-making process.* Englewood Cliffs, NJ: Prentice Hall.

Mares, I., & Carnes, M. E. (2009). Social policy in developing countries. *Annual Review of Political Science, 12,* 93–113.

Marmot, M. G., & Wilkinson, R. G. (2006). *Social determinants of health* (2nd ed.). New York: Oxford University Press.

McGuire, J. (2010). *Wealth, health, and democracy in East Asia and Latin America.* New York: Cambridge University Press.

Mesa-Lago, C. (1978). *Social security in Latin America.* Pittsburgh: University of Pittsburgh Press.

Midgley, J. (1987). Need and deprivation in developing societies: A profile. In S. MacPherson & J. Midgley (Eds.), *Comparative social policy and the third world.* New York: St. Martin's Press.

Muntaner, C., Lynch, J. W., & Smith, G. D. (2000). Social capital and the third way in public health. *Critical Public Health, 10,* 107–124.

Navarro, V., & Shi, L. (2003). The political context of social inequalities and health. In R. Hofrichter (Ed.), *Health and social justice: Politics, ideology, and inequity in the distribution of disease* (pp. 195–216). San Francisco: Jossey-Bass.

Pisani, E. (2008). *The wisdom of whores: Bureaucrats, brothels, and the business of AIDS*. New York: W. W. Norton.

Powell, J. D. (1970). Peasant society and clientelistic politics. *American Political Science Review, 64*, 411–425.

Rothbard, M. (1973). A future of peace and capitalism. In J. H. Weaver (Ed.), *Modern political economy*. Boston: Allyn & Bacon.

Sakwa, R. (2010). Politics in Russia. In S. White (Ed.), *Developments in Russian politics* (Vol. 7). New York: Palgrave Macmillan.

Sandbrook, R., Edelman, M., Heller, P., & Teichman, J. (2007). *Social democracy in the global periphery: Origins, challenges, prospects*. New York: Cambridge University Press.

Sen, A. (1999). *Development as freedom*. New York: Knopf.

Stone, D. (1997). *Policy paradox: The art of political decision making*. New York: W. W. Norton.

White, S. (2010). Classifying Russia's politics. In S. White (Ed.), *Developments in Russian politics* (Vol. 7). New York: Palgrave Macmillan.

WHO. (2000). *World health report 2000—Health systems: Improving performance*. Available online at www.who.int/whr/2000/en/index.html

Wilkinson, R. G., Pickett, K., Trust, T. E., & Foundation, M. E. (2009). *The spirit level: Why more equal societies almost always do better*. London: Allen Lane.

Zwanecki, D. (2001). *Social security arrangements in sub-Saharan Africa*. Regensburg, GP: Transfer Verlag.

CHAPTER 7

A Closer Look at Three Political Economies

China, Kerala, and Chile

KEY IDEAS

- Overall, China's efficiency in implementing its plans is therefore also its potential downfall. Its authoritarian government has been impressive in its ability to lift millions out of poverty and quickly implement policies and programs, but it does not always choose the right ones to implement. Without democratic checks, China also has greater trouble preventing tragic disasters.

- With a long history of public governance aimed at social equality, a relatively efficient government, and multiparty political competition, Kerala has been able to achieve impressive health outcomes and a high quality of living for its citizens. It has recently struggled with trade liberalization, however, especially because it lacks the policy-making powers national governments have.

- After a democratically elected socialist government and a right-wing military dictatorship that implemented neoliberal economic reforms, Chile's recent administrations are centrist by comparison. In combining support-led social policies with market-oriented economic and trade policies, Chile is attempting to achieve higher health outcomes incrementally. Whether it succeeds in sustaining substantive changes via these incremental reforms remains to be seen.

The ideas that drive nations and governments change over time. The United States underwent a progressive era during the Great Depression, turned conservative in the period following World War II, turned left again during the antiwar movement of the 1960s and 1970s, and then right again in the Ronald Regan era. Likewise, China went from a communist model to a capitalist model in 1979 under the leadership of Deng Xiaoping. Chile, like the United States, has wobbled right, then left, then right again. No matter where a nation lies on the globe, right-leaning and left-leaning social policies tend to look familiar, so these changes provide a natural laboratory for understanding how different social policies might affect the health and well-being of a nation.

We also include Kerala as a case study here because of its unusual place on the globe as a very low-income region that has achieved good health outcomes. The other popular example in this category, of course, is Cuba. But we chose Kerala because, similar to the other examples, it has wobbled ideologically over time. We also chose it because it is a democracy, and therefore likely produces somewhat more believable data. We do refer to Cuba quite a bit throughout this textbook, though.

CHINA: SUSTAINABLE STATE OF DEVELOPMENT?

The Chinese government argues that without the Chinese Communist Party, the new China does not exist. "If you ask for democracy," they argue, "you will lose all of your economic prosperity as well—the fancy cars, the Starbucks, the fashionable clothing, the multibedroom apartment." The implicit threat in this statement cuts both ways; China's impressive economic performance is essential to continued political rule. If the country's economic growth begins to falter, its people will revolt.

China has suffered several periods of severe repression in the past half-century. First, there was the Great Leap Forward, an economic experiment that turned into the Great Chinese Famine. Next, there was the Cultural Revolution, a move to solidify the citizens' ideology and to root out troublemakers, which led to widespread torture and violence by the Red Guard. Then there was the Tiananmen Massacre, a student movement for democracy that turned bloody. There have also been a number of smaller-scale catastrophes—mostly modern environmental problems—that might have been averted by a free press and democratic input.

The Health Effects of the Great Leap Forward

Of these episodes, the Great Leap Forward was probably the most deadly. Scholars estimate that the 1958–1961 famine caused the deaths of forty million Chinese people (Wemheuer, 2010). The Great Leap Forward was a plan to industrialize and collectivize Chinese production of foods and goods. Moderates in the Communist Party leadership suggested that collectivizing peasant labor in the countryside should be gradual. In fact, a smaller famine in 1956 had already caused some leaders to suggest that collectivization be halted. These tensions led to a nationwide Hundred Flowers Campaign in 1957, whereby the government invited honest feedback from citizens in order to evaluate the strengths and weaknesses of local policies. Some scholars claim that this was just a ploy to identify potential critics and "troublemakers." Others argue that Mao Zedong launched the subsequent Anti-Rightist campaign only when he realized that there was more opposition to his agricultural policies than he originally thought. Approximately 550,000 people—those who genuinely criticized the government and those who were simply falsely accused of doing so as a measure of self-protection—were persecuted in the 1957–1959 Anti-Rightist campaign (Chang & Halliday, 2007).

Mao Zedong ordered that more drastic changes be enforced quickly and simultaneously so that grain and steel could be the key pillars of China's economic development. In terms of grain, those who engaged in private farming, on their own small pockets of land for sustenance as before 1954, were taken to "struggle sessions," where as many as one hundred thousand people gathered to humiliate and berate members of the "exploiting class." Intellectuals were almost inevitably part of the "exploiting class" so that school blackboards were taken off the walls and hung on the necks of teachers during the struggle sessions. Between April and December 1958, more than twenty-five thousand farm communes of an average of five thousand households were set up.

In terms of steel, too, the Communist Party decided that production would double within the year (and surpass the United Kingdom within fifteen years). Mao encouraged the use of small backyard furnaces in every commune and urban neighborhood. In the race to produce more steel, with a deep mistrust of intellectuals or metallurgy experts and with a culture of fear preventing ordinary citizens from speaking up about their struggles, these backyard furnaces only produced worthless pig iron. Meanwhile, household pots, tools, or anything else deemed to be metal were used to produce this pig iron. There was intense pressure to give up one's worldly possessions in order to meet production quotas, and even parts of some Buddhist temples were melted during this era. This left many without basic cooking implements and tools— their only real assets. Further, more than fifty million workers were added to nonagricultural state payrolls by 1960 to meet these production quotas, double the payroll of 1957. Many of these had been male agricultural, school, and hospital workers. This placed undue stress on the food-rationing system and on grain production.

Although grain production in 1958 was pretty impressive, governmental officials had felt compelled to exaggerate their yields in order to please central authorities. Central authorities, in turn, used these inflated numbers to calculate mandatory exports. This left little food for the peasants themselves. Then, in 1959, river floods led to the deaths of two million people via drowning or crop failure, and a number of droughts destroyed the crops in 1960. The rural provinces that had most enthusiastically participated in the Great Leap Forward were those who suffered the most, and the starvation did not end until central party members abolished exports in January 1961.

Although the years between 1959 and 1962 are locally known as the "Three Years of Natural Disasters," the awful effects were politically constructed. Maybe the floods and droughts would not have wreaked such havoc if agricultural workers had not been forced to produce low-quality steel instead of growing crops. The earlier bumper crop in 1958 would not have rotted in the fields if workers had not been told to abandon their work in the field for their backyard furnaces. Yet, at the height of the famine, there were still twenty-two million tons of grain being stored in public granaries. Top officials ignored reports of starvation and cannibalism, instead ordering that all provincial records of population decline be destroyed (Yang, 2008). In addition to those who starved, at least 2.5 million were beaten or tortured to death for failing to meet their quotas or to feed other villagers, and between one and three million committed suicide. In Hiyang prefecture in Henan alone, over one million people died, sixty-seven thousand of whom were beaten to death by the military. Fuyang, a region with around eight million people in 1958, saw one-third of its population perish in three years (Dikotter, 2010). Over the same period, one-fifth of all Tibetans died (Jones, 2010). In all areas, children, women, and the aged were especially hard hit. To see the impact of these policies on life expectancy in China overall, visit www.gapminder.org, and select China from the list of countries to track over time.

At the same time, Mao claimed that unless central authorities asked for more than one-third of crop yields, the people would not rebel. Those with political connections attended as many official party conferences as possible, primarily because food supplies were consistent there. In "famine-ravaged Guizhou province, 260 cadres spent four days working through 210 kilos of beef, 500 kilos of pork, 680 chickens, 40 kilos of ham, 130 litres of wine, and 79 cartons of cigarettes as well as mountains of sugar and pastries" (Dikotter, 2010, p. 193).

By 1962, moderates within the Communist Party, such as Deng Xiaoping and Zhou Enlai, had taken over economic policies. Mao focused on regaining his prestige and political power. Over the next few years, Mao managed to do this partly by gaining control over the Propaganda Department and the popular press. In early 1966, the government announced the Great Cultural Revolution.

The Health Effects of the Cultural Revolution

The Red Guard troops, mostly made of students, peasants, and Communist Party cadres, were charged with punishing intellectuals and opponents of

Mao's regime. By 1967, nationwide Red Guard troops began to seize weapons from the Army and conduct increasingly violent struggle sessions against counterrevolutionaries. No one held the Red Guards accountable for their actions, especially when the national police chief gave orders such as, "Don't give them [the Red Guards] orders. Don't say it is wrong of them to beat up bad people: if in anger they beat someone to death, then so be it" (MacFarquhar & Schoenhals, 2008, p. 125).

In August and September 1966, Red Guard troops murdered almost two thousand people in Beijing alone, and they tortured and injured many more. The country fell into further chaos as local governments purged more and more officials, and the Red Guard broke into splinter groups, accusing one another of being counterrevolutionaries. Altogether, the Cultural Revolution led to the deaths of roughly eleven million people between 1966 and 1969 alone, though millions more died before the Deng Xiaoping administration introduced "socialism with Chinese characteristics" in the 1980s.

Remarkably, after a great leap backward in life expectancy during the Great Leap Forward (plunging from fifty in 1958 to thirty-two in 1960) and the Cultural Revolution, life expectancy rose dramatically again in 1970, from fifty-two in 1963 to sixty-four in 1971. The country's current life expectancy is around seventy-three, so in the four decades since 1971, it has not achieved the same life expectancy increase of twelve years that it managed to attain in the eight years of pro-public health (albeit antihuman rights) policies after the Great Leap Forward. Remember from previous chapters that programs such as the barefoot doctors and parasite eradication campaigns were institutionalized nationwide in 1968. These programs may have made a great difference.

The Public Health Effects of Tiananmen and Market Reforms

In the late 1970s and early 1980s, Deng Xiaoping's administration reversed many of Mao's policies on property ownership, as discussed in previous chapters, and attempted to implement "checks and balances" in the governance system (Chirot, 1996). These reforms included decentralization of political authority to the provinces, under what is known as the *tiao-kuai* or "branch-lump" system. The "branches" stand for vertical lines of authority stemming from central governmental ministries, whereas the "lumps" stand for horizontally aligned territories of government at the provincial or local level.

Unfortunately, this means that unlike the organizational tree or pyramid federalist systems, the Chinese organizational branch-lump system looks like a loose netting or weaving, where ministerial branches have the same rank as provincial lumps, and governmental units of the same rank cannot set binding rules for each other. Therefore, the environmental, housing, and consumer protection standards that are so essential to the Chinese population's health are often unenforceable because of the tiao-kuai system (Lieberthal, 1997).

Although the Chinese government has recently introduced some parallel economic policy units to overcome this tiao-kuai deadlock, the prevailing system remains one in which each governmental unit bestows on the one below it just enough flexibility to grow economically. There are few coordinated efforts or political reforms. As a result, many township officials are primarily entrepreneurial, and health-related standards and enterprise protections are hard to come by.

A stark example lies in the Henan Province blood scandal, which took place in the early 1990s. Local business owners and government officials worked together as "bloodheads," encouraging villagers to sell blood. The bloodheads acted as intermediaries, selling the blood plasma in bulk to hospitals and companies that made health products. The bloodheads reused needles, failed to screen for diseases, and reinjected red blood cells into peasants (when they returned to sell more blood). As a result of this mass reinjection program, more than thirty thousand people in Henan were infected with HIV, and almost seventy thousand people in China overall. Government officials closed the blood stations in 1995 but then attempted to cover up the scandal. Although the Chinese government has made moves to mandate testing and stop these illegal blood collections, it continues to underfund its public health infrastructure; thus, economic pressures continue to push small-town hospitals and villagers to participate in illegal blood collections. Further, China continues to lack a central tracking or accreditation agency to oversee blood facilities (Anderson & Davis, 2007).

Some of Deng Xiaoping's governance reforms were reversed by Jiang Zemin, who reconsolidated and recentralized power in the "party state" and military. The so-called fourth generation of Communist Chinese leaders, including current president Hu Jintao, have faced increasing civic protests and unrest. In response, they have added to Deng Xiaoping's economic focus a new twin goal of a "harmonious society," one that for the first time aims to address the needs of rural residents (in contrast to past policies, which explicitly favored urban dwellers) and to suppress dissident opinions through heavy censorship and limits to civil liberties.

Indeed, since the 1990s, the government has continued to imprison and repress dissidents, but these targets have generally shifted from "capitalists," as in the sixties and seventies, to journalists, unofficial religious groups, members of ethnic minorities, and human rights lawyers and activists. Falun Gong practitioners have received the most notice; they claim that their mixture of meditation, slow-moving *qigong* exercises, and moral philosophy constitute a spiritual practice. Western scholars usually describe Falun Gong as a religious movement, but the Chinese government labels them a dangerous and heretical cult. Christians who do not belong to the Three-Self Patriotic Movement and the Chinese Patriotic Catholic Association, the only legal Christian churches in China, have also been harassed or possibly imprisoned. With respect to human rights targets, environmental activists and proponents of the Charter '08 have been particular targets. The charter, released on December 10, 2008, the sixtieth of the United Nations Declaration of Human Rights, was authored by more than 350 Chinese intellectuals and activists, including 2010 Nobel Peace Prize winner Liu Xiaobo, and signed by over ten thousand people worldwide. It primarily asks for a legal system independent from the Communist Party, freedom of association, and a multiparty system of governance.

More strikingly, the range of people who are now considered activists has widened considerably. They include not only those who ask for multiparty rule and democracy, but also the parents of children who died in shoddily built schoolhouses after the 2008 Sichuan earthquake that killed over sixty-nine thousand people and left almost half a million injured, other parents who have lost children to scandals in lead-tainted toys and melamine-tainted infant formula, thousands of peasants who have become sick because of extreme environmental pollution and exposure to toxic fumes and chemicals, people who did not wish to relocate for massive projects such as the Three Gorges Dam or new real estate developments in rapidly growing cities, and consumers with grievances against relatively new businesses or local corrupt officials. These activists include Wu Lihong, a machine salesman who served three years in prison for exposing that local officials had allowed factories to pour industrial waste into a lake in Jiangsu Province, and Zhao Lianhai, who sought compensation for parental victims of the tainted milk scandal.

The Chinese Ministry of Public Security cites between eighty and one hundred thousand annual "mass incidents," often taken by foreigners to be street demonstrations and protests; however, it is impossible to present accurate information on just how many protests there are each year. Further, it is difficult to glean the extent to which Chinese citizens are satisfied with their government's social policies because there are few institutionalized means for honest feedback and discussion as well as bottom-up accountability. The government continues to censor or ban many public media outlets (from newspapers to television broadcasts to outline forums and websites) as well as to hire students, nicknamed "little sisters," who shadow "big brothers" to monitor their classmates (French, 2006).

In such circumstances, and with comparatively greater freedoms and media access than they enjoyed before, it is unsurprising that many citizens decide that it is easier to consume readily available Chinese media rather than rock the boat by using illicit, anonymous Internet pathways (often funded by foreign governments as well as decentralized groups) to access censored news sites. The Chinese state's adept practices of governmentality create structural conditions that give the government social control. They render most Chinese citizens indifferent or apathetic or fearful of political participation, and willing to accept the argument that China is an exceptionalist society, one in which citizens thrive most in a Confucian system that respects authority (and authoritarian states). In such a society, political and economic rights are mutually exclusive and not mutually constitutive.

Despite these struggles, China remains largely a health policy success story. Its life expectancy remains higher than India's. Policy makers have begun to go beyond drastic gestures—ordering capital punishment for and executing the top executives of toy and milk companies mired in scandals, for example—to develop new policies that address the deep urban-rural inequalities plaguing the country. For example, the government built two million affordable housing units in the "mid-sized" city of Chongqing alone, just in the year 2012. In 2005, the government also reformed the hukou household registration system that dictates the family's official province of residence, their responsibilities, and their rights. The system previously rendered China's eight hundred million rural residents inferior citizens in what has been called "China's apartheid" because more than one hundred million migrant workers could not access services and jobs in thriving cities without breaking the law. However, scholars have noted that in reality, the government did not abolish the hukou system but rather decentralized it, so that local government approval has become critical in any migrant worker's legitimate existence. Further, the government has continued to deny pensions, education rights for primary school, health care benefits, and other social services to migrant laborers, even bulldozing unauthorized primary schools attended by the children of migrant laborers, *after* reforms (Chan & Buckingham, 2008). China's reforms at the central level, then, are mitigated by its complex federalist structures and lack of implementation at the local level.

In other societies, democracy is messy (as evident in the Kerala and Chile cases) but it also helps governments to avoid major health disasters like the Great Famine, the Cultural Revolution, and on a smaller scale, recent blood, infant melamine, earthquake school construction, and SARS scandals. Overall, China's efficiency in implementing its plans is therefore also its potential downfall.

KERALA: EXPERIMENTS WITH RADICAL DECENTRALIZATION

India is the world's largest democracy, with regular, competitive, multiparty elections and a large and robust civil society since its independence from Great Britain in 1947 (Isaac & Heller, 2003). Currently, more than seven hundred million voters might participate in a general national election, a population roughly twice as large as that of all residents in the United States. Nevertheless, this history of liberal democracy (in which individual votes for representatives and technically governed bureaucracies reign supreme) has not addressed growing social and economic inequalities. According to some estimates, the wealth of just the forty richest people in India equals 30 percent of its trillion-dollar GDP. Meanwhile, 80 percent of Indians continue to live on less than US$2 a day and two hundred million residents are chronically hungry (Reed, 2009). (Yes, US$2 goes much further in India than it does in industrialized countries, but it does not help Indians to rise above the poverty line.)

What does the relationship between governance and these demographic statistics mean? Many Indians point to unequal social policies that do not tax rich corporations, are rife with corruption, or employ clientelistic tactics that reward elites more than ordinary citizens. At the same time, other critics point to ineffective, top-down governmental structures that are unable to respond to the people's needs, even if they mean well. These tensions have only increased with recent economic growth; proverbially, the rising tide of India's economy has yet to lift all boats.

Kerala has had a fairly long history of public health and medical institutions, as described in chapter 5, and it boasts of a long history of civic engagement and social mobilization as well. This track record of an active citizenry, sometimes across class lines, bodes well for the state in many ways. Kerala has the highest per capita number of newspapers in the country, and ordinary citizens regularly protest when policy makers enact laws and programs that the public perceives as contrary to their interests. Two trends stand out: first, civil society groups in the area became strong and worked toward expansive social policies. Second, at the same time, local groups were able to compromise and not fight for market capitalism or pure communism or socialism.

The struggle for Indian independence in Kerala reflected not just locals' desire to free themselves from British colonial rule but also other class and community tensions as well. For example, in the northern part of the state, a specific class of Brahmin landlords received preferential treatment by the British and held disproportionate power over not just poor Muslim peasants but also upper-caste Nair households. Whereas the Congress Party was able to rally support in other parts of India after independence in 1947, Keralans were more likely to support more radical political parties as well. In the southern part of the state, agrarian reforms from 1865 helped to build a stable, prosperous, propertied class of small-scale farmers, who then helped to build home-grown local capital and a middle class. This, in turn, made the area less dependent on British capital. These developments eventually allowed local elites to form associations that not only encouraged further business but also other social goals, such as community-based schools and public services. An anticolonial legacy in the area, the prosperity of lower-caste, middle-class groups such as the Ezhavas, and the growth of an agrarian working class all led to a growth in civil society institutions as well as postindependence social movements that combined missions of democracy, dignity, and redistribution.

This shows that Kerala has a strong civil society and that civil society groups worked toward expansive social policies.

At the same time, unlike earlier communist movements in other parts of India, Kerala's postindependence movement was more pragmatic and flexible, allowing constituents to claim grievances along lines other than orthodox Marxist, class-based ones. Further, even as land reform politics became more contentious in the 1960s and 1970s, they did not devolve into civil war or violence in Kerala precisely because the political system allowed more radical parties to participate. The communist party, for example, has acted as the ruling party in Kerala over the years but only intermittently and never for two consecutive terms. Put simply, all of the regional key players felt as if they were part of the democratic system.

Because of this history, Keralans believe that their government works, that laws are made to ultimately serve them, and that most policies make sense. In other words, they have normalized the "rational-legal state" in Keralan society (Sandbrook, Edelman, Heller, & Teichman, 2007). This is illustrated in their faith in an effective bureaucracy—one that will correct major faults when citizens are informed and read newspapers, write letters of protest, and organize social movements. This trust that bureaucrats are generally effective, professional, and follow the law stands in stark contrast to the (lack of) implementation of anticaste and antidiscrimination laws in other parts of India, and where more than one-fifth of national parliamentary members face criminal charges (*Economist*, 2008). This also means that interest groups are less likely to attempt conflicts via mob violence or protracted strikes in Kerala when they know that they can compromise and meet most of their goals via institutionalized channels.

Finally, Kerala is also famous for its decentralized governance, another important element of their political economy. Starting in 1997, the state of Kerala launched the People's Campaign for Decentralized Planning, its ninth five-year plan for local *panchayats*. The campaign aimed not only to devolve authoritative decision making to local areas but also to provide incentives for community participation and to help create new networks and coalitions of community-based and civil society groups, politicians, and administrative decision makers. The system encouraged participation not just at the district level but also at the even smaller and more grassroots *grama panchayat* or municipality level. (There are 990 grama panchayats, 58 municipalities, 152 blocks, and 14 districts in Kerala state.)

Ordinary citizens are most likely to participate in the *grama sabhas*, or municipal assemblies (kind of like town hall meetings), that take place several times a year. In the first grama sabha, anyone can present a local issue to be addressed (a dangerous intersection, say, or the need for more funds for a certain health clinic) or make a policy proposal. Together, the people prioritize proposals and form subcommittees (called *development seminars*). The elected panchayat members work with subcommittees to conduct feasibility studies and research on the prioritized proposals and present their revised plans in later grama sabhas. At subsequent meetings during the annual cycle, volunteers devote intensive energy and time to selecting, defending, revising, and implementing proposals.

In the first year alone, two million Keralans attended grama sabhas, three hundred thousand delegates attended development seminars, one hundred thousand residents volunteered on task forces, twenty-five thousand volunteers helped to formulate plan documents to present to higher-ups at the municipality and panchayat levels, five thousand volunteers worked on documents to present at the block and district levels, and five thousand volunteer technical experts (such as civil engineers) worked on appraisal committees to draw up the actual blueprints and so forth necessary to have the newly selected roads, schools, clinics, and so on built.

Ideally, this system of participatory governance allows Kerala to develop "stable political orders and workable social compacts," outstripping all other Indian states in performance, responding to demand-side pressures by the people, and largely avoiding the awful caste and sectarian violence that has plagued the rest of the country in the past few decades (Dreze & Sen, 1989; Sandbrook et al., 2007, p. 73).

Kerala's current government, although far from perfect, stands out as a case study of participatory, decentralized governance and strong, equity-supporting social policies in the context of India and middle-income countries overall. It has managed to decentralize enough so that local politicians and ordinary citizens have some decision-making power over the policies and programs that affect them most (such as how their school and health centers are run) but not decentralize so much as to render local planning councils isolated from one another. The latter situation can exacerbate inequalities between different local areas so that the differences between posh neighborhoods and slums worsen and eventually threaten social and political stability, or they can simply make regional planning and coordination more difficult. In that case, many resources would be wasted because local councils might unknowingly replicate or implement overlapping programs even when they are not necessary or leave gaping holes in policy by assuming that their neighboring councils have those services covered.

Decentralization involves devolution of *both* decision-making power and resources, with some centralized oversight and support. In some countries, national governments have told local councils that they now have the power to run all of their own education, police, health, and housing systems, all while giving them none of the state funding they used to receive. In turn, it is not surprising that those "decentralization" experiments did not turn out so well, with central governments lamenting new failed schools and so on. Local residents then complained that the central government in effect gave them the responsibility but not meaningful power to design and implement good local policies.

At the same time, all is not rosy: in this highly politicized context, "schools, cooperatives, shopfloors, and local institutions have all become objects of fierce political competition" (Isaac & Heller, 2003, p. 85). Further, the caste system has been blunted but not eradicated by cross-class coalitions and pro-poor policies over time. These trends, alongside top-down bureaucratic decision making, helped to make Kerala's civil society less robust than it might have been otherwise.

These factors also greatly shape medical care and the social determinants of health in Kerala. Researchers have found that panchayats allocated lower percentages of resources to health programs than the state government did prior to decentralization. This decentralization accelerated in the 1980s, and lower expenditures in direct patient services were particularly acute in areas where primary health centers lacked involved representatives in the local budgeting process and where panchayat participation rates were lower overall (Narayana & Hari Kurup, 2000; Varatharajan, Thankappan, & Jayapalan, 2004).

As we discussed in previous chapters, Kerala has some impressive successes, but it is also struggling to meet the shifting challenges of trade liberalization. For instance, the public distribution system for ration shops, school lunches, and agricultural pensions was widespread and universal entitlements were in the food-deficit state until 1997, when the system became means tested and limited to low-income households. Many of the households that were above the cut-off line but had relied on the system for rice purchases could no longer afford this staple. The prices of major commodities such as rubber and coconut oil, two of the biggest cash exports grown in the state, fell by almost half after trade agreement liberalization in 1994; India's membership in the WTO called for the removal of the remaining trade restrictions (Thankappan, 2001). (The WTO sets international rules for trade, and member nations have to sign on to abide by these rules.)

In response to such changes, many Keralans have left the state in order to try to earn money elsewhere. In 2008, almost 2.2 million Keralans resided outside of the state or country (if abroad, then primarily working in the Persian Gulf nation-states) and sent remittances home (Zachariah & Rajan, 2010). Around 40 percent of households in Kerala have at least one migrant (Thankappan, 2001). These prodigious remittances may help to cushion the blow of welfare retrenchment for many households (indeed, many of the migrants come from poorer households that had relied on more generous social policies) and may even help to revive growth (via consumer demand), especially in the service sector.

Increased private sector capital inflows have not adequately substituted public sector losses. In the meantime, Kerala does not have the negotiating power of nation-states to try to renegotiate trade deals or enforce federal policy. Still, given these circumstances, the state income has been more stable and the number of labor strikes much lower than popular perceptions might suggest. Communications, software, and tourism sectors continue to grow, helping Kerala to move away from low-value-added and unstable commodity sectors, such as rubber. State policy makers hope that decentralized governance reforms will help the state to redirect public funds to areas in dire need and to reduce waste; indeed, there is evidence that local accountability has helped to reduce corruption, increase housing and other goods for the poor, and help the state government to now focus on the quality, and not just the quantity, of public services.

CHILE: A PRECARIOUS THIRD WAY

Chile's brand of the "middle path" came from a history of civil strife and trauma. This also means that Chile's current political economy remains somewhat precarious, especially amid quickly changing global trade policies, volatile markets, and social conditions.

Chile's economic history is marked by copper. When Chile won independence from Spain in 1810, its main exports were wheat and other agricultural products. By the late nineteenth century, however, copper and nitrates dominated the export market. Chile's social investments began expanding greatly at the beginning of the twentieth century, just as they had in the United States and other now high-income countries. When scientists developed synthetic substitutes for nitrates around World War I, Chile's economy became even more heavily dependent on copper exports as the source of roughly 80 percent of government revenues. In the three years after the Great Crash of 1929, Chile's GDP shrank by half.

Because of this traumatic period, Chile's policy makers expanded import substitution economic development programs (in steel, petroleum, and other industries) in the following decades. Still, the domestic enterprises were not always efficient and relied on governmental subsidies, and a large majority of Chile's citizens remained poor, especially in the countryside. In the early 1960s, the Chilean government attempted to pass some agrarian reform laws to help the rural poor as well as the urban middle and upper classes.

In 1964, Chileans elected Eduardo Frei as president, and his administration began large-scale redistributive efforts, especially to help the urban poor and peasants who had not benefited from previous social policies. For example, rural workers began to work at the same minimum wage as urban workers, and education and milk distribution programs expanded. In 1970, Chileans elected the Popular Unity coalition of left political parties and its presidential candidate, Salvador Allende, into power. The continuation of capabilities-building programs improved health outcomes so that infant mortality fell by 63 percent between the 1940s and 1970s (Sandbrook et al., 2007).

Under the Popular Unity government, expropriations of private property peaked under Allende, with the state owning 28 percent of industry assets in 1970 and 69 percent just three years later; public employment almost tripled in the same three years. There were few alliances between leftists and centrists, and the country was severely divided (Sandbrook et al., 2007).

The economy was stagnant and inflation hit 35 percent that year. The government hoped that by increasing real wages, especially for poor people, there would be greater consumer demand and greater productivity so that the economy could grow without exacerbating inflation. Unfortunately, inflation and deficits continued to rise, real wages and governmental reserves fell, and the underground economy grew in response.

The Chilean case contrasted with the Keralan one in that Chileans had few institutional or electoral means to resolve conflicts, as in Kerala, and the left parties' policies were radical enough that they lost the support of most small landowners (unlike the leftist parties in Kerala), with the exception of indigenous Mapuche minifundistas.

On September 11, 1973, the military assassinated Allende and staged a coup. General Augusto Pinochet took over and handed economic policy making to the Chicago boys, so called because they trained under Milton Friedman at the University of Chicago.

Beginning in October 1973, the Pinochet regime violently repressed, tortured, and killed thousands of Chileans who had opposed the coup, were engaged in human rights work, or were simply unlucky. In the first month alone, the Caravan of Death (*la Caravana de la Muerte*), an army death squad, killed ninety-seven prisoners, many of whom had turned themselves into the military, had no history of violence, and posed no violent threat. According to the Valech and Rettig Truth and Reconciliation reports, respectively ordered by later presidents Ricardo Lagos and Patricio Aylwin, Pinochet's military junta was responsible for at least 3,200 "disappearances" or killings, 29,000 political prisoners (many of whom were tortured), and "extreme trauma" for at least 200,000 citizens (many of whom were family members who had not been politically active but wanted to find out what had happened to their children or grandchildren). The frequent "disappearances" of labor leaders, human rights activists, religious leaders, and others continued for many years. Labor rights, such as the right of workers to go on strike without losing their jobs or to voice grievances, were severely curtailed.

The Chilean junta also worked in tandem with other South American right-wing dictatorships, such as that in Argentina, in Operation Condor, a political repression campaign that began in 1975 aimed at eradicating leftist opposition movements. Agents killed at least sixty thousand people on behalf of the campaign, and the United States acted in a supervisory role in the Operation Condor coalition (McSherry, 2002). In more specific cases regarding higher-level opposition politicians, CIA agents such as Michael Townley worked to produce biochemical weapons used in assassinations and biological experiments on prisoners.

Alongside these brutal political policies, markets were liberalized, and national deficits decreased. Poverty levels and income inequalities increased dramatically under Pinochet's reign from 1973 to 1990. Most of the reforms fell in line with neoliberal doctrine: banks were reprivatized and the governments changed rural farm ownership rules once again, favoring small farms in lieu of the large cooperatives established by Allende's administration (which had themselves replaced large *latifundio* concentrated in the hands of a small minority of landowners). By 1978, governmental rights to expropriate land (as in eminent domain cases in the United States) were revoked, ceilings on landholdings were lifted, and all public landholdings had been distributed or auctioned off to private individuals or firms. In education, chasms between poorly resourced public schools and well-resourced private schools widened greatly. School governance was decentralized, but unlike in Kerala, resources were not. Thus, local school officials were supposedly given the decision-making power to make policy, but they did not have the funds to keep up the schools (Taylor, 1998).

General Pinochet's junta banned all of the socialist and leftist parties that had constituted Allende's Popular Unity coalition. In September 1980, the Chilean people voted in a referendum to replace their 1925 constitution with a new one, giving General Pinochet an eight-year term as president. Although opposition political parties stated that there had been evidence of electoral fraud, the popular vote nevertheless paved the way for military control of the government and expanded presidential powers. These changes took effect in 1981.

In 1989, the Chilean people did not reelect Pinochet as president. Before a new administration came into power, lawmakers passed an amnesty law that prohibited prosecution of military personnel for human rights violations, and Pinochet was elected senator for life. This decision, too, effectively prevented prosecutors from ever pressing charges or bringing him to trial. Some of the presidential powers given to Pinochet, such as the power to dissolve the Lower Chamber of Congress, were taken away when Chile transitioned to a democracy in 1990.

It was also during Pinochet's reign that Chile introduced private health insurance companies, called ISAPREs, used by the 15 percent most well-off segment of the population, with the remainder of the population using the public FONASA system. This system exacerbated health inequalities, especially because health care companies discriminated against demographic groups associated with higher health care costs, such as women, the elderly, and those with preexisting conditions. Thus, two people paying the same premium but with different family histories may receive vastly different levels of treatment. (This is similar to the private insurance system in the United States, when insurance companies sometimes consider not just hepatitis B exposure a preexisting condition, but other factors such as being the victim of a rape as well because proper recovery from the rape may involve future treatments.) The Pinochet government also allowed ISAPREs to refuse coverage to potential paying customers with preexisting conditions. For example, all ISAPRE insurance firms denied coverage to HIV-positive people. (As this textbook goes to press, similar provisions in the United States will be overturned by the health care reform passed by the Obama administration in 2010.) Thus, any high-risk (high-risk from the perspective of the insurance company, as in potentially using more medical care) or low-income person turned to FONASA.

Nevertheless, it is important to remember that although civil society groups especially suffered under Pinochet's military dictatorship, popular mobilization did not altogether disappear. Likewise, dramatic trade liberalization certainly occurred under Pinochet's regime but certain social policies— subsidized child care and targeted public investments in nutrition, for example—also existed. In fact, the Pinochet regime introduced some of the first noncontributory social security provisions. All of these programs were means tested for the poorest 10 percent of the population, improving outcomes for the poorest and worsening outcomes for the working poor and near-poor.

Thus, although many economists claim that neoliberal policies and structural adjustments programs led to the "miracle of Chile" and economic growth and improvements in social indicators through the 1980s and 1990s, other economists, such as Amartya Sen, disagree. Sen argues that there was little economic growth in the late 1970s and early 1980s, and that sustained growth only occurred after Pinochet replaced the Chicago boys with more pragmatic economists who relied less on "automatic adjustment" and "invisible hand of the market" policies and more government-led macroeconomic policies, especially in periodic devaluations in the exchange rate. Further, Sen argues that improvements in social indicators and health outcomes such as life expectancy came despite, not because of, neoliberal policies. Instead, improvements in health outcomes came about because of support-led policies that persisted and survived despite overall opposition in the Pinochet regime; these policies included subsidized child care, childhood nutrition, and especially programs to curb infant mortality. For instance, although Chileans' predicted life expectancy at birth increased dramatically, life expectancy for older Chileans did not (Dreze & Sen, 1989).

From 1990 to 2010, the center-left Concertación coalition held majority rule in Chile, trying to tackle the poverty and inequalities left behind by Pinochet's dictatorship and rule with a motto of "growth with equity." The Concertación government kept some of the neoliberal principles of their policy-making predecessors. Grassroots groups complained, for example, that government health campaigns against a cholera outbreak focused on individual-level factors (admonishing women living in slum areas to "keep their area clean" and boil water), ignoring the social determinants of health (that these women lacked adequate housing, that their water supplies were of lower quality than those of wealthy areas, that the cholera outbreak was preventing them from pursuing their livelihoods, and that the campaign rhetoric appeared to suggest that *they* were dirty and deficient rather than their surroundings) (Paley, 2001).

Nevertheless, the coalition's successes were substantive. Per capita income doubled, with a 70 percent rise in the minimum wage, and the poverty rate decreased by more than half from 1990 to 2004. Social expenditures that were universal, not means tested, increased in education and health. Especially notable were a shift toward social determinants of health and preventive health (with an increase in attention on workers' health, for example), and the development of Plan AUGE, which is described in further detail in the feature at the end of the chapter.

Despite more than two decades of democratic elections once again, Chile is not quite the robust democracy Kerala is. Namely, it has a policy process that remains technocratic and unfriendly to civil society organizations and rank-and-file members of political parties, even as it grants business interests access to high levels of government. For example, businesspeople held monthly meetings with the head of the Central Bank and participated in trade negotiations, although labor and civil society groups did not have such unfettered access. Many of the high-level policy makers were traumatized by the Popular Unity experience and feared that "excessive" social mobilization or participation would once again destabilize their society, and others were wary of the experiences of Eastern European countries transitioning from communism to capitalism. Many civil society organizations operate via political parties rather than independently, and in general, there continues to be a "culture of fear" in which everyday citizens fear that speaking up will once again bring the sort of repression rampant during Pinochet's rule.

However, a new, younger generation of activists and civil society organizations—one less scarred by Pinochet's brutality—has also begun to emerge. For example, 790,000 primary and secondary school students took to the streets on May 30, 2006, to demand education reform—not just lower fees for school buses and university exams (similar to the SATs) but a better public education system overall. What is especially remarkable about the "penguin revolution"—so dubbed because most of the students wore black-and-white school uniforms—is that it joined self-identified liberal, primarily lower-income public school students with wealthier, conservative, private school ones. (Of the four key teenaged organizers, two identified as right-wing and two as left-wing. Imagine, in other countries with mass income inequalities, mass protests led by self-identified right-wing students to protest the role of SAT fees and prep courses in exacerbating class-based inequalities.) Days after then-president Michelle Bachelet failed to mention education reform in her state of the union address on May 22, 2006, tens of thousands of public school students went on strike and peacefully occupied school buildings without violence or defacement. By May 26, dozens of exclusive and elite private schools joined the strikes, unraveling banners that declared, "Private but not silent," and "Education is a right, not a privilege" (Vogler, 2006).

During these weeks, more than a million students (or almost 25 percent of all students aged five to eighteen) had participated in the protests, and in June, Bachelet announced a new presidential education commission, grants for university entrance exams, and additional funding for school repairs, meals, and transport (Chovanec & Benitez, 2008). Although the coalition and social movement were not without tensions, their solidarity was nevertheless noticeable.

As Chile continues to grapple with its twin goals of equity and growth, its current "third way" is all the more impressive given the country's turbulent history. This history also suggests that a century of democratic governance and reforms could not be overturned by two decades of military dictatorship, and that the relationship between governance and health-related social policies runs deeper and more complex than that of any single presidential administration or dictatorship (McGuire, 2010). Indeed, the Chilean state has been consistent in its involvement with export-led economic development.

A PLAN TOWARD UNIVERSAL HEALTH CARE?

Plan AUGE presented all Chileans with a list of forty diseases and health conditions guaranteed to be covered by the government, within a certain period of time, with a limit to copayments and guaranteed standards of care. The list of forty in Plan AUGE was chosen according to epidemiologic prevalence rates, the cost-effectiveness of appropriate treatments, as well as a citizen participation process. Of these forty conditions, twenty-five were covered beginning in 2005 and an additional fifteen in 2006.

This citizen participation played an integral role in helping the policy makers make better design decisions regarding the reform, legitimize the program and help to gain popular support, and help publicize how it works. The citizen participation consisted mainly of two stages. In the first stage, the government conducted large-scale surveys on (1) individuals' perceptions of their own health, (2) individuals' perceptions of the health care system, and (3) health care workers' perceptions of the health care system in the public and private sectors. In the second stage, which took place in 2001, three thousand representatives from public and community organizations and stakeholder groups participated in a pilot round of "citizen participation workshops" in forty-eight communities. Together, they discussed questions such as the nation's key health objectives and whether there are some rights to health care that should apply to all people (or all Chileans). After governmental officials developed a better template for these community meetings, an additional twenty-five thousand citizens participated in 250 additional meetings around the country. Then, the government held 199 additional local meetings to draft patients' rights and responsibilities in the legislative bill. This citizen participation was integral to making the Plan AUGE reform the first of its kind and the first to be sent to the legislature in 2002 (Rivas Loria, 2007).

Further, the citizen participation helped to (1) legitimize the criteria outlined by epidemiologists (exposing a much wider public to concepts such as cost-effectiveness and helping to publicize concerns over costs and impact and prevalence rates of disease) and (2) give higher-ups a more nuanced sense of citizens' concerns and demands. For instance, citizens convinced policy makers that although they agreed that conditions with high prevalence rates and known cost-effective measures should be the first ones to be covered, they also wanted to make some exceptions. They explicitly asked that childhood cancers and HIV/AIDS be covered, even if treatments for childhood leukemia are often risky and expensive, and they were willing to pay higher taxes for this. The citizen participation then gave reform advocates additional political clout in arguing that those who were against the reforms were against these citizens' wishes and essentially for withholding treatment from these children. The citizen participation was thus essential not just to civic education about the health care system and proposed reforms but also to shaping guiding principles in the reform, facilitating a less politicized discussion, mediating between conservative and liberal politicians, and building political support.

Still, although President Lagos's administration did attempt to reach out to new civil society groups in the citizen participation process, many smaller and grassroots groups complained that the process was overly technocratic and really catered to long-standing partners and interests. These tensions were serious enough so that some working groups broke down and had to be reassembled in the 2001–2002 participation process. Questions remain, then, on the extent to which the process was substantively inclusive and participatory (Missoni & Solimano, 2010).

Policy makers were also careful to keep a dialogue open with unions so that they did not feel threatened and to keep debates open on the senate floor. In combination with the citizen participation, Plan AUGE helped to pave the way for major health care reforms that finally went into effect in 2004. The five bills that together constituted health system reforms in Chile were as follows: (1) restructured the Ministry of Health, regional offices, and health services so that regulatory bodies were separate from service providers, (2) provided the Plan AUGE universal access that necessitated a new governing health authority, (3) governed private insurance companies (ISAPRES) so that patients would not suddenly pay much more or face discriminatory costs because of natural occurrences such as pregnancy or old age, (4) financed for the greater coverage via a 1 percent increase in the VAT, and (5) wrote a new social contract on patients' rights and health care professionals' responsibilities. The policy makers were quite politically adept in first introducing popular measures that paved the way for subsequent bills; it is less likely that they could have reformed the health care system in one take. The executive branch (with presidents Lagos and Bachelet) was unwavering in its support for the reforms and in the use of human rights discourse in the campaigns.

In addition, the Chilean government launched publicity campaigns to promote the passage of the reforms, increase public awareness of their new free services and patients' rights, and attribute differences in care to these specific reforms. They have been successful enough so that an additional sixteen conditions (including dental emergencies and detached retinas) became covered in 2007, and another ten conditions (including Parkinson's disease and hepatitis B) in 2010—for a total of sixty-six conditions for which all Chileans can receive free treatment (Missoni & Solimano, 2010).

Plan AUGE managed to introduce a notion of solidarity into health care in Chile—whereby one's need, rather than one's ability to pay, is paramount, and rich folks and poor folks are treated similarly. In 2006, public health expenditures outstripped private health expenditures for the first time in over a decade, even as health expenditures overall as a percentage of GDP decreased (in sharp contrast to patterns in the United States). A large percentage of the Chilean population has now received some treatment for free under Plan AUGE, making it quite popular across all income levels. At the same time, more low-income households have made use of AUGE than have high-income households; this has also helped the government to work toward its goal of reducing health disparities.

However, this is not to say that Plan AUGE has been an unmitigated success. There have been quite a few implementation snags along the way so that patients whose doctors recommend other procedures are not covered by Plan AUGE and resources have not always kept up with demand. Therefore, waiting times have at times been longer than ideal, though the government has been able to address this issue over time.

Substantively, critics also note that the important notion of solidarity applies only to people suffering from one or more of the sixty-six conditions; those who are unlucky enough to suffer from an ailment not covered by Plan AUGE may still face severe challenges with health insurance companies or not be able to afford treatment. The women's health movement has argued that most of the prioritized conditions that disproportionately affect women, such as osteoporosis, sexual violence, sexually transmitted diseases, and reproductive health conditions, have all been excluded (Dannreuther & Gideon, 2008; Missoni & Solimano, 2010).

Overall, Plan AUGE is better at addressing disparities in treatment than at addressing the social determinants of health or promoting preventative policies that could help Chile minimize health disparities in the first place. Some scholars have also noted that the criteria for condition prioritization (rule of rescue, costs, prevalence, burden of disease, social preferences, etc.) sometimes operate in contradictory ways and that, significantly, the government has not been very transparent in how, exactly, it parses these different criteria (Vargas & Poblete, 2008). There are also no protocols for appeals or revising decisions, no set of guarantees for participating citizens, and no plans for social monitoring or further citizen participation, even as the laws continue to evolve and become implemented.

When Plan AUGE was first implemented, only 40 percent of the beneficiaries in the public system were aware of their new benefits, whereas 98 percent of private health insurance holders were aware of their new Plan AUGE benefits. In other words, Plan AUGE was not successfully reaching as many of the clients who needed the most help. More recent surveys show that, even though so many Chileans have benefited from Plan AUGE, an overwhelming majority of Chileans still do not know the sixty-six conditions covered by the plan (Missoni & Solimano, 2010).

SUMMARY

No matter what the social policy, it likely has an impact on the health of a given nation. Food safety, environmental protection, and universal education are examples of nonhealth policies that tend to be associated with the political left. These policies probably have hugely affected population health over time. Likewise, reducing red tape to starting and running a businesses, opening up borders to free trade, and reducing taxation are all policies that free up financial resources and stimulate economic growth. Such policies have probably led to epidemiologic transitions in countless nations, producing large increases in life expectancy by lifting the poor into the middle class.

But there can be a paradoxical relationship between regulations on businesses (e.g., occupational safety regulations) and economic growth. It is difficult to state where lines should be drawn and in what contexts. Many economists believe that India's economy would be greatly helped by reducing regulations on doing business, allowing foreign investment, and so forth. Many health experts also believe that the accompanying growth that would lift many millions out of poverty would also benefit the nation's health. But, as we see with China, lifting millions out of poverty does not always boost life expectancy. However, it seems that the socialist governments of Chile and Kerala both did quite well in boosting health without much in the way of economic growth. Did the "middle path" leaders of modern Chile get the mix right? One answer to that question is "maybe, given their political economy."

DISCUSSION QUESTIONS

1. What two to three characteristics do you think are most important in describing China's health care situation? Kerala's? Chile's?

2. Do you think China will be able to sustain its current path of development? Will it avoid population health crises? Why or why not?

3. What do you think the main factors are in Kerala's current success? Do you think this success can be maintained? Is Kerala's model replicable elsewhere?

4. What will Chile's health care system look like in ten years? Do you think it will be universal? What are the key factors that determine whether Chile will have universal health care?

5. What is the role of democratic institutions in these three case studies?

FURTHER READING

Missoni, E., & Solimano, G. (2010). Towards universal health coverage: The Chilean experience. WHO. *World Health Report Background Paper,* No. 4. Available online at www.who.int/healthsystems/topics/financing/healthreport/4Chile.pdf

The Wall Street Journal. (2012, August 29). Report: China's health care system deeply sick. Available online at http://blogs.wsj.com/chinarealtime/2012/08/29/report-chinas-health-care-system-deeply-sick

REFERENCES

Anderson, E., & Davis, S. (2007). *AIDS blood scandals: What China can learn from the world's mistakes.* New York: Asia Catalyst.

Chan, K. W., & Buckingham, W. (2008). Is China abolishing the hukou system? *The China Quarterly, 195*(1), 582–606.

Chang, J., & Halliday, J. (2007). Mao: The unknown story. *The China Quarterly, 189,* 187–228.

Chirot, D. (1996). *Modern tyrants: The power and prevalence of evil in our age.* Princeton, NJ: Princeton University Press.

Dannreuther, C., & Gideon, J. (2008). Entitled to health? Social protection in Chile's plan AUGE. *Development and Change, 39*(5), 845–864.

Dikotter, F. (2010). *Mao's great famine: The history of China's most devastating catastrophe, 1958–1962.* London: Bloomsbury Publishing.

Dreze, J., & Sen, A. K. (1989). *Hunger and public action.* New York: Oxford University Press.

Economist. (2008, 11 December). The democracy tax is rising: Indian politics is becoming ever more labyrinthine. Available online at www.economist.com/node/12749771

French, H. W. (2006, May 9). As Chinese students go online, little sister is watching. *New York Times,* p. 9.

Isaac, T. M., & Heller, P. (2003). Democracy and development: Decentralized planning in Kerala. In A. Fung & E. Wright (Eds.), *Deepening democracy: Institutional innovations in empowered participatory governance.* New York: Verso Books.

Jones, A. (2010). *Genocide: A comprehensive introduction.* New York: Routledge.

Lieberthal, K. (1997). China's governing system and its impact on environmental policy implementation. *China Environment Series, 1,* 3–8.

MacFarquhar, R., & Schoenhals, M. (2008). *Mao's last revolution.* Cambridge, MA: Belknap Press.

McGuire, J. W. (2010). *Wealth, health, and democracy in East Asia and Latin America.* New York: Cambridge University Press.

McSherry, J. P. (2002). Tracking the origins of a state terror network: Operation Condor. *Latin American Perspectives, 29*(1), 36–60.

Missoni, E., & Solimano, G. (2010). *Towards universal health coverage: The Chilean experience*. Geneva: WHO.

Narayana, D., & Hari Kurup, K. K. (2000). *Decentralization of the health care sector in Kerala: Some issues*. Thiruvananthapuram, Kerala: Centre for Development Studies.

Paley, J. (2001). *Marketing democracy: Power and social movements in post-dictatorship Chile*. Berkeley: University of California Press.

Reed, A. M. (2009). *The reality of mass poverty and social exclusion: "How is India?"* Montreal: Centre for Research on Globalization.

Rivas Loria, P. (2007). *The steering role of the National Health Authority in action*. Washington, DC: USAID.

Sandbrook, R., Edelman, M., Heller, P., & Teichman, J. (2007). *Social democracy in the global periphery: Origins, challenges, prospects*. New York: Cambridge University Press.

Taylor, L. (1998). *Citizenship, participation and democracy: Changing dynamics in Chile and Argentina*. New York: St. Martin's Press.

Thankappan, K. R. (2001). Some health implications of globalization in Kerala, India. *Bulletin of the World Health Organization, 79*(9), 892–893.

Varatharajan, D., Thankappan, R., & Jayapalan, S. (2004). Assessing the performance of primary health centres under decentralized government in Kerala, India. *Health Policy Plan, 19*(1), 41–51.

Vargas, V., & Poblete, S. (2008). Health prioritization: The case of Chile. *Health Affairs, 27*(3), 782.

Vogler, J. (2006). Chile: The rise of the penguin revolution. *Upside Down World*. Available online at http://upsidedownworld.org/main/content/view/330/34

Wemheuer, F. (2010). Dealing with responsibility for the Great Leap Famine in the People's Republic of China. *The China Quarterly, 201*, 176–194.

Yang, J. (2008). *Tombstone: A record of the great Chinese famine of the 1960s*. Hong Kong: Cosmos Books.

Zachariah, K. C., & Rajan, S. I. (2010). *Migration monitoring study: Emigration and remittances in the context of surge in oil prices*. Trivandrum, Kerala: Ministry of Overseas Indian Affairs (Government of India) Research Unit on International Migration at Centre for Development Studies (CDS).

CHAPTER 8

Global Governance
and Health

KEY IDEAS

- Global institutions such as the UN, IMF, and World Bank influence health outcomes.

- The WHO works to coordinate health policies worldwide.

- The WTO is the only global governance organization with the ability to truly enforce its rules, which have tremendous public health implications, but it is currently not democratically governed.

- Increased global trade, combined with advanced technology, can help participating countries to increase their health and wealth, but they can also unleash negative health consequences.

In chapter 1, we mentioned that the end of World War II ushered in a new era of global governance. The UN, IMF, World Bank, and other major global institutions were supposed to foster peace, prosperity, and health. Recall that the UN is meant to work like a mega-parliament for all nations of the world. The IMF is supposed to prevent major economic disasters, such as the Great Depression, by addressing economic crises as they arise. The World Bank was charged with rebuilding the world after World War II and helping poor nations develop economically.

The process of building an effective global government was derailed in part by the Cold War, which effectively polarized the world into two superpowers. With no clear way forward, global governance was delivered a major setback.

We will first visit the WHO, which is explicitly charged with keeping the world healthy. We will look at the WTO, which is the first major post–Cold War global governance institution. The WTO plays direct roles in health by, for example, influencing a nation's ability to use and produce drugs, and indirectly by affecting economic development (Pollock & Price, 2003). We then revisit the tour of global governance that we started in chapter 1, exploring what it might have become in the post–Cold War period.

THE WORLD HEALTH ORGANIZATION

The **World Health Organization** (WHO) is the most prominent global health institution and is an agency within the UN. It was established in 1948 and inherited the same mission and mandates that guided its antecedent, the Health Organization of the League of Nations. The WHO is charged with monitoring and responding to the world's global health needs. However, its budget is so small that it would not qualify as a top-tier multinational corporation—coming in at under $5 billion depending on voluntary contributions. (General Electric had revenue of $150 billion in 2011 and an operating income of $20 billion.)

The WHO works in four primary areas: (1) it helps to declare and co-ordinate efforts to contain pandemic and epidemic outbreaks (as it did with SARS and the H1N1 virus), (2) it develops evidence-based minimum practices to recommend to all member states, (3) it implements campaigns to make headway on global health issues in ways that individual foundations or nation-states cannot (such as in setting guidelines for good preventive policies and individual healthy behaviors), and (4) it attempts to increase the capacity of individual countries to research and address national health issues.

The WHO is based in Geneva, Switzerland, but it also has six regional offices around the world that operate with quite a bit of autonomy as well as an additional dozen or so specialist liaison offices. The WHO also works with external organizations such as NGOs, the Bill & Melinda Gates Foundation, and pharmaceutical companies.

Some of these ties have proven controversial because influence from companies and others outside of the government may stand to profit from WHO actions and recommendations. But the WHO is essentially hamstrung by a lack of funds and has to rely on revenue from other sources.

THE WORLD HEALTH ORGANIZATION 195

FOR HEALTH OR PROFIT?

The 2009 decision by the WHO to declare H1N1—the "swine flu"—an emergency was based on sixteen emergency committee panelists. These panelists advised the director general, Margaret Chan, but their identities were kept confidential. An investigation found that three of the advisors held ties to Roche and GlaxoSmithKline. These companies make the antiflu drugs oseltamivir and zanamivir, and they benefited financially from the epidemic. (Further, there is significant controversy surrounding whether these drugs work at all and whether they are cost-effective [Doshi, 2009; Godlee & Clarke, 2009; Muennig & Khan, 2001].) The WHO and individual countries stockpiled these drugs, which were never used because the pandemic (thankfully) never became widespread (Cohen & Carter, 2010). As a result, critics have called for greater transparency in WHO decision making (Godlee, 2010).

The swine flu debacle illustrates how, as with other large institutions with a range of stakeholders, the WHO is a political organization. As a result, recommended practices are sometimes driven by outside priorities rather than the best scientific evidence. These priorities are usually set by member states' political concerns rather than private interests, but both probably influence decision making at the organization.

Of course, the WHO often does make decisions based on hard scientific evidence not biased by private entities. But, similar to those of other UN agencies, the WHO's resolutions are usually nonbinding. Member states must separately sign on to specific conventions, such as a 2003 convention on tobacco control, and often have to fund these initiatives themselves.

This relative lack of power makes it that much harder for the WHO to make sure that policy recommendations are followed in coordinated, comprehensive, and efficient ways (Pisani, 2008). For example, the WHO has met resistance from the Vatican on the role of condoms in the battle against HIV/AIDS. At the end of the day, the Vatican wields substantially more power to prevent condom use in Catholic nations than the WHO has to promote their use. Likewise, South Africa, under the former leadership of Mbeki, declared that HIV/AIDS was not caused by a virus at all and refused to engage in prevention and treatment efforts at the national level. Unlike the WTO, the WHO cannot hand out penalties to nations that fail to implement good preventive practices.

That does not mean that the WHO is completely subservient to donors. For instance, the WHO has engaged in debates with major funders such as the Bill & Melinda Gates Foundation on the usefulness of intermittent preventive therapy for malaria (McNeil, 2008). Other recent fierce debates surrounded its ban on flavoring additives to cigarettes, which some tobacco groups claimed would strip 3.6 million African farmers of jobs. It was also hamstrung on actions surrounding **female genital mutilation,** a cultural practice in which women's external genitalia are surgically removed, usually around the time of puberty. (This most often includes the clitoris.) Finally, it debated the ethics of **assisted reproductive technologies,** which involve medical intervention in human pregnancy (Hornos, 2010; Keck & Sikkink, 1998; Vayena, Rowe, & Griffin, 2002).

Debate is obviously healthy; if the WHO could enforce its mandates, your authors would probably be griping instead about all the top-down decisions it makes without input from its constituents. But it should probably be more engaged in the global health problems that really matter. For instance, the WHO is ill prepared to deal with the next global epidemic. It doesn't really even fully have the capability to monitor it. Sadly, only after massive deaths are we likely to get a more effective WHO.

PRIVATE EFFORTS AT PREVENTING EPIDEMICS

Lacking a comprehensive command-and-control initiative on the part of the WHO designed to prevent the next infectious disease epidemic, private organizations have stepped in to fill the gap. One example is Biodiaspora (www.biodiaspora.com), a project aimed at mapping infectious agents and their contacts on flights. This dataset contains global flight patterns. If public health experts detect a new infection, they can also easily identify where it will spread by mapping flights out of the area of infection as well as connecting flights. Biodiaspora can also be used to identify the comings and goings of people on a flight on which a known infectious patient has traveled. Google has also embarked on projects to track the spread of infectious disease. One such project helps identify unusual Internet search activity for key words such as *influenza* or its symptoms (www.google.org/flutrends). (Google's project operates partly by tracking people who are infected and who search for these terms when they become ill.) With such tools, average Internet users may also guess whether a flu outbreak has reached its peak and whether it's worth it to go get a flu shot or mask (as in figure 8.1).

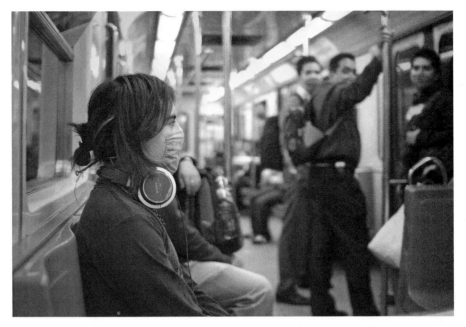

Figure 8.1. Citizens of Mexico City wear masks to prevent the spread of influenza.

Source: Eneas De Troya. Available online at www.flickr.com/photos/eneas/3471986083/.

THE WORLD TRADE ORGANIZATION

Global financial governance institutions tend to hold much more policy-making power than other global governance institutions. Although the WHO would have a difficult time withholding vaccines from a country that did not develop its health system as it should, a bank can penalize a nation for not making loan payments on time. If a nation does not abide by the rules of global finance organizations—for instance, for not playing by trade agreement rules—it can be excluded from lucrative global trade.

The **World Trade Organization** (WTO) is the most important global institution created in the post–Cold War period. As mentioned previously, the WTO sets international rules for trade, and member nations have to sign on to abide by these rules. Exclusion from the WTO means that it becomes difficult to sell the things that your nation produces. For this reason, nations are careful to abide by the rules, even if doing so can have negative effects on population health (see figure 8.2).

What, specifically, are anti-WTO protesters complaining about? First, critics argue that many of the products being imported into global south countries, often in the name of "free" markets, are extremely dangerous to people's

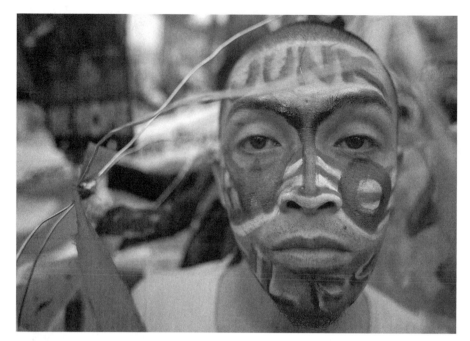

Figure 8.2. An anti-WTO protestor demonstrates in Hong Kong in 2005.
Source: Copyright © Paul Hilton/epa/Corbis.

health. For example, some WTO agreements state that a country must prove that a product is extremely and directly harmful to human, animal, or plant life before prohibiting its entry, and the threshold for proving that the product is harmful is quite high. In fact, there has been only one successful court case regarding this. In this case, the French had banned asbestos products, which are known human carcinogens, but the Canadians sued them in the courts because their asbestos was similar to glass fibers that the French did allow, so the French were not allowed to ban their asbestos. The French lost (Labonté, 2003). In the end, little becomes banned, and low-income countries lack the resources to keep out products sold by multinational corporations from rich nations. Ironically, many of these products are banned in the high-income countries exporting them. Critics want the WTO to reinstall the precautionary first-do-no-harm principle that supposedly governs health care. According to the precautionary principle, corporations should prove that a product is safe before exporting it rather than forcing poor countries to spend so much money and time keeping out unsafe products.

Second, other WTO agreements also tend to take power away from national governments, especially over the manufacture of goods or provision of services that could be provided by private businesses. As we discussed in chapter 5, high-income nations tend to have some public financing and administration and private delivery of health care. WTO agreements force many low-income and middle-income countries to play by a different set of rules: these poorer countries must have both private for-profit financing and private delivery (Shaffer et al., 2005). If these countries eventually build the tax bases needed to expand their public education and health care systems, they must pay "compensatory damages" to the WTO and the foreign companies who might subsequently lose business (Labonté, 2003). In short, many WTO agreements make it difficult for poorer countries to implement the sorts of support-led policies that Amartya Sen advocates.

BRAZIL, AIDS, AND THE WTO

The WTO works in part to protect intellectual property. This includes drug patents, such as those protecting large pharmaceutical companies that were charging US$12,000 for a yearlong supply of a drug that cost just US$100 to US$200 to produce. Most countries were afraid to violate these laws even though thousands of their citizens were dying because the drugs used to treat HIV/AIDS were out of reach. Brazil used a clause in the prevailing international trade agreement at the time and declared HIV/AIDS a public health emergency that required violation of patent laws. Accompanied by popular protest and international outrage, Brazil's moves eventually led pharmaceutical companies to lower the price of their drugs. This opened the door to universal treatment programs that have made a dramatic impact on the global death rate due to HIV/AIDS.

Although they are not charged with governance, there are a large number of regional banks that do have an influence on health and economic policy. These banks, such as the Inter-American Development Bank, operate with similar missions as the World Bank. That is, they mostly tend to loan money for development projects but also provide technical assistance and even grants. The difference is that they work on a more local level.

Even such local institutions tend to operate from the top down with Western ideals and no local input or consideration. For instance, the World Bank and IMF continue to push an agenda of **economic liberalization** without a whole lot of attention to local circumstances. Economic liberalization refers to a concerted push by international institutions to privatize government services and to open nations to free trade.

WHAT IS FREE TRADE, ANYWAY?

The term *free trade* implies that governmental intervention and borders should be removed from any international business dealings. When businesspeople want to do business with another country, they have to fill out paperwork, pay taxes, and make sure that the products that they are trading meet local regulations (which can range from protection of the consumers using the products to bans that protect the local economy).

These bureaucratic and transaction costs associated with selling goods across borders, such as import tariffs, are referred to as **trade barriers.** Trade barriers make it more difficult to sell goods and more expensive to buy them, thus reducing business globally. By reducing trade barriers, free trade can, in theory, make medicines easier to get, make food cheaper, and improve economic conditions, thus reducing hunger.

Free trade can help move an economy forward by facilitating business transactions. But some call *free trade* a misnomer because truly unregulated markets exist only in theory. In real life, markets at the very least have some laws protecting property rights by private individuals, firms, nonprofit institutions, and the state. Workers and consumers need to be protected, too. In the end, even laws stating that types of tariffs should be banned or that set up processes for money exchanges and commercial transactions (to make sure that firms do not just take other firms' money and then leave without fear of retribution) usually constrict some entities' property rights and expand others'.

AN EVOLUTION OF GLOBAL GOVERNANCE

In chapter 1, we pointed out how global governance suffered a major setback with the onset of the Cold War. This was partly because poor nations were sometimes used as proxies through which battles were waged or dictators were installed. We now take some time to dig more deeply into how history has shaped the institutions that set policies across international borders.

Some experts felt that the end of the Cold War would bring an "end of history." That is, it could have ushered in a new era of democracy and health. First, many dictators were kept in place by the United States or the Soviet Union so that their military and political objectives could be maintained worldwide. The end of the war lowered the use of such dictators. Second, in current dollar terms, many trillions of dollars were spent on the war effort. Therefore, some saw the end of the Cold War as a new dawn in which less military expenditures would usher in an era of domestic social welfare expenditures in rich nations and ample aid to poor nations.

Unfortunately, history did not exactly unfold that way. Internal politics in the United States prevented large reductions in military expenditures. Post-Soviet countries such as Russia actually reported *declining* life expectancy rates (from seventy in 1989 to sixty-four in 1994, though this began to rise again by 2008). This decline in life expectancy was probably due to the sudden dismantling of former Soviet health, transit, and welfare programs coupled with a massive wave of alcoholism and drug use. In addition to losing life-saving services, the citizens of former Soviet countries underwent a rapid decline in their quality of life. At this textbook goes to press, some post–Cold War Eastern Bloc nations such as Hungary still have a lower life expectancy than before the fall of the wall.

Income inequalities also grew within former Soviet economies along with many low-income nations in the 1990s. Economic and political factors seem to be the most important determinants of conflict in middle- and low-income nations (Blattman & Miguel, 2010; Collier et al., 2003; Ross, 2006). Many nations directly or indirectly supported by the Soviet Union faltered. Instability and civil conflict proliferated globally. By 1991, nearly 30 percent of the world's states were engaged in some sort of warfare (Gleditsch, Wallensteen, Eriksson, Sollenberg, & Strand, 2002). In the face of all of this instability, HIV/AIDS took a strong foothold, especially in sub-Saharan Africa.

The massive life expectancy gains realized between 1900 through the 1990s had stalled or even declined in many places, and not just in former Soviet economies. In some sub-Saharan African nations, life expectancy dropped even more precipitously due to HIV/AIDS. In the United States, a silent change had occurred in which life expectancy began to decline in some counties, and people's perception of their health started to decline sometime in the early 1990s. The only nations whose health continued to grow solidly were those of Western Europe and recession-laden Japan.

We point all this out because a coordinated effort across nations could have provided the economic and intellectual infrastructure to address these health and economic problems, but most nations were simply concerned with events occurring within their own borders. In fact, although much attention was paid to the collapse of the Soviet Union, internal civil conflicts received less attention. The power vacuum left by rapidly exiting dictators fueled some of these conflicts, and there was no one to step into the void.

The Promise of Peace

It was also thought that the economy of the United States and its allies would climb as military expenditures fell in the post–Cold War period. This is because military expenditures are thought to come with a massive **opportunity cost.** That is, every dollar spent on the military would probably produce much more economic growth if it were spent on another social good, such as education.

From an economic standpoint, this is because a good deal of money in the military is spent on goods and services that one hopes will never be put to use or are wasted in bureaucracy.

Military expenditures may also come at a huge opportunity cost with respect to health. That is, money spent on the military could reduce mortality if spent on something else because the use of military goods and services produces a net loss of life. Of course, military spending also has a preventive role as well; the United States and the Soviet Union never actually came into direct warfare perhaps in part because the expensive nuclear build-up both nations took part in could have meant total nuclear annihilation. But military strength also emboldens strong nations to invade weaker ones, as exemplified by the two Gulf Wars.

Even if democracy did not happen, the hope was that by engaging in international global commerce, nations would become so economically intertwined that they would no longer be able to engage in conflict without mutually assured economic destruction. This, it was thought, would produce a huge disincentive for warfare.

WAR, IDEOLOGY, AND PUBLIC HEALTH

Public health is a broad field, including any area of study that might affect human health. One major area is war and war prevention. One leader in this area is Victor Sidel, who helped place the prevention of war squarely on the public health agenda. (His organization, which won the Nobel Peace Prize, partly forwarded simple solutions such as placing heavy objects on top of nuclear silos in former Soviet countries to prevent rogue leaders from easily launching them.) Other disciplines, such as political science, philosophy, and economics, also include the study of prevention of war. Some argue that war is best prevented by international political collaboration and democracy (an argument that probably more public health experts would be inclined to make) and others believe that war is best prevented by international economic collaboration.

Can Money and Scissors Save the Day?

The 1980s and 1990s brought in a new era of global governance, but it almost entirely took the form of economic governance. Some nations, such as India, had become deeply mired in protectionism, bureaucracy, and government-run industries. They needed to be freed from the chains of government red tape and corruption if they were to create the kind of economic growth that would lift citizens out of poverty. By scissoring away some of this red tape, India began a two-decade economic rise that produced reductions in absolute poverty.

This basic "economic liberalization" agenda was similar to the policy prescriptions forwarded by the IMF and the World Bank. But because these prescriptions were universal, nations where public services were working also saw pressures to liberalize. In some places, water was being delivered effectively and cheaply to people's homes by the government. Privatization of these services meant that people could no longer afford water. Left with little choice but to riot or die of thirst, many citizens took to the streets.

The IMF and the World Bank pressured governments to privatize rather than improve the management of their existing services. Moreover, many industries in many nations, such as health care (described in chapter 5), are left to the market when they probably should be left to the government. This led many to argue that the "prescription" should be tailored to local governments and should involve improvements in management rather than wholesale cuts in government services (Tendler, 1998).

THE IMF'S STANDARD PRESCRIPTION

When financial crisis hits, the IMF is there to come to the rescue with a package of loans. However, to get the loans, the IMF often recommends that the recipient devalue its currency (this makes exports cheaper, thus fueling a return to growth), reduce its spending (so that it can pay off its debt and balance its budget), and liberalize its trade with other nations (to make transactions more efficient and compete in the global economy).

This standard package of advice may be well and good for some nations in some circumstances, but it can also make the beneficiary fall into greater financial trouble than it had before the IMF showed up at its door. To make currency devaluation worthwhile, a country had better be sure to have a lot of exports. If its debt is in dollars, it should also have very little debt. Because loans are usually valued in dollars, a drop in the value of the recipient's currency can artificially increase its debt overnight. For instance, say the country's currency is 10 pesos to the dollar and it owes US$100. If it devalues to 20 pesos to the dollar, its exports will be cheaper but it will suddenly owe US$200.

Cutting spending on government programs not only means fewer schools and health clinics but also larger numbers of unemployed people. In reducing trade barriers, the country needs a big domestic market because it will risk a sudden inflow of cheap foreign goods that its domestic industries will have to compete against. Often, countries are better off not taking any money from the IMF at all. When Argentina's economy collapsed, some attributed the collapse to the IMF's advice.

One cornerstone of this economic liberalization carried out in the 1990s was **free trade.** Free trade involves reducing barriers to the exchange of goods and services across borders. Wealthy nations benefited from heavy agricultural subsidies and mechanization and managed to exempt themselves from many of the provisions for free trade in international agreements. Without barriers, poor nations could not protect themselves from inflows of cheap (and subsidized) agricultural products, such as corn and milk from the United States. As a result, **trade liberalization** shocked local economies, leaving farmers and other citizens alike without gainful employment. This, in some cases, *increased* hunger. Still reeling from the structural adjustment programs of the IMF, the median per capita growth in low- and medium-income countries shrank from 2.5 percent between 1960 and 1979 to 0 percent between 1980 and 1999 (Easterly, 2001).

Unlike their predecessors, rapidly industrializing nations must attempt to provide their citizens with rights in the face of pressures from coalitions of still wealthier nations. They have been forced to treat their HIV/AIDS cases with unnecessarily expensive drugs and to open their domestic markets quickly to competition. At the same time, there is little by way of punishment doled out by such nations for massive, transborder pollution. The reasons for this are largely political. Although the WTO can give out punishment for failure to play fair economically, it rarely exerts its power to mandate good environmental practices. Thus, our main achievement in post–Cold War governance—the WTO—has still not managed to deliver much by way of governance that might improve global health.

Democracy in Governance

Last but most certainly not least, democracy itself did not flourish in the post–Cold War period quite in the ways that many expected. Many countries in Latin America, Africa, and Asia remained autocratic. With notable exceptions such as Singapore, less-than-robust democracies and authoritarian states are less likely to pursue the balance of economic growth and social policy that helps their people to thrive (McGuire, 2010).

The WTO has been the only major player added to the global governance landscape in the past few decades. Its rules and agreements may have a greater impact on global public health than any other single entity, but it is not considered a health organization. Because of this, some policy scholars have argued that environmental, health, education, and labor ministers should attend WTO talks alongside the trade ministers (Stiglitz, 2006).

Further, the WTO has well over 150 members, constituting the majority of the world's nations, but it is not democratic; the most powerful nations exert undue influence over less powerful nations. Although decisions are supposed to be made via a voting system in which each country gets one vote, no votes have actually been taken. Instead, most WTO negotiations happen informally, in small and exclusive meetings. These meetings are often called "green room" negotiations, after the color of the WTO director-general's office in Geneva. Members from low-income countries are often left out of the green room. It doesn't help that, until recently, the United States alone employed over 250 full-time and part-time negotiators, whereas over one hundred countries could not afford to send a single negotiator (Labonté, 2003). Although some scholars note that low-income country participation has begun to increase in the current round of development negotiations, most state that further reforms are direly needed (Jones, 2009).

Like the WTO, some would argue that the UN is also not fully democratic. Some nations have veto power, for instance. It is also widely seen as hamstrung by bureaucracy. To many, working for the UN means writing reports that no one is given the authority or resources to execute.

When the **Asian financial crisis**—a major economic downturn in Asia which was precipitated by speculation that Asian economies had grown too fast for their weak financial institutions to keep up—hit in the 1990s, only the IMF, never governed by a citizen of any Asian nation, was there to lend money and step into the fray. The IMF prescribed the same sorts of economic liberalization, austerity cuts, and structural adjustment programs that it had been recommending since the 1980s. China, the world's largest nation with respect to population, chose to ignore their advice and was the only nation in the region to come out of the crisis unscathed. Instead of cutting social programs, it began to use its massive cash reserves to reinvest in them.

CHINA AND SOCIAL DEVELOPMENT

To fully open its markets, the Chinese government thought it was necessary to dismantle its social programs, such as the barefoot doctor's program and many public health and education programs. As it grew, China reinvested in such programs to a much greater extent than was previously possible. (The Chinese economy was reportedly so broke in the late 1970s that the government did not have enough money to fly international delegates to visit other countries.) But it is important to remember that China's growth came on the heels of earlier investments in education that left a highly literate workforce. It also came at the sacrifice of environmental regulations, health care investments, and safety regulations that just might account for the dramatic slowdown in its life expectancy gains since market reforms were enacted. Even thirty-two years after the market reforms, it has not managed to make much of a dent in the environmental damage caused by its industrialization. Still, it is undoubtedly true that most of the roughly half-billion people who have been lifted out of poverty over this period would prefer modern China to that of the China of 1979.

Thus, although many expected that massive health and economic benefits would be reaped by the end of the Cold War, the 1980s did not go so well. Still, as we saw in chapter 1, many of the largely ignored and unseen health and economic problems of the early 1990s seemed to slowly resolve themselves by the end of the decade.

A New Era of Health and Democracy

As mentioned in chapters 1 and 4, private aid took off in the first decade of the twenty-first century, with many billionaires leading other wealthy world citizens to donate to social programs. Although aid remains highly controversial, many less economically developed countries are now experiencing rapid industrialization and democratization. It is as if, despite a lack of global governance, the hope of the post–Cold War era is finally starting to be realized.

Much of this growth, ironically, came on the coattails of China, the world's wealthiest nondemocratic government. China's hunger for ore and energy took it to countries that wealthy nations did not invest in to the same extent. Many of the contracts that China signed obliged it to help build roads and schools. Although China's move toward capitalism was accompanied by some reforms— it even allowed Premier Wen Jiabao, a reformer, into its third highest governmental position for a spell—it remains a repressive state.

Nevertheless, China is also interesting because Washington pushed these nations toward market liberalization for decades with very little economic progress. (Some have even argued that the Washington Consensus moved these nations backward economically.) Yet, with small pushes, nations in Latin America and sub-Saharan Africa began to economically flourish.

Whether democracy follows wealth, education, or culture is a topic of great debate. The sociologist T. H. Marshall divided citizenship rights into three components, each with its own new age of glory: civil rights in the eighteenth-century revolutions, political rights and mass enfranchisement in the nineteenth century, and social rights and the development of a comprehensive welfare state with adequate unemployment and health insurance, worker protections, safety laws, adequate housing, public education, and a basic, universal safety net in the twentieth century (Marshall, 1963). Although industrialized countries varied quite a bit in the sorts of welfare states they ended up with, they largely followed this pattern, with each component slowly evolving concurrently. As they developed socially and economically, they faced challenges. For instance, most modern wealthy economies became wealthy through exporting goods, so they had to regulate industrial pollution even as their production of goods increased. Income inequality and other problems associated with industrialization also had to be addressed.

WHICH COMES FIRST, THE CHICKEN OR THE DEMOCRACY?

Democratization occurs when governments shift from authoritarian regimes and dictatorships to allowing citizens to participate in selecting political leaders and informing public policies on a regular basis. This can happen gradually—as when a semidemocratic government slowly allows more participation. But more often, it happens abruptly, as by revolution (removing existing leaders by mass will) or by removing semi-democratic regimes by ballot (as happened when the Liberal Democrats were removed from office in Japan after decades of rule). Some have argued that the general trend toward democracy arises from wealth and that wealthy countries have much more stable democracies (Przeworski, 2000).

However, it is also the case that countries with a good deal of mineral or energy resources often have a difficult time establishing democracy, a trend referred to as the **resource curse,** described in much more detail in chapter 10. (Democratic leaders are sometimes overthrown when weakly governed nations strike oil.) Another possible antecedent to democracy is that mass literacy naturally leads to a well-educated populace that ultimately demands democratic reform. A variety of other factors have also been cited, such as growing social capital (recall from chapter 2 that this refers to resources such as social connections with others). For instance, many governments, including the British government managing the United States colonies, banned coffee consumption because coffee houses facilitated conversations on politics and the need for democracy. Culture, modernization, and a large plethora of other factors have also been cited, and most ultimately were disproved. For instance, many "experts" referred to oppressive Arab dictatorships in Arab nations as a "cultural norm." That is, there is something inherent to Arab culture that requires a dictator to hold things together. Then, injustice inflicted on a single fruit vendor in Tunisia led to a series of democratic revolutions throughout the Middle East. So much for the experts.

Today, low- and middle-income countries follow different paths and are sometimes able to leapfrog over certain stages of economic development (Perkins, 2003). That is, newer technologies already developed by rich nations make it possible to bypass inefficient old ones. The concept of leapfrogging is not just limited to economic development; there are many social welfare programs globally that nations can learn from. Some aspects of management science, occupational safety methods, and environmental health are global concepts, largely free from patent protection and available to any nation or business that wishes to adopt them.

Even through the Great Recession, the HIV/AIDS epidemic statistics have ameliorated a bit. Educational attainment and literacy are improving, especially for girls. Maternal and infant mortality is on the decline and life expectancy is rising. Governments have moved from measuring well-being in terms of economic development to a measure in which overall well-being is emphasized. (This started with a measure of life expectancy, literacy, and economic growth, known as the human development index [HDI], and is moving to more complex measures of well-being.) This trend toward a global hug fest is called *convergence*.

CONVERGENCE!

Although there were some setbacks along the way, including the HIV/AIDS epidemic and the difficult transitions following the fall of the Soviet Union in the 1990s, the overall picture of the post–World War II era to 2013 was hopeful. Educational attainment and literacy in low-income nations has grown consistently, as has life expectancy. In fact, most nations are becoming healthier, wealthier, and wiser over time. The global population explosion is leveling off, and the world population is projected to level off in a few decades. Sub-Saharan Africa, recently bleakly portrayed in the media as a hopeless continent, is now considered the next economic equivalent to China. So, whatever we are doing—providing aid, allowing China to grow economically, working toward global democracy—seems to be working. This trend toward better statistical indicators across nations is called *convergence*, implying that all nations' statistics will look like Sweden's at some point in the future.

SUMMARY

Through much of the twentieth century to the present day, global governance has taken place in the bureaucratic corridors of the United Nations, which sets the bulk of the global political agenda. Other institutions include the World Bank, the International Monetary Fund, and the World Trade Organization. It could be argued that because the World Bank, the IMF, and the WTO exert great control over money, they have much more meaningful enforcement capabilities than the UN. In practice, organizations such as the WTO probably could exert more influence on public health policies by imposing loan or trade restrictions on nations that fail to comply. Most of these organizations promote trade liberalization, representative electoral democracy, and so-called "good governance" (intended to limit problems such as the resource curse). However, it is not clear that interference in other nation's governance structures is usually or even often a good practice.

KEY TERMS

Asian financial crisis
assisted reproductive
   technologies
convergence
democratization
economic liberalization

female genital
   mutilation
free trade
opportunity cost
resource curse
trade barriers

trade liberalization
World Health
   Organization (WHO)
World Trade
   Organization (WTO)

DISCUSSION QUESTIONS

1. What aspects of health policies and health outcomes are unlikely to be addressed via national social policies? Which of these tend to be addressed by global health institutions such as the WHO?

2. What is globalization? In what key ways are diseases less likely to be caused by or affect trends in just one country compared to earlier periods in history?

3. Should WTO regulations be reformed to improve population health? If so, what is needed to implement these reforms?

4. What sorts of provisions in trade agreements are most relevant to public health? Can these be addressed at the international level?

5. Among the WHO, IMF, and WTO, which intergovernmental institution do you feel most profoundly shapes health outcomes in low-income countries? Why?

FURTHER READING

Hans Rosling on HIV: New facts and stunning data visuals. (2009, February). TEDTalks. Available online at www.ted.com/talks/hans_rosling_the_truth_about _hiv.html

Labonté, R., & Schrecker, T. (2007). Globalization and social determinants of health. Globalization and Health, 3(5). Available online at www.globalizationandhealth .com/content/3/1/5

REFERENCES

Blattman, C., & Miguel, E. (2010). Civil war. *Journal of Economic Literature*, *48*(1), 3–57.

Cohen, D., & Carter, P. (2010). Conflicts of interest: WHO and the pandemic flu "conspiracies." *BMJ*, *340*, c2912.

Collier, P., Elliott, V. L., Hegre, H., Hoeffler, A., Reynal-Querol, M., & Sambanis, N. (2003). *Breaking the conflict trap: Civil war and development policy*. Washington, DC: World Bank and Oxford University Press.

Doshi, P. (2009). Neuraminidase inhibitors: The story behind the Cochrane review. *BMJ*, *339*, b5164.

Easterly, W. (2001). The lost decades: Developing countries' stagnation in spite of policy reform 1980–98. *Journal of Economic Growth*, *6*(2), 135–157.

Gleditsch, N. P., Wallensteen, P., Eriksson, M., Sollenberg, M., & Strand, H. (2002). Armed conflict 1946–2001: A new dataset. *Journal of Peace Research*, *39*(5), 615–637.

Godlee, F. (2010). Editorial: Conflicts of interest and pandemic flu. *BMJ*, *340*, c2947. doi: 310.1136/bmj.c2947.

Godlee, F., & Clarke, M. (2009). Why don't we have all the evidence on oseltamivir? *BMJ*, *339*, b5351.

Hornos, C. (2010, November 10). World health officials debate new tobacco controls. Reuters. Available online at http://af.reuters.com/article/worldNews/idAFTRE6AE2SI20101115

Jones, K. (2009). Green room politics and the WTO's crisis of representation. *Progress in Development Studies*, *9*(4), 349–357.

Keck, M. E., & Sikkink, K. (1998). *Activists beyond borders*. Ithaca, NY: Cornell University Press.

Labonté, R. (2003). Globalization, trade and health: Unpacking the linkages, defining the healthy public policy options. In R. Hofrichter (Ed.), *Health and social justice: Politics, ideology and inequity in the distribution of disease.* San Francisco: Jossey-Bass.

Marshall, T. H. (1963). *Class, citizenship, and social development*. Chicago: University of Chicago Press.

McGuire, J. W. (2010). *Wealth, health, and democracy in East Asia and Latin America*. New York: Cambridge University Press.

McNeil R., Jr. (2008, February 16). Gates Foundation's influence criticized. *New York Times.*

Muennig, P. A., & Khan, K. (2001). Cost-effectiveness of vaccination versus treatment of influenza in healthy adolescents and adults. *Clinical Infectious Diseases*, *33*(11), 1879–1885.

Perkins, R. (2003). Environmental leapfrogging in developing countries: A critical assessment and reconstruction. *National Resources Forum*, *27*, 177–188. Available online at http://personal.lse.ac.uk/PERKINSR/NRF_Leapfrogging_27%202003.pdf

Pisani, E. (2008). *The wisdom of whores: Bureaucrats, brothels, and the business of AIDS*. New York: W. W. Norton.

Pollock, A. M., & Price, D. (2003). The public health implications of world trade negotiations on the general agreement on trade in services and public services. *Lancet*, *362*(9389), 1072–1075.

Przeworski, A. (2000). *Democracy and development: Political institutions and well-being in the world, 1950–1990* (Vol. 3). New York: Cambridge University Press.

Ross, M. (2006). A closer look at oil, diamonds, and civil war. *Political Science*, *9*(1), 265.

Shaffer, E. R., Waitzkin, H., Brenner, J., and Jasso-Aguilar, R. (2005). "Global trade and public health." *American Journal of Public Health*, *95*(1), 23–34.

Stiglitz, J. (2006). *Making globalization work*. New York: W. W. Norton.

Tendler, J. (1998). *Good government in the tropics*. Baltimore, MD: Johns Hopkins University Press.

Vayena, E., Rowe, P. J., & Griffin, P. D. (2002). *Current practices and controversies in assisted reproduction*. Geneva: WHO.

PART THREE

Key Challenges in Global Health

CHAPTER 9

Poverty

KEY IDEAS

- Different nations have different standards of poverty for individuals, and these standards are usually based on individual or household income.

- Poverty has been called the main underlying cause of poor global health because it plays a complex role in many different areas of health, such as infectious disease, crime, and unsafe housing.

- In low-income countries, poverty is tied to health because it can prevent individuals from attaining necessary nutrients.

- Poverty can also prevent households from attaining other goods—safe housing to weather the elements, transportation, and so on—that are essential to health.

Poverty is without a doubt a leading global killer. In low-income nations, it is the root cause of hunger and death from infectious disease. In all development contexts, it is a major contributor to crime, unsafe housing, and a large number of other "deadly deprivations" that bring lives to an untimely end. If the poor could somehow magically be elevated to middle-class status, billions of years of life would be gained globally. About 544 million years of perfect health are lost to poverty within the United States alone, relative to 149 million years of perfect health from obesity (Muennig, Fiscella, Tancredi, & Franks, 2010). The UN has essentially declared poverty to be the number one enemy in all matters of international or global health. From this viewpoint, poverty is one risk that spins out most diseases.

But is it really safe to say that *poverty* is the cause of all of these things? Or is it merely just one other link in a large chain of problems linking social conditions to disease?

INCOME AND HEALTH ACROSS NATIONS

It has been said by many that "economic policy is health policy." (So many people have said this, in fact, that our research assistants have not definitively tracked the first person to say it.) Countries that are economically developed tend to have less disability and morbidity and have the longest life expectancies.

If so, why not just focus on economic indicators? Money is easy to track, and more or less gets us the same information as complex health statistics, right? Not exactly. To equate economic growth with health would be a mistake. The United States of America—the wealthiest country overall and one of the most wealthy on a per capita basis—has a life expectancy that is on par with many countries most people would consider low-income nations. Costa Rica, Chile, Cuba, and Dominica are but a few such countries. Moreover, some still wealthier nations (e.g., Qatar) are doing even worse than the United States on life expectancy. Democracy also does not always follow from economic development. This has led some leading thinkers to question whether we as a global society should be focusing so much attention on economic indicators, suggesting instead a capability approach to thinking about economic development.

THE CAPABILITY APPROACH IN PUBLIC HEALTH

We first described the capability approach in chapter 5 in our discussion of health systems. Recall that although many measure a nation's progress in terms of GDP, the capability approach forwards the idea that people also highly value things such as longevity, literacy, and free speech, so these indicators should also be tracked. The problem is that different capabilities do not always all go hand in hand. Singapore is one of the most highly educated and longest-living societies in the world, but one cannot speak freely about the government there. China, up to the time of press, has done amazingly well in terms of maintaining economic growth but quite poorly on most other measures Sen mentions (Sen, 1999). Another problem is that it is difficult to measure national progress on some capabilities.

One index that is commonly used is the HDI, a combined measure of economic growth, literacy, and life expectancy, introduced in chapter 2. Taking a cue from the HDI, the American Human Development Project (www.measureofamerica.org) presents similar measures for individual US states and congressional districts. Yale University's Environmental Performance Index (http://epi.yale.edu) presents scales half composed of "ecosystem vitality" measures, such as fisheries and climate change, and half composed of environmental health measures, such as air pollution and sanitation. Meanwhile, Freedom House presents measures of democracy and capabilities of expression and democratic participation in its annual reports (www.freedomhouse.org/).

As we pointed out in chapter 2, economic growth and longevity are linked together only to the point that a nation's average per capita GDP exceeds about US$4,000 per person per year in standard international dollars. After that, all bets are off—there is no relationship between a nation's income and longevity. What is true of longevity is also true of health more broadly and even happiness. After people's basic needs are met, it turns out, the relationship between wealth and health disappears into the night.

So why does the relationship exist for poor countries but not wealthy ones? As more than alluded to previously, one idea is that very poor countries tend to have nonexistent public health infrastructure—the clean water, sanitation, and vaccines that account for twenty to forty years of life expectancy. Once this is in place, infectious diseases can be overcome. But, of course, eating is one core ingredient of survival, and this cannot be done without money to buy food, so this is almost certainly another reason why money matters for health in very poor nations.

But there is more to the picture than that. Countries with very low per capita income often have terrible governance, have nothing to sell, or both. By nothing to sell, we mean that they have no infrastructure for manufacturing, little by way of human capital, and few natural resources. As a result, there is no money for people to buy food or for governments to buy public health infrastructure.

According to a UN report from the Conference on Trade and Development, integrating such nations into the global economy had produced very little benefit by the mid-2000s. The poorest countries have indeed become more integrated into the world economy. Yet, by 2004, their incomes had sunk to 1990 levels (UN, 2004). Various strategies are typically sought to create an economy in this setting when at all possible. Common strategies include tapping into textiles or cash crops in the hopes of jump-starting some industry. For better or worse, three of the countries in that older UN report have since started exporting oil. But most of this money has ended up in official's pockets, and very little has gone to creating infrastructure or jobs.

One of the biggest problems in low-income nations is a lack of a functioning education system. An unskilled workforce is unlikely to be able to grow crops or make textiles very well; therefore, even with lower wages, factories built in nations with highly unskilled labor are not often competitive in higher yield markets. China continued to be an export powerhouse through 2013 even as wages skyrocketed. (Although skyrocketing wages will ultimately destroy any export market, it is remarkable that China manufactures most of the world's goods with low-end wages that are considerably higher than in neighboring countries.) Another problem is that developed nations do not trade fairly. In 2003, the average European cow received US$2.50 in subsidies, nearly twice what the one billion poor people of the world earn in a day (Bearak, 2003). This makes it difficult for the poorer nations to catch up.

Of course, if the governments of these poor nations were capable of it, it would theoretically be possible to channel all available resources into clean water, sanitation, food guarantees, vaccinations, and education. This is what has led to health successes in Cuba and the Indian state of Kerala despite abject poverty. Though Cubans are often heard complaining that they "live like poor people but die like rich ones," it is probably a much preferable fate to living like poor people and dying like poor people.

Whatever is done, these very low-income nations, although lagging among other racehorses, will probably eventually also slowly converge with the rest of the global economy to become wealthier and healthier. Conditions among many of these nations may be inching toward improvement, as wages rise in China and elsewhere, raising the global price of labor. Eventually, prosperity has to spill over. So one day, all nations will pass the magical $4,000 per capita GDP threshold and money won't matter at all. At least, that is, when comparing average incomes across nations. Within nations, poverty will still matter for health, and will probably continue to matter for a long, long time. This raises the cortical question of why poverty matters within nations but not across them. To begin to understand this, we must first understand what poverty is in the first place.

DEFINITIONS OF POVERTY

Every nation has a different **standard of poverty**. In the very poorest nations, poverty is typically defined as the number of folks who make very, very little money—less than 1 international dollar per day. The international dollar is a unit of currency that is supposed to buy roughly the same amount of goods in Thailand as it does in Switzerland. This is accomplished via the miraculous adjustment factor called *PPP*. PPP takes differences in the cost of living and inflation rates between nations. For instance, a yummy vegetarian tali meal in India will typically run about 25 rupees in a bus stop and about US$15 in an urban restaurant in the United States. At the time of press, 25 rupees amounted to a little over US$0.50, so one could buy twenty-four tali meals in India for the price of one in the United States. (The ones in India usually come with refills, making the deal all the sweeter.) Using PPP-adjusted international dollars, though, both should *in theory* come out to be roughly the same. In practice they do not because PPP is adjusted based on some goods and services but not *all* of them. Individual items flux a lot depending on where they were produced (locally or globally) and how (for example, food requires cheap labor and India has lots of that).

MEASURING THE POOR

The 1990 edition of the World Bank's annual *World Development Report* estimated the number of people living on US$1.00 per day to be about one billion. This definition of poverty stuck, mostly because it was simple to remember and cite (1 billion on 1 dollar). This "dollar" became the standard measure for poverty. In 2005, the standard was revised to US$1.25. But that same year, a massive effort was undertaken to improve our understanding of price variations in 146 countries. It was found that, lo and behold, the cost of living is much higher than previously thought. (Anyone outside of the World Bank—a place that offers heavily subsidized gourmet food for lunch—could have told them that.) Therefore, the number of poor people was adjusted upward to 1.4 billion. The economic crisis of 2008 and 2009 worsened this figure substantially (World Bank, 2013).

In practice, what one is buying and where one buys it matters. For instance, after PPP corrections, the meal will still seem cheap in India, but a television will be outrageously expensive, even by Western income standards. On average, the corrections are certainly better than nothing. (One alternative is the Big Mac Index, which uses differences in pricing of the ubiquitous Big Mac sandwich. It is difficult to choose the "basket of goods" that most universally represent the core needs and costs of households around the world to be used in PPP calculations, and the Big Mac serves as one reliable benchmark.)

Typically, earnings of 1 international dollar per day or less qualify as extreme poverty, and an income of 2 international dollars per day is considered very poor. If any of the readers are enthusiastic about performance art, you can try living in any part of the United States for US$1 per day (or the new standard of US$1.25 per day). You will probably find that it is a bit of a challenge to meet caloric needs on this budget. In fact a quick search on the web will produce many misinformed blogs detailing the writers' experiments from living on $1 per day in Ecuador, Guatemala, or Sierra Leone. But the reality is that $1 per day is significantly higher than the PPP-adjusted living costs that families are really tied to.

About 1.4 billion people meet the **extreme poverty** criterion of $1.25 per day and about 3 billion people meet the more general poverty criterion. At the time of press, three billion people constituted just over 40 percent of the world's population. Although progress has been made in alleviating poverty, poverty is difficult to control because most of the world's population growth is occurring among its poorest inhabitants. A high birth rate is generally seen among poor people in developed and low-income nations.

Extreme poverty not only correlates with high birth rates but also with poor health outcomes. The vast majority of the world's illness occurs among those earning less than 2 international dollars per day. Of course, Cubans who earn INT$365 dollars per year live to be seventy-nine years, way ahead of fifty-eight years for Native American males in South Dakota who make INT$27,000 per year (Murray et al., 2006). Despite such exceptions, one can link poverty to poor health as a general rule.

Indeed, if one were only to look at their health statistics, we would certainly call low-income Americans "extremely poor." Americans living at less than 200 percent of the poverty line have a life expectancy on par with Nicaraguans (Muennig et al., 2005). It is also the case that very poor people in some very poor countries will far outlive poor Americans. Yet what most people consider "poor" in the United States looks very different when measured in terms of purchasing power. *Some* Americans living under 200 percent of the poverty threshold (a common definition of *poor* in the United States) can afford a car and three meals a day.

Therefore, if one is tempted to link poverty and health, it is clear that a definition based on how much one can buy in a given day is wholly inadequate. Because poverty is relative (the "poor" must be compared to "nonpoor" people in any given country), the face of poverty looks very different from place to place. Many welfare-dependent "poor" people in Sweden or Norway may be difficult to distinguish from some chief executive officers of Scandina-

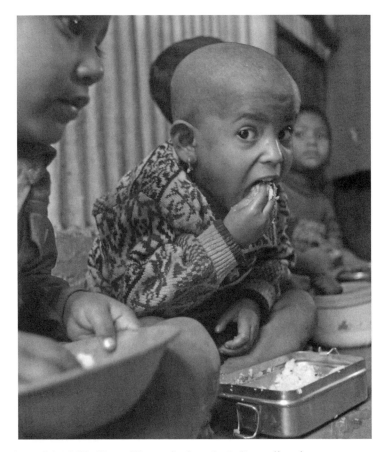

Figure 9.1. This child, like millions of others in India, suffers from extreme poverty and hunger.

Source: Copyright © Rajanish Kakade/AP/Corbis.

vian corporations, at least in terms of one's standard of living. They might dress similarly, drive similar cars, and have at least somewhat similar homes. In that case, the major distinguishing feature of poverty may be additional life stressors, somewhat worse health outcomes, and a few billion fewer Kroner in the bank account. In fact, so many Scandinavian executives live such middle-class lives that they have been reportedly quite upset to be "outed" within their mixed-income communities by *Fortune Magazine* as billionaires. So, poverty obviously looks very different in Sweden than in India (figure 9.1).

Some countries, such as the United States, have an explicit poverty line, a threshold below which people are considered poor and therefore eligible for **means-tested governmental benefits.** In the United States, this poverty line is calculated by putting together an essential **basket of goods,** researching how much this basket of goods costs and adjusting it for household size. In 2011, the poverty line for a family of four was approximately US$22,000, regardless of whether they lived in rural Montana or New York City. This sort of system assumes that there is an important **absolute poverty line.** Other countries, such as Sweden, tend to have **universal benefits** rather than means-tested benefits so that people are eligible regardless of income. (For example, all US citizens are eligible for Medicare, a universal program for the elderly, but only certain individuals are eligible for Medicaid.) Instead, some industrialized countries determine who is poor according to a **relative poverty line,** such as whoever makes less than half of the national median income distribution. According to such a definition, the person would be considered poor even if they could buy an essential basket of goods, partly because they would be so different from most of compatriots that they would likely face **social exclusion.** Policy makers therefore differ on the extent to which they emphasize **material deprivations** or social exclusion in responses to poverty.

There is one consistent trend among the poor. They always have worse health status than wealthy people within their own countries.

WHY DO WE WORRY ABOUT POVERTY IN PUBLIC HEALTH?

Those living in extreme poverty (less than US$1.25 per day) and regular poverty (less than US$2.00 per day) suffer the majority of disease and disability in the world, even though they make up just one-third of the world's population. The average person living in Swaziland, Angola, or Zambia will not see his or her thirty-eighth birthday. For citizens of these countries, the term *living wage* takes on a whole new meaning because many cannot afford food, clean water, vaccinations, or basic health care.

It is no coincidence that the number of people worldwide who earn less than one dollar a day (let's use the old one dollar a day metric to keep things simple) and the number of people worldwide who go hungry on a regular basis is the same (one billion). Money not only buys the calories needed for sustenance but it also buys nutrient diversity. One of the greatest problems in public health is the lack of **micronutrients.** (The term *micronutrient* is used in health because it has significantly more syllables than the term *nutrient*.) The major micronutrients in question include iodine, iron, and vitamin A.

Iodine and iron deficiency are major contributors to lost intellectual function. The WHO estimates that about six hundred million people suffer from goiter, the most common effect of iodine deficiency. In goiter, the thyroid gland becomes greatly enlarged as it works to produce hormones needed for regulating the body's metabolism. When a fetus is deprived of iodine, intellectual impairment occurs. The most extreme form of impairment is cretinism, a severe physical and mental stunting.

Unlike the effects of iodine deficiency, the effects of iron deficiency are much more subtle. But iron deficiency's very high prevalence—4.5 billion people or two-thirds of the world's population—makes it a much greater public health problem. Children who are iron deficient may suffer from moderate lifelong deficits in intellectual functioning. The loss of a few IQ points may not seem like a big deal. After all, many a college student has lost significant gray matter to alcohol. But over the lifetime of entire populations, iron deficiency can take a serious toll on an economy. Less cognitively endowed workers make for a less favorable business environment for investors, for one. And iron deficiency also leads to extreme fatigue, making it difficult even for laborers to provide for their families. Finally, because of menstruation, iron deficiency disproportionately affects females, the group from which the benefits of a strong education system are most strongly realized (Browne & Barrett, 1991; Subbarao & Raney, 1995). (As mentioned previously, schooling reduces fertility among females, and females are much more likely to pass knowledge on to their offspring than are males.)

Whereas iodine and iron deficiencies affect intellectual functioning, vitamin A affects the immune system. Vitamin A deficiency is a major cause of blindness worldwide. In addition to its role in vision, vitamin A appears to play a major role in immune function. As a result, people, especially children, who are deficient in vitamin A are at significantly greater risk of death when they contract infectious diseases, especially measles.

Many other micronutrient deficiencies are prevalent in the world, but they all have one thing in common. Be it through increasing disease, impairing cognitive development, or leading to extreme fatigue, all micronutrient deficiencies keep poor people in poverty.

In its extreme, poverty can lead to famine. The economist Amartya Sen points out that famine does not arise simply from a lack of food in an area; it arises from the lack of money to buy food (Sen, 1999). When commodities are fairly easily distributed (as is true in the case of food, in contrast to, say, railroad lines), markets are very good at responding to need. So, if there is a crop failure, food can travel quickly through global supply chains to replenish local supplies. So, famine is typically caused by a local economic shock rather than an actual shortage of food. This shock can certainly take the form of crop failure, but flooding or simple recession are common causes as well. This shock results in the inability to purchase food (because income is low, food prices are high, or both). The best, more sustainable treatment is not food aid but jobs. When there are no jobs, people die of hunger, even when there is food available.

Two conditions are typically seen in extreme hunger or famine. One is **protein energy malnutrition,** in which the body can no longer make the proteins it needs to help regulate electrolytes in the blood. As a result, water

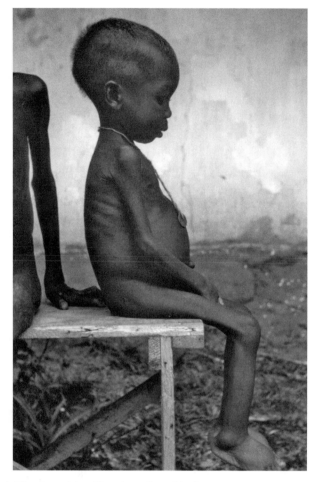

Figure 9.2. A Nigerian girl suffers from kwashiorkor.

Source: PHIL, CDC/Dr. Lyle Conrad. Available online at http://phil.cdc.gov/PHIL
_Images/20050210/efb926ea658c4cd58c629d5c712c01cd/6901.tif.

leaks from blood vessels into body cavities. This results in kwashiorkor, the paradoxically bloated belly seen in malnourished children who aren't getting enough protein (see figure 9.2). (Rarely do aid organizations show the adults on television, but people of all ages are subject to this condition.)

The other form of severe malnutrition is **wasting,** or **marasmus.** In this condition, the body begins to break down muscles once it has depleted the body's fat reserve. This leads to an emaciated appearance (see figure 9.3). Both conditions overlap and both occur over prolonged periods of less-

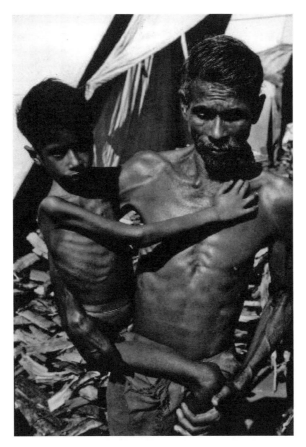

Figure 9.3. In India, a father and child suffering from marasmus.

Source: PHIL, CDC/Don Eddins. Available online at http://phil.cdc.gov/phil/details .asp?pid=1702.

than-sustainable caloric intake. (This is about 1,800 calories per day for a seventy-kilogram person.)

Like vitamin A deficiency, hunger and starvation increase one's susceptibility to infectious disease. Energy is needed to fight off disease, and those who have less caloric intake are much more likely to succumb to infectious disease. Of course, poverty itself places people at greater risk of exposure to infectious disease. The poor often live in crowded housing, usually have no access to clean water or vaccines, and commonly lack basic toilets, often resorting to defecating on the ground.

Infectious diseases, in turn, can contribute to micronutrient deficiencies. Hookworm, for instance, is probably the leading cause of iron deficiency

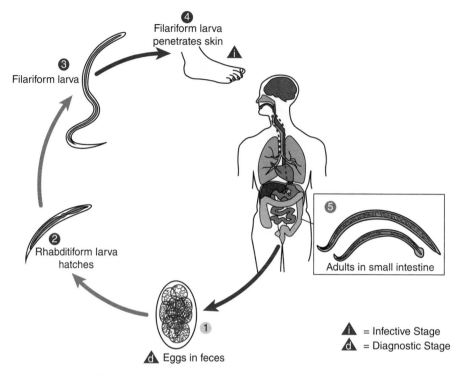

Figure 9.4. The life cycle of the hookworm parasite.

Source: CDC. Available online at www.dpd.cdc.gov/dpdx/images/ParasiteImages/
G-L/Hookworm/Hookworm_LifeCycle.gif.

anemia worldwide (see figure 9.4). Hookworm is one of many intestinal parasites that live in soil contaminated by human feces. When a person walks
outside barefoot to do his or her business, the worm's larvae burrow into the
skin on the foot. From there, they pass into the circulation, finding their way
into the lungs, where they mature. Once enough larvae enter the lungs, one
develops a cough. Thus, the worms are coughed up, swallowed, and enter into
the intestinal tract, where the life cycle is completed. While there, they latch
onto the intestine, causing internal bleeding and, ultimately, the loss of iron
through the loss of blood.

In these cases, policy solutions might include shoes to prevent the spread
of hookworm, new diet pyramids (or dinner plates) and food aid, iodized salt,
and other specific remedies, but none of these policy solutions would address
the root causes of health risks or address them in sustainable ways. Intermedi-
ary policy solutions might include better sanitation systems, school lunches,

and other types of infrastructure that help a larger number of people to prevent disease.

Pathways Between Poverty and Health

Of course, extreme poverty is linked to many health risks besides malnutrition and infectious disease. No money for medical care, poor housing, unsafe jobs, dangerous transit, and crime are a few of the dangers that poor people in poor countries face. Wealthy people in poor countries can avoid these problems by purchasing safe housing, medical care, and so on. In many wealthy countries, the poor are provided with these goods by the government.

But these are obvious problems that poor people in underresourced countries face. Let us take a deeper look at education, and explore why not being able to afford school might pose major health risks. Poor countries rarely offer adequate schooling. When they do attend school, hungry children with iron deficiency anemia do not learn much. Still, education is critically important for breaking the cycle of poverty. Education not only increases future earnings and survival but, as mentioned previously, also reduces female fertility (Browne & Barrett, 1991; Subbarao & Raney, 1995). Researchers hypothesize that this is because educated women have greater access to and knowledge of family planning and contraception, that they have greater decision-making power within the household (regarding the allocation of budgets, for example), and that they have more access to jobs that can raise household incomes.

This higher income, in turn, also means that their children are more likely to receive adequate nutrition, become educated themselves, and survive childhood. Higher child survival rates, in turn, change the household calculus. Women who expect all of their children to survive and thrive usually have fewer children because they know that their few children will be able to care for them in their old age. Thus, education is one of the key components of breaking the chain of poverty and building instead a virtuous cycle. Without adequate schools, poor people are further embedded in their social and economic circumstances. Poor girls are often the last in the family to get fed, the last to receive medical care, and the last to be enrolled in school. Thus, financial limitations have huge implications for gender inequalities in health.

Because education in childhood can break the chain of poverty in adulthood, education opportunities probably play a large role in explaining why very small changes in a poor nation's per capita income lead to very large increases in life expectancy in poor countries.

Education is important over the long run, but hunger and malnutrition are probably still the most important reasons for why poverty predicts poor health. After all, good schools take a generation to work.

Sometimes, halfway measures go a long way. In Thailand, for instance, the government only bothers to regulate the purity of ice—tap water remains usually unfit for consumption. Nevertheless, rates of infectious disease are relatively low because most families know to drink from wells or to order home delivery of clean water. If China, Chile, and Kerala had similar policy contexts, we might expect China (with a GDP per capita of just over US$3,744 in 2009) and Chile (US$9,644) to greatly outstrip Kerala (US$839 in 2008) in terms of eradicating poverty and promoting life expectancy and health outcomes. But as previous chapters have suggested, Kerala has managed to have lower poverty levels and better health than other places with similar levels of GDP per capita. That is, Kerala's policies blunt the effects of low average income on poverty and health.

POVERTY IN LESS-DEVELOPED NATIONS

Recall that we opened the chapter this way:

> Poverty is without a doubt a leading global killer. In low-income nations, it is the root cause of hunger and a major contributor to the global burden of infectious disease, crime, unsafe housing, and a large number of other "deadly deprivations" that bring lives to an untimely end . . .

But, we could have started the chapter this way:

> Poor governance is without a doubt a leading global killer. It leads to weak educational opportunities, lousy job opportunities (if any), and massively inadequate government safety net programs, leading to high rates of poverty. In its extreme, it means poor sanitation, lack of basic vaccination provisions, and unclean water, leading to infectious disease. The high levels of poverty in poorly governed nations result in high rates of infectious disease, crime, unsafe housing, and a host of other things that bring lives to an untimely end.

Dovetailing with chapters 6 and 7, then, poverty can be seen as a completely preventable social condition, one dynamically engaged with a country's governance and political economy. It is not necessarily the ultimate root cause of loss of life. In fact, we could have told a story about how inadequate education leads to poverty or, if we wished, how inadequate international aid is the problem. These phenomena are so irrevocably intertwined that it is difficult to assign a hierarchy of causalities. Whatever the story, the poverty-related policies and institutions in place within a country make the difference between life and death. The poor are more likely to get sick, but only if they are left to fend on their own.

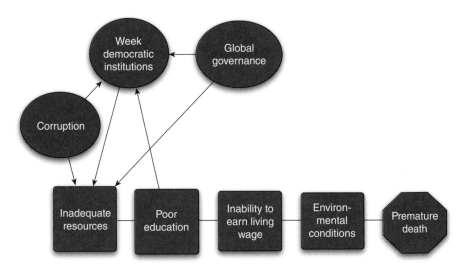

Figure 9.5. A diagram outlining the potential connections between poverty and health. We see that inadequate resources are linked to poor education, low wages, and poor environmental conditions (boxes). However, these factors are in turn caused by a confluence of poor governance and historic circumstances (among other factors).

This brings us to **upstream causes of disease** and **downstream causes of disease.** That is, if we see disease as being like a river, then different sources contribute to the health of the water stream as it flows along toward the sea of death. Suppose that, at the end of the river, we encounter death due to malaria. Along the way, we see that a lack of access to malaria medicines because of poor health care delivery services was a problem. Mosquitoes are the vector for malaria transmission (see chapter 4), and nations that do a poor job of controlling mosquito populations tend to produce this upstream cause of disease. Poverty certainly contributed because areas with wealthier folks are more likely to be sprayed and wealthier households are more likely to have purchased mosquito nets. So, poverty might be thought of as further "upstream" than medical care. At the source, we could argue that bad policies started the flow of disease—vector control is not terribly expensive, especially in countries where the human labor costs of draining stagnant water sources are low. Or maybe corruption is the cause of bad policies. Or maybe a long history of colonialism led to the corruption, which led to the poor policies.

In figure 9.5, we see a very incomplete but illustrative picture of how a weak government contributes to factors such as corruption and otherwise limits the resources made available for social goods such as schools. With few educational opportunities, people cannot develop the skills needed to open stores, invent things, or otherwise meaningfully contribute to the local or global economy. This means that there are fewer jobs for everyone and the jobs that are around are lousy. Without cash, it becomes difficult to access clean water, safe housing, or basic technologies such as vaccines or mosquito nets. Worse, without adequate education, people might not even understand that these basic things are even needed for survival.

From this, it should be clear that poverty is a side effect of weak or poor sets of policies and institutions. Appropriate remedies can come in the form of wisely designed and implemented global aid, improved governance, or coordinated grassroots activities, that improve local conditions. These remedies are not mutually exclusive, but they must always be systemic. One-off, small-scale, or pilot projects will not do. All of this should reinforce the idea that economic development alone (one good way of reducing poverty) might not be the best way to improve measures of human development that are more important, such as health. (In the end, yes, health is more important than wealth. Ask any dead wealthy person.)

In chapters 4 and 7, we saw how global aid policies might help or hinder a nation's economic or social development by either strengthening infrastructure or weakening institutions. Such larger debates are unlikely to be solved in the near future. Many interesting local proposals, though, do hold promise for strengthening policies that will help make poverty look more like it does in Sweden than in Angola.

From these examples, we draw several conclusions. First, poverty means very different things in different development contexts. Second, poverty—whether measured internationally or within countries—usually but not always means higher premature mortality. Third, in places where poor people thrive, protective public health and social policies are usually well established.

Therefore, the poverty-health relationship is only really useful to talk about within a given local context. Poor people in wealthier countries may benefit most from entitlements, such as improved schools, redistributive policies, and universal health care. When we talk about policies that reduce poverty in the name of "global public health," though, we are usually talking about policies concerning those folks earning less than US$2 per day who are living in countries on the low end of the GDP scale. For meeting this definition of poverty, the appropriate intervention is sometimes clean water, vaccinations, and health knowledge. For others, agricultural training and fertilizer may be just as important or more important. Some medical interventions can radically alter people's lives at very little cost, such as obstetric fistula repair or maternal health care.

OBSTETRIC FISTULA REPAIR AND THE HEALTH OF THE POOR

When women go into labor, the baby is sometimes unable to pass through the vagina, a process called **obstructed labor**. As a result, the baby's head presses against the wall of the vagina for a long time, causing a hole to form. This hole, called an **obstetric fistula,** can open up into the rectum, causing feces to be released through the vagina. (Technically, a fistula is just a connection between two organs.) The result is that the baby's father often abandons the mother. The mother is often socially excluded because of the smell and incapacity associated with the fistula. The good news is that a fistula is very easy to repair surgically. In many countries, providers with as little as a few years of primary school education are trained in fistula repair. Aid agencies focusing on fistula repair are present in most of the least-developed nations, but funding is often inadequate.

Countries That Grow Too Much

For wealthier countries, life expectancy really depends more on basic lifesaving regulations than fancy technological robots in the hospital. Countries that have good schools, stringent workplace safety requirements, income protection programs, a high quality of life, and strong medical systems will have a higher life expectancy. But not all wealthy countries choose to invest in such things.

Sometimes, even when they do come up with the cash, countries make poor investments. In the United States, for instance, school funding is based mostly on property taxes. As a result, schools in localities with low housing values (also known as poor neighborhoods) tend to be vastly underfunded. In the United States, there are reports of schools with no working toilets, students who have to wait for hours to pass through metal detectors, and classrooms that are so overcrowded there are not enough desks for all the students or room in the cafeteria to eat. In one school in the Bronx, lunch begins at 9:40 and passes in half-hour shifts throughout the day until 3 PM, because the small cafeteria cannot accommodate all of the students. These examples contrast with virtually gilded schools in wealthier neighborhoods, where teachers include some PhDs giving lessons in more intimate settings.

Recall from chapter 3 that primary and secondary education play a much larger role in population health than does health insurance. Add to that the effects of antipollution regulations, traffic safety measures, and social safety net programs and we are possibly accounting for the huge gulf in life expectancy between the United States and Sweden.

POVERTY AND HEALTH AMONG WEALTHY NATIONS

The health effects of poverty look different in wealthy nations. As we discussed in chapter 5, factors such as education can be thought of as the nonmedical determinants of health. Variations in life expectancy between nations are often attributed to factors such as demographic diversity, a high prevalence of behavioral risk factors, a lack of a social safety net, violence, or a car culture.

We bring this up again here because they are also thought to explain **health disparities** by income or race in wealthy nations. That is, although we think of dirty drinking water as a major nonmedical determinant of health in the least-developed countries, we tend to think of much more subtle policies, such as **income redistribution,** as nonmedical determinants in wealthy nations.

WHITHER INCOME REDISTRIBUTION?

Income redistribution means that the government transfers resources from wealthier citizens to less wealthy ones. In chapter 6, we mentioned progressive taxation as one form of income redistribution. For example, in Sweden, at the time of press, the wealthiest citizens paid up to 65 percent of their income in taxes, and these tax dollars are then used to pay for things such as universal health care and schooling. Because the poorest members of society do not have to pay taxes at all, the wealthy are effectively paying all of the costs of health care and schooling for the poor. In the United States, redistributive programs work both ways. For instance, homeowners (like one of your authors) get to deduct the interest they pay on the loan for their primary home. This money to buy a home comes from everyone paying taxes, including the poor. So, in the United States, the poor are effectively buying housing for the rich. Given that there is no universal health care in the United States and the schools for the poor are not great, poor redistributive policies may explain why the poor are so much healthier in Sweden than in the United States, the difference in life expectancy being about ten years in the United States but just a few years in Sweden (Muennig et al., 2005).

So, how is it that a nation's redistributive policies might have such a large impact on the health of the poor? The idea is something like this: one's inability to access social goods, such as quality schools or universal health care, can translate into a wide variety of social deprivations over the course of an individual's life. These deprivations can, in turn, determine one's health and longevity. For instance, those without quality schooling may be unable to get a good job or earn a living wage. These deprivations not only lead to lower access to lifesaving resources, such as health insurance, but also to psychological stress, a breakdown in social ties, and disruptions in social capital (one's connections with others, as discussed in chapter 2).

Psychosocial factors, in turn, are thought to cause wear and tear on the body, leading to premature mortality. These material and psychosocial deprivations suffered by disadvantaged groups appear to be major contributors to health disparities in the United States.

GOING PSYCHOSOCIAL

The word *psychosocial* is a combination of *psychological* and *social.* These two concepts are mushed into a compound word in health because they are very difficult to tease apart in the real world. For instance, our friends (the social part) give us psychological support. We have talked about social capital being important for health. Psychological stress may also matter. For instance, biological measures of cell aging show that very stressed people have white blood cells that indicate that they are biologically ten years older than those with less stress (Epel et al., 2004). When a group of people is randomly infected with the cold virus or given saline, those who have very high levels of stress are much more likely to catch a cold than those with low levels of stress (Cohen, Tyrrell, & Smith, 1991). What does all of this have to do with poverty? Those who live in crappy housing, live in a high-crime neighborhood, or work two jobs to support themselves tend to have a higher-stress life than those who do not.

In theory, if access to a social good (e.g., health insurance, a park, or high-quality housing) is good for one's health, then providing more of that good in low-income or minority communities should have the effect of reducing health disparities (Adler & Ostrove, 1999; Levin & Belfield, 2007; Muennig et al., 2009; Woolf, Johnson, Phillips, & Philipsen, 2007). Some researchers have suggested that it would be much more cost-effective to reduce health disparities by reducing disparities in access to social goods than improving access to medical care (Schoeni, House, Kaplan, & Pollack, 2008; Woolf et al., 2007).

However, we must be very careful when we speak of the nonmedical determinants of health as major factors accounting for variation in life expectancy *between* nations. Although many researchers believe that they are of major importance—and many studies suggest that they are—they are not proven as such. This is because it is very expensive to conduct randomized trials of housing, neighborhood characteristics, schooling, or other **social determinants of health.** That is not to say that this has not been tried, but when it has the evidence is not conclusive (Attanasio, Meghir, & Schady, 2010; Lagarde, Haines, & Palmer, 2009; Leventhal & Brooks-Gunn, 2003; Muennig, Johnson, & Wilde, 2011; Muennig et al., 2009; Ozer, Fernald, Manley, & Gertler, 2009; Wilde, Finn, Johnson, & Muennig, 2011). Many more studies are needed to sort out this story. In the meantime, we can only go by less-definitive study techniques and common sense.

WHY ARE RANDOMIZED TRIALS SO IMPORTANT?

There have been thousands of studies suggesting that families or individuals with low income have poor health and a lower life expectancy than people with higher income. But correlation does not mean causation. If people become sick in the United States, for instance, they are likely to incur huge medical bills and may lose their job. Therefore, when we go back and see that low-income people are very sick, we do not know whether they are sick because of their income or whether their income is low because they are sick. Thus, the real problem may be a lack of adequate disability and health insurance to protect income.

If we could randomly assign families to different levels of income, we could be sure that any of the changes in health we observe years down the line are due to changes in income itself.

The effects of social factors on health have been and can be studied in a lot of different ways. Quantitative analyses try to establish patterns on the size of effects (and, ideally, causal connections) usually using large amounts of survey data collected over time. Qualitative analyses explore the logical pathways of how and why something happens using extensive, personalized interviews with smaller numbers of participants. The methods employed in quantitative analyses range from those with fairly weak power of inference (correlations) to those with fairly strong power of inference (randomized controlled trials). For example, quantitative studies often attempt to do the following:

- *Examine variations in life expectancy across nations.* Such studies generally find that education, particularly female education, is one of the most important determinants of life expectancy (Browne & Barrett, 1991; Subbarao & Raney, 1995). Social programs also seem to be important. Of course, this is a very messy way of digging up the social determinants of disease. For instance, Sweden nearly always comes out close to the top of health, social, and economic indicators, probably in part because it has outstanding social programs. But some researchers claim that it takes a small, socially cohesive, compassionate society to enact and effectively operate such social programs. This social capital (see chapter 2) could be the actual "determinant" of health. That is, we cannot tell whether welfare programs are good for people's health or whether people who are likely to vote for welfare programs are healthier than those who do not. Moreover, many Asian countries with high life expectancy, such as Singapore, might have among the best schools in the world, but they are hardly shining examples of Scandinavian-style social democracy. (One alternative explanation is that Singapore, Hong Kong, and Macao, three of the world leaders in life expectancy, are also full of immigrants, who tend to be healthier than native-born people.) Researchers can attempt to qualitatively analyze all of these quantitative data to come up with some hypotheses, but in the end it is difficult to prove anything. There is always an alternative explanation unless randomized trials occur or other causal models are used.

- *Look at which factors are responsible for the most disease within a given society.* The United States serves as a great case study because the health data are high quality and because life expectancy is so bad. One burden of disease analysis found that the wide spread of income in the United States was responsible for most life years and health lost, followed by smoking, dropping out of high school, racial inequality, alcohol consumption, and the high numbers of uninsured (Muennig et al., 2010). This list is, by necessity, highly incomplete. Other studies that looked at more traditional risk factors have also found that toxic exposures and transit policy were very important (Mokdad, Marks, Stroup, & Gerberding, 2004; Tengs et al., 1995).

- *Exploit the fact that international life expectancies tend to change over time.* For instance, the United States was once one of the top performers in terms of life expectancy, but it has consistently fallen in rank since the 1970s. This allows one to see how factors such as obesity, smoking, violence, traffic accidents, and cultural diversity change along with the decline in life expectancy relative to other industrialized nations.

- *Use naturally occurring changes in policy as experiments.* One study looked way back at compulsory schooling laws to see what effect education might have had on health in the United States. This study was repeated in many other nations. These teams of researchers found that compulsory schooling laws increase longevity and income and decrease teenage birthrates by increasing the time that people spend in school (Black, Devereux, & Salvanes, 2008; Lleras-Muney, 2005). Casino earnings on one Native American reservation in the United States were found to have mixed but generally positive effects on mental illness and substance abuse (Costello, Erkanli, Copeland, & Angold, 2010). Of course, people who earn their money could have very different health outcomes than those who have it handed to them (either by their parents, by a welfare state, or by the reservation). This is one of many problems with randomized trials—you never know whether what you are studying will generalize to social policies. A much better way of exploring these factors would be to randomize children to families of differing wealth. One clever researcher figured out how to mimic just a study. This involved looking at children who were adopted into families of different wealth very close to birth. Although this study did not follow the children until they were old enough to have later-life health problems, the family environment had huge effects on drinking behavior (Sacerdote, 2004).

- *Use randomized controlled trials.* There are very few randomized trials of the effects of income, education, or employment on health. Of course, scientists cannot just randomly keep kids out of school, but they can study the health effects of programs that might improve educational outcomes. The problem with such studies is that you never know whether you are actually studying the long-term effect of improving education on health or the long-term effect of the program that improved health in the first place. For example, two such studies tried to improve parenting while providing poor children with inten- sive preschooling. Studies of these programs showed that children randomized to intensive preschooling versus no school or community-based schooling did much better in school and were healthier than those in the control group as adults (Muennig et al., 2011; Muennig, Schweinhart, Montie, & Neidell, 2009). However, another study of reduced class size versus regular class size found that kids randomized to small class sizes did much better in school but had higher mortality as adults (Muennig, Johnson, & Wilde, 2011). Studies of welfare supplements and welfare reform have had mixed effects (Elesh & Lefcowitz, 1977; Kehrer & Wolin, 1979). One standard welfare program was found to reduce anemia and improve cognition among children in Ecuador, and two programs in the United States to end welfare were associated with higher mortality (though these did not reach statistical significance). Conditional cash transfer programs, which we talk about a lot in chapter 12, are programs that provide cash to families in exchange for meeting basic requirements, such as making sure that their children are vaccinated and go to school. These programs have been quite successful in improving health in some places (Lagarde, Haines, & Palmer, 2009).

Although there is not much of a relationship between per capita GDP and longevity when comparing one wealthy country to the next, the same cannot be true of the folks that live *within* these nations. Where researchers have looked, they have always found a wealth-health gradient, the sort we first described in chapter 2. That is to say that the poor tend to have the shortest lives, the middle class longer lives, and the wealthy have the longest lives. The wealth gradient holds some surprises. One is that people who are pretty well off—people who have nice houses, health insurance, and so on—tend to have shorter lives than those of higher social status. Once again, it is important to make the distinction between the income-longevity connection *between* countries and the income-longevity connection *within* countries.

In the United States, for example, health disparities in life expectancy have been increasing, alongside rising income inequalities. Although most public health researchers talk about the effect of low income on health, some researchers wonder about reverse causality—whether sick people become poor because they cannot earn lots of money (Deaton, 2002). Although the latter trend certainly exists, longitudinal studies suggest that the effects of income on health are quite significant. The remaining puzzles, then, lie in how and why income shapes health in such pronounced ways in the United States when there is plenty of food to go around, a public education system, advanced medical technologies, and all of the accouterments befitting the world's only remaining (albeit precariously so) superpower.

For instance, health insurance status highlights many of the disparities in the United States today, especially between those who have some sense of security in life and those who are an accident away from bankruptcy or fore-closure. It does not help, however, to adequately account for the massive health disparities according to race, income, and region in the United States. For example, the gap between the life expectancy of African American males in high-risk urban areas and Asian American females was 20.7 years in 2001. Asian American women in the Northeast live to an average of ninety-one years, whereas Native American men in the Dakotas live to an average of fifty-eight years—a thirty-three-year gap in life expectancy. These differences largely persist after holding constant health insurance status and excluding HIV and homicide. Further, the ten leading risk factors (smoking, obesity, high blood pressure, illicit drug use, unsafe sex, etc.) cumulatively account for only 30 percent of disease among men (Murray et al., 2006). What else is going on?

The Role of Inequality?

Although the wealth-health gradient exists as a correlation, researchers are still searching for definitive causal mechanisms to explain why, exactly, wealthier folks within a society tend to live longer, and some have turned to income inequality as an explanation. High-income white Americans tend to live a lot longer than low-income African Americans, but on average, American whites still live *less healthy* lives than low-income English whites (Banks, Marmot, Oldfield, & Smith, 2006). Researchers such as Richard Wilkinson and Michael Marmot argue that more just societies overall bring more social cohesion, solidarity, better governance, interdependence, and, in the end, lower stress, more happiness, and longer, healthier lives.

This problem of income inequality is currently most striking in high-income, industrialized countries because we know that they can do better. It also applies to middle-income countries such as China, Chile, and India, however. All three of this book's case study countries suffer from high-income inequalities—in the cases of China and India, precipitously dangerous levels of inequality alongside their explosive levels of growth since the 1990s.

At the very least, large income inequalities—especially in contexts where GDP growth often surpasses an astounding 5 percent a year, as it does in India and China—suggest that the country's middle class is smaller than it should be, that their tax-based coffers may be in jeopardy, and that there may be political instability if the government cannot contain the poor masses' resentment or improve their living conditions. By some estimates, there are over two hundred mass street protests per day in China that go unreported in world news. Mass inequalities and divisions within the national population also render it incredibly difficult for governments to prioritize public services and public spending well because *what* they spend money on depends so greatly on *who* the dominant political actors are.

Dramatic income inequalities might also matter in more subtle ways. Researchers focused on the relationship between income and health are still disentangling just how income inequality might shape health (Marmot & Wilkinson, 1999; Wilkinson & Pickett, 2009). Is it via more education and better jobs and wages? Is it via social status? In diverse societies, income inequalities are also often marked by region (think of northern versus southern Italy or urban versus rural China), race or tribe, or other factors. Are income inequalities somehow a reflection of the people? Whereas few public health researchers would forward a "culture of poverty" thesis in which it is the poor people's fault that they are poor, the real-life mechanisms through which poverty and inequality shape health are quite complex. Wilkinson and Pritchett (2009), for example, argue that societies with greater inequality tend to have less social capital and social cohesion, be associated with poorer mental health and higher illicit drug-use population rates, and have greater levels of obesity (in industrialized nations), teenage births, violence, and imprisonment. Are these correlations causal and, if so, in what direction? After all, societies where citizens cannot relate to their neighbors (let alone folks on the other side of the tracks, town, or country) are also less likely to share resources with them, and this perpetuates inequality. The evidence on the primacy of inequality in some policy fields is spotty at best; in others, such as physical violence and domestic abuse, it is a little stronger.

For the purposes of this book and this chapter, the problem of inequality makes the field of health economics even trickier in three crucial ways. First, economic analyses tend to focus on individuals, firms, or geographical units (states, provinces, countries) as interchangeable units of analysis, and the whole point of inequality is that these units are not interchangeable. Even if we discover a health intervention that is cost-effective for a specific person or an entire population, not everyone will receive that intervention.

Second, in terms of policy implications, paying serious heed to issues of inequality may require policy makers to jump-start more fundamental, but diffuse initiatives such as restructuring the tax-financing formulas for public education funding rather than well-defined pet pilot projects with specific missions, outcomes, and ribbon-cutting photo ops.

Finally, redistributive policies such as progressive taxation incur what economists call *dead weight loss*—a loss of economic efficiency that occurs when policy makers use tools such as taxes, minimum prices, or subsidies, and the market is not at the "equilibrium" it would achieve in a "free market." Again, policy makers must weigh this inefficiency against other naturally occurring inefficiencies, such as externalities and spillover effects, as well as competing policy priorities and political considerations. The Nordic countries have pulled this magic off by offering a mix of low corporate tax rates, help for companies to meet regulatory targets, and less paperwork for business while still investing heavily in education, health, and other welfare programs. One secret to their success has been a remarkable lack of partisanship. Instead, they seem to shoot for what works, whether the idea comes from the political right or the political left.

Whereas poverty remains the primary culprit for health policy puzzles in low-income nations, and inequality one of the main ones in high-income nations, middle-income nations must simultaneously grapple with both, in equal measures.

THE COMPLEXITIES OF POVERTY

Between countries, *poverty* has little substantive meaning. Whether in the United States or the Congo, poor people have a shortened life expectancy. But poor people in the Congo may need more caloric intake for survival whereas very poor people in the United States may need less caloric intake.

Hunger and infectious disease probably explain why the poorest countries generally have a much lower life expectancy than wealthier countries. Evidence that the poorest people in some poor countries enjoy high life expectancies suggests that even poor countries can attain high life expectancies with good governance and appropriate public health and social policies in place. Although many international agencies identify poverty as the most important underlying health problem, poverty is often a proxy measure for failing governance and poor social policies.

SUMMARY

Poverty has been called the "spider in the web of causation," meaning that it is the root problem of all of our social and health ills. If so, there are a number of ways that one might improve health by reducing poverty, such as progressive taxation. But poverty can't explain why some rich people smoke or abuse their children. It also can't explain why some of the wealthiest nations on earth do not make the top-twenty lists in terms of life expectancy. We believe that the "root cause" of disease and disability is probably related more to the ability of a nation's government to enact rational, cost-effective policies that improve education and health delivery systems. Programs that purely redistribute income may be helpful, but other forms of social investment are important, too. Finally, although it is not our business to worry about such things, all of these social expenditures need to be done in a rational way that does not get in the way of other important human capabilities. This includes having a robust economy in a nation that is not weighed down with debt. Although small, the Nordic countries have shown that a pro-business, pro-health policy environment is possible.

KEY TERMS

absolute poverty line

basket of goods

downstream causes of
   disease

extreme poverty

health disparities

income redistribution

marasmus

material
   deprivations

means-tested
   governmental
   benefits

micronutrients

obstetric fistula

obstructed labor

protein energy
   malnutrition

psychosocial factors

relative poverty line

social determinants of
   health

social exclusion

standard of poverty

universal benefits

upstream causes of
   disease

wasting

wealth-health gradient

DISCUSSION QUESTIONS

1. Why is poverty considered the main underlying cause of disease and ill health? Do you agree? Why?

2. How does poverty tend to affect the health of individuals in low-income countries? In high-income countries?

3. What sorts of policies might policy makers advocate to address poverty and its health consequences in low- and middle-income countries?

4. Why might the wealth-health gradient exist within countries but not between them? Do you think poverty and income inequality play a role in health inequalities within a country? Why or why not?

FURTHER READING

Hans Rosling: New insights on poverty. (2007, March). TEDTalks. Available online at www.ted.com/talks/hans_rosling_reveals_new_insights_on_poverty.html

The rise of the $1 a day statistic. (2012, March). BBC. Available online at www.bbc.co.uk/news/magazine-17312819

REFERENCES

Adler, N. E., & Ostrove, J. M. (1999). Socioeconomic status and health: What we know and what we don't. *Annals of the New York Academy of Sciences, 896,* 3–15.

Attanasio, O., Meghir, C., & Schady, N. (2010). Mexico's conditional cash transfer programme. *Lancet, 375*(9719), 980.

Banks, J., Marmot, M., Oldfield, Z., & Smith, J. (2006). Disease and disadvantage in the United States and in England. *JAMA, 295*(17), 2037–2045.

Bearak, B. (2003, July 13). Why people still starve. *New York Times.*

Black, S. E., Devereux, P. J., & Salvanes, K. G. (2008). Staying in the classroom and out of the maternity ward? The effect of compulsory schooling laws on teenage births. *The Economic Journal, 118*(530), 1025–1054.

Browne, A. W., & Barrett, H. R. (1991). Female education in sub-Saharan Africa: The key to development? *Comparative Education, 27*(3), 275–285.

Cohen, S., Tyrrell, D. A., & Smith, A. P. (1991). Psychological stress and susceptibility to the common cold. *New England Journal of Medicine, 325*(9), 606–612.

Costello, E. J., Erkanli, A., Copeland, W., & Angold, A. (2010). Association of family income supplements in adolescence with development of psychiatric and substance use disorders in adulthood among an American Indian population. *JAMA, 303*(19), 1954.

Deaton, A. (2002). Policy implications of the gradient of health and wealth. *Health Affairs, 21*(2), 13–30.

Elesh, D., & Lefcowitz, M. J. (1977). The effects of the New Jersey-Pennsylvania negative income tax experiment on health and health care utilization. *Journal of Health and Social Behavior, 18*(4), 391–405.

Epel, E. S., Blackburn, E. H., Lin, J., Dhabhar, F. S., Adler, N. E., Morrow, J. D., et al. (2004). Accelerated telomere shortening in response to life stress. *Proceedings of the National Academy of Science of the United States of America, 101*, 17312–17315.

Kehrer, B. H., & Wolin, C. M. (1979). Impact of income maintenance on low birth weight: Evidence from the Gary experiment. *Journal of Human Resources, 14*(4), 434–462.

Lagarde, M., Haines, A., & Palmer, N. (2009). The impact of conditional cash transfers on health outcomes and use of health services in low and middle income countries. *Cochrane Database of Systematic Reviews, 4*, ref. no. CD008137.

Leventhal, T., & Brooks-Gunn, J. (2003). Moving to opportunity: An experimental study of neighborhood effects on mental health. *American Journal of Public Health, 93*(9), 1576–1582.

Levin, H., & Belfield, C. (2007). *The price we pay: Economic and social consequences of inadequate education.* Washington, DC: Brookings Institution Press.

Lleras-Muney, A. (2005). The relationship between education and adult mortality in the United States. *Review of Economic Studies, 72*(1), 189–221.

Marmot, M., & Wilkinson, R. (1999). *Social determinants of health.* London: Oxford University Press.

Mokdad, A. H., Marks, J. S., Stroup, D. F., & Gerberding, J. L. (2004). Actual causes of death in the United States, 2000. *JAMA, 291*(10), 1238–1245.

Muennig, P., Fiscella, K., Tancredi, D., & Franks, P. (2010). The relative health burden of selected social and behavioral risk factors in the United States: Implications for policy. *American Journal of Public Health, 100*(9), 1758–1764.

Muennig, P., Franks, P., Jia, H., Lubetkin, E., & Gold, M. R. (2005). The income-associated burden of disease in the United States. *Social Science Medicine, 61*(9), 2018–2026.

Muennig, P., Johnson G., & Wilde, E. T. (2011). The effect of small class sizes on mortality through age 29 years: Evidence from a multicenter randomized controlled trial. *American Journal of Epidemiology.* doi: 10.1093/aje/kwr011.

Muennig, P., Robertson, D., Johnson, G., Campbell, F., Pungello, E. P., & Neidell, M. (2011). The effect of an early education program on adult health: The Carolina Abecedarian Project randomized controlled trial. *American Journal of Public Health, 101*(3), 512–516.

Muennig, P., Schweinhart, L., Montie, J., & Neidell, M. (2009). Effects of a prekindergarten educational intervention on adult health: 37-year follow-up results of a randomized controlled trial. *American Journal of Public Health, 99*(8), 1431–1437.

Murray, C., Kulkarni, S., Michaud, C., Tomijima, N., Bulzacchelli, M., Iandiorio, T., et al. (2006). Eight Americas: Investigating mortality disparities across races, counties, and race-counties in the United States. *PLoS Medicine, 3*(9), 1513–1524.

Ozer, E. J., Fernald, L. C., Manley, J. G., & Gertler, P. J. (2009). Effects of a conditional cash transfer program on children's behavior problems. *Pediatrics, 123*(4), e630–e637.

Sacerdote, B. (2004). *What happens when we randomly assign children to families?* National Bureau of Economic Research. Working paper no. 10894.

Schoeni, R. F., House, J. S., Kaplan, G. A., & Pollack, H. (Eds.). (2008). *Making Americans healthier: Social and economic policy as health policy.* New York: Russell Sage Foundation.

Sen, A. (1999). *Development as freedom.* New York: Oxford University Press.

Subbarao, K., & Raney, L. (1995). Social gains from female education: A cross-national study. *Economic Development and Cultural Change, 44*(1), 105–128.

Tengs, T. O., Adams, M. E., Pliskin, J. S., Safran, D. G., Siegel, J. E., Weinstein, M. C., et al. (1995). Five-hundred life-saving interventions and their cost-effectiveness. *Risk Analysis, 15*(3), 369–390.

UN. (2004) *The least developed countries report, 2004.* Available online at http://unctad.org/en/pages/PublicationArchive.aspx?publicationid=132

Wilde, E. T., Finn, J., Johnson, G., & Muennig, P. (2011). The effect of class size in grades K–3 on adult earnings, employment, and disability status: Evidence from a multi-center randomized controlled trial. *Journal of Health Care for the Poor and Underserved, 22*(4), 1424.

Wilkinson, R., & Pickett, K. (2009). *The spirit level: Why greater equality makes societies stronger.* New York: Bloomsbury Press.

Woolf, S. H., Johnson, R. E., Phillips, R. L., Jr., & Philipsen, M. (2007). Giving everyone the health of the educated: An examination of whether social change would save more lives than medical advances. *American Journal of Public Health, 97*(4), 679–683.

World Bank. (2013) Poverty headcount ratio at $1.25 a day. Available online at http://data.worldbank.org/indicator/SI.POV.DDAY

CHAPTER 10

The Physical Environment and Disease

KEY IDEAS

- The field of environmental health concerns not only damage to the natural environment but also some aspects of the built environment.

- Infectious diseases are often easy and relatively inexpensive to treat but remain leading killers in very poor countries.

- To address most infectious disease, a few simple components are needed: (1) basic public health infrastructure, such as latrines and clean water; (2) vaccination programs; (3) eradication programs; and (4) functioning governance structures.

- By addressing infectious disease, it is possible to rapidly move a country through the epidemiologic transition from high mortality to high longevity.

- Chronic diseases can also be addressed with core changes to the environment, such as improvements in city planning and architecture.

When we think of environmental health, many of us tend to envision glowing mounds of fluorescent green waste piling up outside of factories and people walking around with huge tumors. But environmental health is a very broad field, one that extends far beyond the side effects of industrial development. For example, the most important predictors of a long life for poor people include a means of human waste disposal, clean water, adequate housing, and disease vector control. All of these important factors, not all of which are directly correlated with the intersection of built and natural environments, are considered central to environmental health.

245

In this chapter, we focus on the major infectious diseases that rob people of long, healthy, productive lives in countries that have not undergone an epidemiologic transition. We focus on environmental policies that facilitate or hinder the transmission of these diseases, including lack of sanitation and clean water. We then focus on other important environmental conditions and phenomena that shape health: **air pollution, outer-ring development** of major urban areas, and global **climate change.**

INFECTIOUS DISEASE AND DEVELOPMENT

In chapter 3, we outlined the basic burden of disease because of some of the common infectious causes in different development contexts and why their elimination should be prioritized over medical management of chronic diseases. (That reflects medical management as opposed to nonmedical management through policies that promote healthy lifestyles.) We learn that about 25 percent of the world's morbidity and mortality (measured in DALYs) is due to diseases related to undernutrition coupled with poor waste infrastructure.

In most violent conflicts, many more people die of infectious disease than of war wounds, mostly because food becomes scarce and people must huddle together in unsanitary conditions (Burnham, Lafta, Doocy, & Roberts, 2006; Kuzman et al., 1993; Murray, King, Lopez, Tomijima, & Krug, 2002). By destroying basic infrastructure and economic exchange, the two US wars in Iraq cost many more lives than its deposed dictator, Saddam Hussein, would likely have taken in his lifetime (Burnham et al., 2006). This happened despite the fact that every effort was made to minimize civilian casualties in the air and on the ground. This is because functioning rural and urban infrastructure— clean water, functioning food markets, and so forth—are needed to keep people from being exposed to germs. When this basic protective infrastructure is destroyed, people become exposed to infectious agents at the same time that their immune systems are weakened by hunger.

This is a shame, because also in chapter 3, we touched on some of the basic policies needed to reduce the burden of infectious disease and learned that such solutions are quite inexpensive and simple. In this chapter, we focus on what these diseases are and how they are transmitted. We emphasize how infectious diseases interact with the larger social conditions that created them, as in the example of how malnutrition can greatly increase one's risk of death due to infectious disease.

In this section, we focus on diarrhea, intestinal parasites, and malaria as examples of important infectious agents. The other major infectious diseases typically covered in global health textbooks include HIV, tuberculosis, and pneumonia. In this book, pneumonia is covered in the built environment section later in this chapter, and HIV and tuberculosis (two diseases that too often go together) are covered in chapter 11 because they are prevented with changes to the social environment and social institutions.

Diarrhea

If you ultimately decide to work in poor nations, you may find yourself openly discussing your gastrointestinal problems in graphic detail with complete strangers—not just your personal physician or nurses at the local hospital but also new acquaintances you meet over lunch. And no one will stop eating. This is because diarrheal illness is extremely common in countries with inadequate sanitation, water filtration, and food safety. So common, in fact, that it tends to become a part of daily conversation. Human feces are everywhere in poor countries, and even the most careful aid worker will spend many painful hours in the privy.

Diarrhea takes roughly 2.6 million lives a year, with 1.5 million of these occurring in children under five. It is the second-leading cause of death in this age group. These lives can be saved in the short term by keeping the victim hydrated and keeping body salts in balance. This is not always as easy as it sounds; it can be extremely unpleasant to drink salty water when sick, and diarrhea is often accompanied by vomiting in young children.

Diarrhea can be caused by the entire spectrum of pathogenic organisms: bacteria, viruses, and parasites. But no matter what the cause, the vast majority of these cases can be prevented with widespread use of simple pit latrines. When such latrines are not available, people must defecate on the ground. When near waterways, the feces, accompanied by viruses and bacteria, can wash into the water, causing illness or death, downstream.

Another major source of water contamination comes from untreated or incompletely treated sewage systems in towns and cities. In too many cases, sewage flows into nearby waterways, from which people subsequently drink.

In inland regions, human feces are still deliberately used as fertilizer for vegetable crops in some places, placing the crops' end consumers and farmers alike in great danger. Human feces are sometimes fed to livestock, or meat is handled by workers who have not washed their hands. When the animal is butchered, the meat can contain human and animal feces laced with human pathogens. Finally, soap and running water are relatively uncommon near toilets, meaning that anyone who goes on to handle food after using the toilet can potentially spread their intestinal germs to many others.

Prevention and Treatment

As mentioned previously, the most basic preventive measure is the simple pit latrine. But regardless of the level of development, sewage systems of some sort are critical in villages, towns, and cities, even if the sewage is only partially covered and incompletely treated. Although better than nothing, incomplete treatment comes at great risk, especially if the sewage enters waterways. Sometimes, untreated sewage can enter into groundwater (the water extracted using wells and pumps) that people assume is safe.

In many middle-income countries, septic systems are used in rural areas and proper sewage treatment plants are used in towns and cities. But not all of them make these basic investments. You can easily locate the ones that do not make these investments by scanning WHO lists of under-five child mortality rates. Much less common in middle-income countries are food-handling standards in restaurants and the broader food industry. This can also be true of hospitals. The next most basic preventive intervention, then, is hand washing.

Once the illness has taken hold, hydration and salts are the most common and most appropriate treatments for diarrheal illness. Antibiotics are important in cases where the infection is more serious. Some human pathogens, such as the organism that causes typhoid fever, must be treated with antibiotics because they can eventually kill the person who is infected and because some people can carry the infection and spread it to others. One simple policy—pharmacist training—can greatly facilitate the proper management of infectious diseases. Most poor countries have pharmacies, but those who sell drugs often lack some of the most basic elements of training, such as knowing to prescribe antibiotics for diarrhea only when a high fever is present.

It is especially important to become judicial in treating bacterial illnesses such as diarrhea because **drug resistance** can develop when an antibiotic is overused. Drug resistance occurs when large numbers of pathogenic bacteria are exposed to a drug. This leads to the natural selection of only the fittest bacteria for survival. Eventually, those bacteria go on to infect the next person. This is a major problem, particularly for antibiotics, because pharmaceutical companies do not make a good deal of profit from antibiotics, so new drug development is not keeping up with new super strains of bacteria. When penicillin was first developed, it could be used to treat most common bacterial infections. Now, it is only effective against a handful. This issue is addressed in more detail in chapter 11.

TYPHOID MARY

Mary Mallon was a cook who lived in New York City in the late part of the nineteenth and early part of the twentieth centuries. She was a healthy carrier of *Salmonella typhi*, the bacteria that causes typhoid fever, and the first such known person in the United States. Like many healthy carriers, she may have once had the disease and recovered but continued to shed the disease when she went to the bathroom. Although it is not pleasant to think about, people often walk around with fecal material on their hands. When they cook food, it can spread into the food. After a heroic epidemiologic investigation, Mary Mallon was found to be the source of various typhoid fever outbreaks. As hard as the authorities tried to prevent her from being a cook, she continued to evade the authorities. She probably did so in part because discrimination against the Irish was prevalent in her day, and she had a very poor regard for the authorities, including the health official who was pursuing her. As a result, she probably believed that she was not, in fact, a carrier. Ultimately, she infected at least fifty-three people and two of them died. Was it systematic discrimination, callous officials, or blatant disregard for others' well-being that led to the tragedy? We will never know ("Mary Mallon [Typhoid Mary]," 1939).

Intestinal Parasites

More than one-third of the world's population is infected with one or more of the three common **intestinal parasites,** *Ascaris*, hookworm (see figure 10.1), and *Strongyloides* (Mascie-Taylor & Karim, 2003). These three parasites have very similar life cycles (see figure 9.4). They are introduced into soil when a person evacuates on the open ground. They then crawl through the soil, and they can live there for quite a while. People defecate quite frequently, of course, particularly when sick. So, the area around a house—and ultimately throughout an entire village—can have soil that is teeming with these parasites. When people walk around with bare feet, the worm burrows into the skin. It then enters the bloodstream, where it makes its way to the lungs. When the victim coughs and swallows the phlegm, the parasite then enters the digestive system, where it matures and prepares for release back out into the environment.

Ascaris (*Ascaris lumbricoides*) can block the intestines and Strongyloides (*Strongyloides setercoralis*) can cause a massive invasive infection in a person who is immunocompromised. The most important of these three parasites is hookworm (a parasite that comes into bodies via various species), which causes intestinal bleeding. This bleeding leads to anemia by lowering the body's iron reserves. Recall that iron is a critical micronutrient that is also lacking in the diets of many poor people. (See chapter 8 on micronutrient deficiency and health.) The anemia, in turn, causes weakness and difficulty

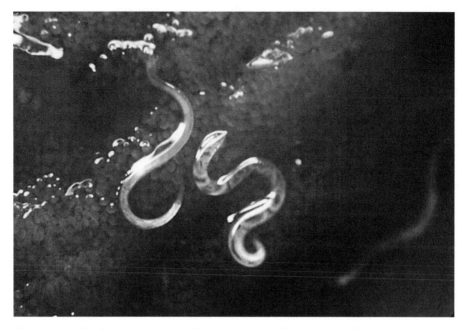

Figure 10.1. Hookworm is one of the most frequently encountered parasitic infections in the world.

Source: Centers for Disease Control and Prevention. Parasite Image Library. Available online at www.dpd.cdc.gov/dpdx/HTML/ImageLibrary/Hookworm_il.htm.

concentrating (Hotez et al., 2004). Because it is difficult for anemic children to learn, anemia produces a devastating effect on academic performance. Of course, poor academic performance in youth will adversely affect that person throughout his or her life.

Adults are also affected. When hookworm infects adults, the weakness arising from anemia reduces one's ability to work productively, so income also drops. This drop in income, in turn, often leads to a vicious downward spiral in which the worm causes anemia, the anemia reduces one's ability to work, and the reduced ability to work worsens the underlying malnutrition.

Prevention and Treatment

As with diarrheal illness, parasitic infections can be treated with medications or prevented altogether with pit latrines or sanitation systems. Parasitic infections can be treated using a safe and effective broad-spectrum medication (albendazole or mebendazole depending on which parasites are dominant in the area). Because the prevalence rate is relatively high and the drug costs are fairly low, this treatment is cost saving even among most immigrants to wealthy countries (Muennig, Pallin, Sell, & Chan, 1999). Providing iron as a dietary supplement and antiparasitic medication can cost as little as US$2 per child. This simple combination therapy greatly increases school participation and academic performance.

PETS OR PEOPLE?

In wealthy countries, the development of new drugs comes as a great monetary cost. But the research and development costs of new drugs can produce large profits, provided these drugs are sold for hundreds or even thousands of dollars for a treatment. Tropical countries tend to have a high prevalence of infectious diseases that are rarely seen in wealthy countries, but they also tend to have small economies. Were companies to develop such drugs, it would not have much of a market. Most of those infected are the very poor—people who earn less than US$1 to $2 per day. As a result, there is no market for drugs to combat these diseases. Any pharmaceutical company that developed a drug to combat **malaria,** leschmaniasis, or intestinal parasites would certainly lose money on the venture (though addressing this precise market-based policy challenge is one of the key drivers of the Bill & Melinda Gates Foundation).

It so happens that animals in developed countries often do contract parasitic infections. Because people in high-income nations tend to invest heavily in their pets' health (and the agricultural industry in the health of livestock), a market for antiparasitic drugs has long existed for animals in wealthy nations. It turns out that the drugs developed to fight parasitic infections in animals also work for people. As a result, we now have a way of treating the billions of people infected with intestinal parasites worldwide (Geary & Thompson, 2003).

MALARIA AND OTHER MOSQUITO-BORNE ILLNESSES

Malaria is a parasite that probably infects roughly 250 million new people a year. About three million of these people die from their infection. Malaria is carried by mosquitoes, which suck blood from mammals. Though many people believe that mosquitoes bite for their own nourishment, it is actually only the females that suck blood, and then only to feed their offspring. (When said that way, who can blame them?) There are many types of mosquitoes, but it is the *Anopheles* genus that transmits the malaria parasite (Wormser & Steffen, 2010). Other mosquitoes do transmit viral diseases, such as dengue fever.

There are four common strains of malaria that cause disease in humans and some are more fatal than others. Part of the parasite's life cycle occurs within red blood cells. When the parasites enter red blood cells, they damage the wall of the cell and explode. (Red blood cell explosions are called *hemolysis* to help prevent people outside the medical field from becoming informed about such things.) This, in turn, causes fever and anemia and can cause joint pain, kidney failure, damage to the eye, and death. The parasites like to conduct their acts of hemato-terrorism at coordinated times during the night, causing the fever to occur in a classic cyclical fashion.

SICKLE CELL ANEMIA AND MALARIA

Humans, similar to all animals, constantly evolve to meet environmental challenges. This helps us ensure that our genes will continue to survive under adverse environmental circumstances. In tropical areas where malaria is prevalent, people with a mutation in their blood hemoglobin, called *HbS,* became partially resistant to the effects of malaria infection (Wellems, Hayton, & Fairhurst, 2009). One-third of all people native to sub-Saharan Africa carry such a gene because their predecessors were more likely to recover from malaria. The mutation works by changing the environment in the red blood cell, reducing malaria's ability to live there and to lyse the cell. This mutation usually occurs on one of two genes that contribute to the coding for hemoglobin in the blood. This mutation has helped people inhabit highly malarious regions by greatly lessening the severity and symptoms associated with malaria. Unfortunately, it is possible to inherit not just one protective HbS gene but two. When this happens, the blood cell can collapse onto itself, forming a rigid sickle shape when the person with **sickle cell anemia** becomes dehydrated or put under stress. An extremely painful crisis ensues because the blood cells cannot pass normally through capillaries. Organ damage can occur. As a result, those with both HbS genes—those who have sickle cell anemia—have greatly shortened life spans (Platt et al., 1994). Americans of sub-Saharan African descent have much higher prevalence rates of sickle cell anemia than other Americans. But HbS pays off overall in survival because not everyone with the gene develops sickle cell anemia (sufferers must inherit one copy from their mother and one from their father for sickle cell anemia to develop).

The mosquito contracts malaria when it bites an infected mammal. When she bites, she spits out a wad of anesthetic saliva so that the victim does not feel the bite, and she then sucks up blood that has the parasite in it (Talman, Domarle, McKenzie, Ariey, & Robert, 2004). The parasite enters into the mosquito and is then transmitted to a new host when the mosquito again needs to feed and spits the parasite back into the new victim. If this sounds disgusting, well, think of all of the other things that a mosquito might spit back inside you. In fact, the mosquito spreads all sorts of nasty viruses this way as well, including dengue fever, Japanese encephalitis, and yellow fever. Fortunately, HIV and hepatitis do not appear to be spread this way.

Prevention and Treatment

Anopheles prefers to bite at dusk and it then continues to do so through the night. This is why mosquito nets for beds are so important for the prevention of malaria. Mosquitoes reproduce in stagnant water, so removal of stagnant water can also help prevent the disease by reducing the number of mosquitoes around to bite people. This can happen naturally when careful planning is set in place during economic development. When the United States built the Panama Canal, it first rid the area of malaria by sending out armies of workers to remove stagnant water from every source it could find. Spraying chemicals on still water is the lazy person's way of reducing mosquito populations. In some areas, however, it remains the only practical way of doing so.

Fortunately, effective treatments also exist, and treating people can not only reduce mortality but also help prevent disease. (By reducing the total pool of infected people and the number of mosquitoes in the environment, it is actually possible to rid an area of malaria.) It is also possible to prevent the disease over the short term (e.g., among aid workers or travelers) using lower doses of oral medications. Unfortunately, many strains of malaria parasites are becoming resistant to the drugs used to prevent or treat malaria. For example, on the Thai-Burma border, there is only one reliable drug to prevent malaria (doxycycline). There are some candidate drugs that could one day be used to prevent malaria (e.g., azithromycin), but it is possible that one day the parasite will become resistant to all known preventive medicines and treatments. **Counterfeit drugs**, which use a fraction of the active ingredients necessary for the drugs to be effective, especially exacerbate the situation. This is unfortunate, because there is little market for antimalarial drugs, and drug resistance threatens to set back the progress that has been made against this organism.

The Policy Implications of Infectious Disease

Infectious diseases take lives and sap economic productivity in the short term and the long term (Sachs & Malaney, 2002). Infectious diseases can kill in the economic prime of one's life. In cold economic calculus, twelve years of government-funded education and parent-funded living costs are lost for every young adult who dies unnecessarily. Thus, not only is human health affected, but a nation's economic development also can be affected.

But also in cold economic calculus, infectious diseases can be a huge economic bonus for wealthy countries. Diseases such as influenza (with the exception of the Spanish flu) and pneumonia tend to kill the very young and very old. These are the two groups that are most expensive for society to sustain. School children require large sums of money to educate, house, and feed while giving little back but a touch of cuteness and love. Likewise, elderly people tend not to contribute via the workforce, but they draw on pension systems and national health systems. As a result, infections tend to reduce the economic burden placed on government safety net systems (*Economist*, 2003).

Of course, no one would advocate killing the young and old in the name of economic progress. Nor would most advocate shutting down our government schools and pension systems. We bring this up once again to reinforce the notion that if the goal of development is to improve well-being, a greater balance between economic development and other forms of human development needs to be achieved. Many textbooks will present litanies of estimates of the economic benefits of eliminating this disease or that (we are guilty of this in the very textbook you are reading), but this should all be taken with a grain of salt. Infectious diseases should be eliminated because they can be eliminated. That this can be done efficiently (i.e., in a very cost-effective manner) is certainly a bonus.

In fact, although considering economic impacts alone can have perverse effects on health (e.g., mass treatment of infectious disease might be cost-effective but can also lead to antibiotic resistance), a cost-effectiveness lens on economic development will not. Over the lifetimes of most students reading this textbook, infectious diseases will drop to low levels in poor nations, and most of the world's disease and disability will instead stem from chronic diseases and accidents. Diabetes and heart disease are major killers worldwide—even in poor countries. We definitely need to tackle these diseases by encouraging healthy communities and healthy lifestyles. There is a growing emphasis in public health on lifelong treatment of these diseases with medications. If this comes at the expense of aggressive infectious disease treatment, many people will die unnecessarily in the prime of their lives. This is because, although the prevention, treatment, and even elimination of many infectious diseases is available given enough resources and political will, chronic diseases are much more difficult to tackle. We can do a lot to begin to reduce many chronic diseases now, but this will require major changes in the way that we manufacture goods, design cities, and design buildings.

AIR POLLUTION AND HEALTH

With factories and personal automobiles come air pollution, occupational accidents, and traffic fatalities. In fact, as we saw from chapter 3, pneumonia (for which air pollution and smoking are major risk factors) and traffic accidents are among the leading causes of death in most middle- and high-income countries.

Air pollution, such as cigarette smoke, enters the body through the lungs and circulates through the blood stream from there, increasing one's risk of heart disease, premature aging, and cancer (Pope et al., 2004). The risk of heart disease and cancer in remote areas of the body, such as the bladder, occurs because the harmful components of smoke enter the bloodstream via the lungs and circulate through the body, causing widespread damage. These harmful microscopic particles include polyaromated hydrocarbons, which are at least as scary as they sound. These chemical compounds tend to slip between DNA strands, causing mutations that can lead to cancer. They also damage the lining of arteries, causing plaques to form, and ultimately resulting in clogging. This, in turn, can increase one's risk for heart disease, stroke, and also death from other diseases, such as the blindness that comes with macular degeneration.

But the lungs themselves are most affected (Lave & Seskin, 1970). When pollution is inhaled, it irritates the lining of the trachea (the pipes leading into the lungs from the throat) all the way down to the alveoli (little sacks at the end of the trachea). This irritation can affect the body's ability to clean out bacteria and debris and can also inhibit the immune system, leading to asthma, emphysema, and pneumonia. Each of these problems is serious, but pneumonia presents an unusual challenge to low-income countries without functioning health systems. Pneumonia is not only very common, but it also can be lethal if left untreated. Many of the bacteria that cause it are becoming resistant to antibiotics. In very poor countries, people often depend on untrained pharmacists to obtain antibiotics, and as treatment becomes increasingly complex, people are often given the incorrect antibiotic.

WHERE THERE IS NO DOCTOR

In some poor nations, people without access to medical care simply die of their disease. In others, they go to the pharmacist. Many nations have largely unregulated pharmaceutical markets in which the pharmacists act as doctors. This system can work well in instances when the pharmacist is trained. Unfortunately, they too often have little or no training. They also tend not to have access to testing. Thus, they often prescribe the wrong drugs, leaving the patient to die either from illness or from the side effects of drugs that should never have been given in the first place.

One of your humble authors, Peter Muennig, has a medical degree and a good deal of travel experience. While traveling, he has been offered cold medicines that carry a risk of psychosis and antibiotics that can permanently shut down one's ability to make blood cells from bone. Many unaware travelers and citizens alike undoubtedly were given these inappropriate drugs, and some probably died from them. (To make sure I was not being hyperbolic, I took a quick look at a number of cold medicines from where I am writing this in China in 2013, and most of the ones I looked at contained an anti-influenza medicine that can produce psychosis.)

Air pollution takes many forms. Diesel particulate matter embeds itself deep in the lungs and can also pose a major risk for lung cancer (Lave & Seskin, 1970). When gasoline or window paint contains lead or factories smelter lead, the lead is inhaled or ingested and can cause brain damage in children. In fact, it probably creates a unique type of brain damage that not only reduces children's ability to learn, but also can lead to violent behavior later in life by disrupting the neural mechanisms that usually give us impulse control resulting in lower IQs (Bellinger, Leviton, & Waternaux, 1989; Bushnell & Bowman, 1979). Crime and lower educational attainment associated with childhood lead poisoning not only present major public health problems but also in turn take a major toll on the economic and social functioning of a society (Muennig, 2009).

Of course, it does not have to be this way. A third path to development can involve regulations on pollution, on private automobile ownership, and on occupational safety standards. Paying for these regulations may slow growth in the short term, but the regulations probably pay for themselves in the long run.

Prevention and Treatment

Air pollution can be prevented with simple regulatory policies, such as mandating smog controls on vehicles and factories (see figure 10.2). Carbon trading schemes (whereby factories emitting fewer emissions can "sell" their emission rights to factories emitting more) can greatly help, though the evidence on whether they are sufficient on their own is mixed. When carbon emissions are reduced, other forms of pollution tend to follow. In the ideal, such schemes

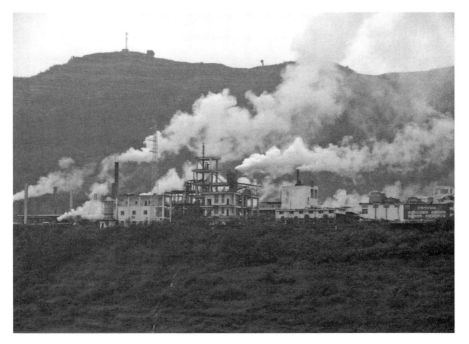

Figure 10.2. A factory in China on the Yangtze River.
Source: Wikimedia Commons/High Contrast.

require polluters to pay a tax. The grand idea is that multiple nations agree to tax their industries for carbon emissions. This tax can be traded so that factories that are especially clean end up being rewarded for their socially responsible pollution control investments. In theory, they can also be used to prevent deforestation. Countries that protect their forests and prevent slash-and-burn farming techniques could potentially be rewarded for their deeds (see figure 10.3). (All this is very difficult to implement in practice because of surveillance issues, lobbying by industry, and the usual policy-making concerns. It is even more difficult to get the nations that are the biggest polluters to come to the table because they are the ones that have to pay.)

Investments in public transit not only clean the air, but they also greatly reduce traffic accidents and reduce other chronic diseases (because one generally has to walk to public transit).

One of the most overlooked sources of global pollution is slash-and-burn farming. Smoke from slash-and-burn farming covers most of Asia in the dry season, causing countless deaths. It is also a major contributor to global warming (though this had not been clearly demonstrated until recently). Changing farming practices in nations that practice slash-and-burn farming could go a long way toward reducing global deaths and rising waters. Although

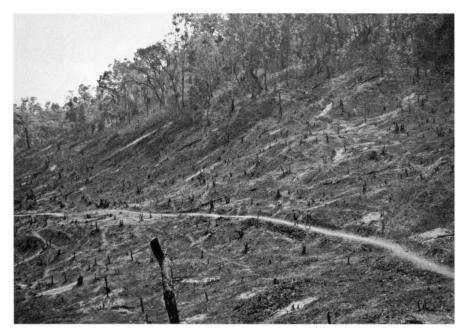

Figure 10.3. Slash-and-burn agriculture is a common form of farming in developing countries. It is also a major contributor to air pollution.

Source: Flickr/mattmangum.

changing such practices is technically simple, getting people to change is very difficult. But it is critically important and rarely discussed in the global media as a way of addressing global air pollution and global warming.

Another related problem is forest fires, many of which are set off by slash-and-burn farming, or by future farmers who wish to clear a little bit of forest for agriculture. A simple and politically viable approach to reducing smoke during the dry seasons of tropical nations is to improve firefighting capabilities in low- and middle-income nations. This carries the additional benefit of increasing the forest canopy, further reducing carbon dioxide in the air.

AIR POLLUTION, CIGARETTES, AND DEVELOPMENT

In wealthy nations, it is often the case that people denounce smokers when they develop lung problems. After all, they only have themselves to blame. But smoking was partly a by-product of social norms generated in part by tobacco companies. Even after epidemiologic studies pointed to the dangers of smoking, doctors continued to advertise cigarettes. And because tobacco is highly addictive and highly profitable, public health officials in wealthy countries had to battle cigarette companies in parliaments and congresses, the courts, and in the public, where pro-smoking norms were dominant. Now, tobacco companies have unleashed onto low-income countries many of the very same products, tactics, and campaigns now banned in industrialized nations. These include marketing tobacco to minors, suppressing information on the ill health and addictive effects of tobacco, and targeting low-income people by selling single cigarettes. Many low-income households spend 10 percent of their income on tobacco. Its use also correlates with malnutrition, lower educational attainment, higher health care costs, and premature deaths *beyond* the effects directly attributed to tobacco (www.who.int/tobacco/health _priority/en). The WHO also estimates that by 2030, more than 80 percent of deaths from tobacco use will occur in low-income countries.

The battle against air pollution is in some ways even more complicated. Transportation and commerce are central to human well-being, and the automobile industry is significantly larger than the tobacco industry. Of course, the public health ideal would be to move everyone making land trips into trains and onto bicycles. But even regulating private automobile emissions is an uphill battle because such regulations greatly increase the cost of an automobile. In poor nations, such regulations put automobiles out of reach of the average person. They also put commercial vehicles out of reach of the small businessperson and hinder economic growth. With the neighboring building barely visible out of the window of most high-rises in virtually any Chinese city, the economic versus human development question is put into stark relief.

OUTER-RING DEVELOPMENT AND HEALTH

In 2010, the world went from having more people living in rural areas to one in which more people live in cities. Economic growth renders a rural agricultural lifestyle less attractive (Davis, 2004). For one, mechanization of farms means that it is much less profitable to run a family farm than a large farming business. The lack of economic opportunities in the countryside and the draw of an urban life will ultimately draw the vast majority of the world's population to its cities.

When people arrive in large cities, they often find that it is unbearably expensive. And the arrival of many people before them means that jobs tend to be scarce. Thus, the urban newcomers sometimes settle in **slums** around the urban periphery, where costs are significantly lower. It is sometimes even possible to build a ramshackle hut with hardly any resources whatsoever save for the time it takes to build it. This way, slum developments tend to form around the outer rings of urban areas. Very roughly one billion people live in urban slums, whether outer ring or otherwise (UN, 2010).

WHAT IS A SLUM, EXACTLY?

According to UN Habitat, "A slum household [lacks] one or more of the following five amenities: (1) durable housing (a permanent structure providing protection from extreme climatic conditions); (2) sufficient living area (no more than three people sharing a room); (3) access to improved water (water that is sufficient, affordable and can be obtained without extreme effort); (4) access to improved sanitation facilities (a private toilet or a public one shared with a reasonable number of people); and (5) secure tenure (de facto or de jure secure tenure status and protection against forced eviction)" (UN, 2010).

This outer-ring development takes different forms in different places. Still, one characteristic common to many outer-ring slums is that they tend to be overcrowded and lack sanitation systems or clean water (UN, 2010). As a result, they also are good places to pick up a parasite, tuberculosis, or a bug that causes diarrhea. Many of the benefits of living in the city are absent, whereas many of the harms are present. For instance, there tends to be little by way of schools, sanitation, or medical care in outer-ring slums but pollution levels tend to be nearly as high as in the urban center. Traffic fatalities can also be high and poorly built housing can collapse. Without a fire department, fires sweep through shoddy, flammable structures. (A fact sometimes exploited by property developers wanting to rid an area of a slum.) It is all too easy to fall through bridges into the rivers of sewage that run through such communities. (Your authors have done this more than once.) These outer-ring slums can thus be quite dangerous places to live not only because of accidents and infectious disease but also because of crime. Without a police force, locals often have to take law enforcement into their own hands, which is a recipe for injustice, including wrongful conviction. As a result, they tend to be associated with very low life expectancies.

Although about two hundred million people were probably upgraded from slum living conditions between 2000 and 2010, the total number of poor people far outstripped this figure, leaving more people in slums than ever before (UN, 2010). This is simply because the highest fertility rates in most places paradoxically tend to occur amongst the poorest members of the society. By UN Habitat's reckoning, more than 95 percent of some habitants—such as those in Ethiopia—live in slums. (Of course, if you visited these places, you might disagree.)

There are also mega slums, such as most of Lagos, Nigeria, where millions live in poverty. Slums can even form around aid agency camps. In Cambodia, it is common to see giant, glistening mansions protruding from slum settlements. These "wedding cake" houses, so called because they are decorated with intricate columns in pastel colors, tend to house the development officials from bilateral donor projects. People camped outside in the donated mosquito nets form a surreal smattering of what look like spider webs growing on the outside of the walled-off compounds.

Similar to so many other public health problems, slums are best addressed with democracy and good governance (Davis, 2004; Sen, 1993). Social movements can also help and can come at very low cost. In Karachi, Pakistan, good governance is not exactly abundant. The government had neglected to build sewers in large swaths of Karachi slums. Thus, people in one community took it on themselves to build their own sewage system to serve houses in their slum. With collective organization, they managed to accomplish their task, much to the health and longevity of their community. (See figure 10.4 for an

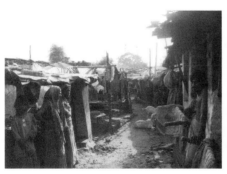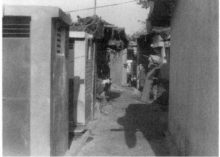

Figure 10.4. Slum upgrade in India. One approach to improving the quality of life in slums is to formally recognize them as neighborhoods within urban centers and to then install critical infrastructure, such as sewage, sidewalks, electricity, and in some cases, even improving the quality of the housing itself.

Source: Parikh, P., Parikh, H., & McRobie, A. (2012). *Role of infrastructure in improving human settlements.* Proceedings of the Institution of Civil Engineering, Urban Design and Planning. Available online at http://duncanmarasanitation .blogspot.com/2008/06/slum-networking-in-india.html.

example of a slum upgrade.) On a larger scale, however, such local initiatives have limited effects. For better or worse, it remains up to the state to coordinate collective efforts and ensure that public interests outweigh private ones in land use planning and policy.

Prevention and Treatment

The Chinese and Latin American approaches to alleviating slums represent contrasting policy models. In China, restrictions are placed on human migration into cities. Policies aimed at restricting human movement range from strict laws banning human movement out of an area to placing heavy incentives on staying put (such as failing to issue driver's licenses or providing health insurance for people who are not in their proper place). However, these policies invariably meet with limited success because people go to where the money is good and enter into the informal economy when needed. This description of China's policies is an oversimplification, of course. In a nation that builds large, heavily planned ghost cities and then simply waits for them to fill up, nothing is simple. Enforcement of China's *hukou* system (named after the document that identifies your geographic location) is highly localized.

In parts of democratic Latin America, outer-ring slums have been seen as giant blocks of untapped voters. As a result, incumbent politicians sometimes make sure to invest heavily in such areas, turning them into livable, healthy communities. This has not always worked perfectly, as in the case of Brazil's *favelas* lining Rio de Janeiro. There, the high concentrations of poverty coupled with shotgun-like slum development projects tended to result in organized crime activity. It took Brazil decades to even begin to address the gang problems. But even Brazil is making a little headway in successful slum conversion (in part thanks to improvements in community policing). Likewise, in the United States, the policy has been to upgrade housing while doing little to address the underlying poverty with day care, job programs, and proven schooling interventions. This, too, has resulted in concentrations of poverty and crime within slums.

Still, "slum upgrades," when coupled with good schools, empowering social service programs, community policing programs that ensure that the police are not themselves criminals, and local democratic institutions, can produce dramatic effects on the health and well-being of the poor.

CLIMATE CHANGE AND HEALTH

Industrialization and population growth—the hallmarks of economic and social development—have brought with them the production of greenhouse gases and deforestation. Industry and deforestation too often go hand in

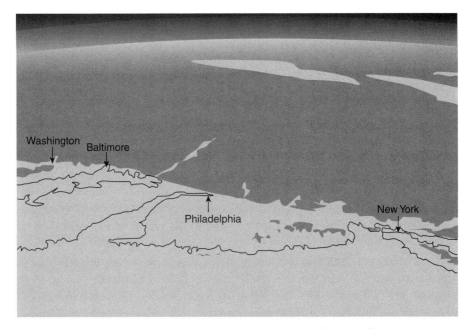

Figure 10.5. Potential land loss due to polar melting. The black outline represents the current landmass above sea level. With sufficient global warming, we can expect New York, Washington, DC, Baltimore, and Philadelphia to be under water.

hand—the destruction of the world's forests reduces the uptake of carbon dioxide, even as industries (such as agriculture) that burn and cut down the forests produce more such gases. These gases work like a one-way shield encircling the earth, permitting heat from the sun to enter but not to escape. As a result, the average temperature is slowly increasing worldwide and the polar ice caps are beginning to melt, causing sea levels to rise (see figure 10.5).

But this oft-repeated description is quite simplistic. In reality, global climate change is producing different effects in different areas of the planet. It is probably contributing to more extreme, and possibly more frequent, weather conditions in some regions of the world. These effects are highly variable and localized; in some areas, it is thought to contribute to droughts and in others to floods.

If humans and all other animal species could just pack up and move to the ideal climate whenever theirs changed, global climate change would not necessarily represent a problem. There would be less landmass among current coastal areas, but all of northern Canada would open up for colonization. However, it is exceptionally difficult to move entire cities. If the current models are correct (those suggesting a greater acceleration of global warming than previously thought), New York City will be completely under water in the lifetime of the average reader's children, as will Bangladesh in its entirety. The mere threat of global climate change will probably soon wreak havoc on national economies. Why would you invest in an apartment in New York if it were to soon be located in Atlantis? Many species are dependent on local environmental conditions for survival, and many have gone extinct as a result of global climate change already.

Further, global warming is only a small part of the threat of global climate change. Human encroachment on forests, the pollution of rivers and seas, and air pollution pose much more immediate threats. Some of the haze that renders California's sunsets brilliant is derived from giant Chinese dust storms and air pollution on the other side of the world. Fish at the top of the food chain, such as tuna, are unsafe for human consumption because they tend to contain high concentrations of methyl mercury and PCBs—by-products of industrial production. (You read that correctly. You should not be eating all those cheap cans of tuna that maintain your student budget. This is particularly true if you are a female of reproductive age as most public health students are. More instant noodles, anyone?) The pollution of rivers that cross national boundaries is causing crossborder tensions and may eventually lead to regional wars.

Water and Health

Clean, potable water is essential to the treatment of diarrheal diseases and for sustaining human life overall. According to the WHO, improving sanitation and water supplies and management would decrease the global burden of disease by 10 percent (Prüss-Üstün, Bos, Gore, & Bartram, 2008). Currently, roughly one billion people lack access to safe drinking water, most of them in sub-Saharan Africa and East Asia, and around one-third of people worldwide are affected by water scarcity (McCornick & Pasch, 2011). Fresh water constitutes only 3 percent of all water on the planet, and in the meantime, climate change, pollution, and mass consumption all exacerbate current water shortages.

The politics of water and health are complicated by several factors. First, there are large inequities in water consumption. According to the OECD, the average American uses approximately two thousand cubic meters of water per year, four times the average German, and ten times the average Dane. This complicates the politics of redistribution, how existing resources should be shared beyond national borders, and how much water should be guaranteed. Forestry, mining, agriculture, and manufacturing all use immense amounts of water. Meat—especially beef production—leads to mass water consumption for hay and grain, irrigation pasture, and carcass processing. On average, one kilogram of beef requires an average of 15,500 liters of water. It takes two hundred times more water to produce one kilogram of beef than it does one kilogram of potatoes. (See www.waterfootprint.org for other statistics and their calculation methodologies.)

Second, crop irrigation has simultaneously disastrous effects on the environment and positive effects on poverty eradication. Each dollar generated by irrigated crop production tends to trigger another two dollars in indirect economic development in India, and women and poor households in particular tend to benefit (Molden & de Fraiture, 2004). In Yemen, agriculture uses 93 percent of the usable water; the crop *qat* (a mild stimulant, a bit like tobacco) alone uses 40 percent of all potable water (Almas & Scholz, 2006; Boucek, 2010). At current usage rates, the country will run out of water by 2020. Yet, because qat is a cash crop that provides peasant farmers with their best hopes for economic sustenance, Yemenis continue to grow qat at the expense of lower-water vegetable crops, causing devastating land degradation. Without interventions at the regional and national levels, what is needed to feed and provide livelihoods to poor people now has far fewer benefits in the long run.

Likewise, major sources of industry-related income generation are also associated with water pollution. In Obuasi, Ghana, a century of machine-driven gold mining has severely contaminated local soil and water with arsenic, killed all nearby marine life with chemicals, and flooded local schools with overflow from local rivers. With increasing urbanization, many farmers use untreated urban wastewater to irrigate crops, worsening public health conditions.

Third, water crosses borders, leading to contentious **hydropolitics** over distribution and spillover (downstream) effects of pollution. India and Bangladesh have argued over the Ganges River for decades, for example. For years, India used a barrage to divert water that would have gone to Bangladeshi mangroves to feed Calcutta's water reservoirs instead. Both countries are worried over the depletion of the Gangotri glacier and deforestation in the Himalayas. In Southeast Asia, six countries attempt to share data and study the implications of industry and hydro-development (especially China's upstream dams) on the area. In northern Africa, ten countries attempt to adjudicate irrigation needs, pollution, dams, and other conflicts over the Nile River via a complex system of colonial treaties, bilateral and regional agreements, and international laws. In the Middle East, usage rights in the Jordan River basin is a signature issue in the Arab-Israeli and Palestinian-Israeli conflicts.

Finally, many countries suffer from poor water management as well as decreasing water supplies. For example, as much as 40 percent of water carried by pipes in Mexico City leaks before reaching its destination. In response, some policy makers have argued for **water privatization,** or private sector provision of sanitation and water services.

Proponents of water privatization argue that governments often only provide water to politically connected and middle-class people, whereas poor households are left unconnected to water mains. They point to cities such as Guayaquil, Ecuador, and Manila, the Philippines, as success stories.

On a closer inspection, the Manila case provides a mixed picture: after the World Bank–headed 1997 privatization of Manila's water supplies led to 81 percent price hikes in some neighborhoods, for example, many poor households lost access to water. Some researchers cite this development as correlated with the cholera outbreak that ravaged those neighborhoods in 2003. Still, after the concession in western Manila went bankrupt in 2003, a new owner in 2007 improved performance. The percentage of households with twenty-four-hour access increased dramatically, from 32 percent in 2007 to 71 percent in 2011.

Opponents argue that privatization reifies, rather than addresses, unequal access to safe water, and that the profit motive can sometimes corrode safety and affordability missions associated with public good. They point to Dar-es-Salaam, Tanzania, and Cochamamba, Bolivia, as failures.

In Cochamamba, the government handed water services concessions to the multinational Bechtel conglomerate. Although tariffs increased by 35 percent, access to water decreased by 40 percent, and supply existed only for four hours a day. The protests eventually led to Bechtel's departure, and water services are once again under public management. Nevertheless, more than half a million residents remain without water. One of the protest leaders lamented that they "were not ready to build new alternatives" (Forero, 2005).

To address the coming water scarcity, policy proposals include (1) lowering consumption by influencing diets toward less water-consuming foods; (2) improving management by increasing food trade from water-abundant countries to water-short ones (trading "virtual water"), promoting on-farm wastewater treatment, introducing safer and more efficient irrigation, upgrading rain-fed systems, and taking action to isolate pathogens; (3) planning and adjudicating distribution more fairly via intergovernmental institutions and multilateral agreements; and (4) regulating industry to prevent further pollution and climate change.

Prevention and Treatment

To reduce the impact of global climate change on human populations, a few relatively painless steps can be taken today. In the 1970s, there was great worry about holes developing in the earth's ozone layer as a by-product of the use of certain industrial chemicals, such as chlorofluorocarbons. As a result, international treaties were enacted to phase out the use of these chemicals and investments were made to find substitutes. This is one oft-forgotten success story of global cooperation on regulating industry. As it turns out, carbon dioxide is just one of many compounds contributing to global warming.

Although released in much smaller concentrations, other industrial chemicals are much more powerful contributors to global warming. Similar to the chemicals that contributed to depletion of the ozone layer, the production of these chemicals can be limited via international treaties. In addition, as mentioned previously in this chapter, reductions in slash-and-burn farming and forest fires can make a dent.

Unless some radical new technologies are developed, the current picture suggests that global warming will sink nations. We cannot prevent this from happening. But we can delay it. And just maybe, if we delay it long enough, the right technology will come along to prevent it altogether.

The real trick is to simply get the global regulatory environment in balance. With regulation, there will always be winners and losers, so implementing anything is a major challenge. As human civilization advances and grows economically, it is not difficult to envision a day when there are global regulations on automobiles and factories, just as wealthy countries impose today.

SUMMARY

Infectious disease was the leading cause of premature death globally until very recently. Nations with extremely high rates of infectious disease can have a life expectancy of just thirty to thirty-five years. Nations with very low rates of infectious disease tend to have a life expectancy greater than seventy-seven years. Infectious diseases are typically addressed with sanitation and clean water projects. The leap in life expectancy that accompanies reductions in infectious diseases is known as the epidemiologic transition. Even simple latrines can greatly reduce the incidence of infectious disease. In many cases, though, more aggressive interventions are needed, such as upgrading slums with sewage systems. Mosquito nets, vector elimination programs, and basic medicines are also important weapons in the war against infectious disease.

KEY TERMS

air pollution	*hydropolitics*	*sickle cell anemia*
climate change	*intestinal parasites*	*slums*
counterfeit drugs	*malaria*	*water privatization*
drug resistance	*outer-ring development*	

DISCUSSION QUESTIONS

1. How do malaria and internal parasites get spread? What three to four policies do you think might best address these infectious diseases? What key factors are you considering in your answer?

2. What do you think is the chief reason these preventable diseases continue to take so many lives?

3. What are some ways in which new manufacturing plants in a port town might lead to new health challenges for the local area? What do you think the local policy makers' priorities should be? The national policy makers' priorities?

FURTHER READING

Radiolab. *Parasites.* Available online at www.radiolab.org/2009/sep/07/

REFERENCES

Almas, A., & Scholz, M. (2006). Agriculture and water resources in Yemen: Need for sustainable agriculture. *Journal of Sustainable Agriculture, 28,* 55–75.

Bellinger, D., Leviton, A., & Waternaux, C. (1989). Lead, IQ and social class. *International Journal of Epidemiology, 18*(1), 180–185.

Boucek, C. (2010). Yemen: Avoiding a downward spiral. In C. Boucek & M. Ottaway (Eds.), *Yemen on the brink.* Washington, DC: Carnegie Endowment.

Burnham, G., Lafta, R., Doocy, S., & Roberts, L. (2006). Mortality after the 2003 invasion of Iraq: A cross-sectional cluster sample survey. *Lancet, 368*(9545), 1421–1428.

Bushnell, P. J., & Bowman, R. E. (1979). Effects of chronic lead ingestion on social development in infant rhesus monkeys. *Neurobehavioral Toxicology, 1*(3), 207–219.

Davis, M. (2004). Planet of slums: Urban involution and the informal proletariat. *New Left Review, 26*(Mar.–Apr.), 5–34.

Economist. (2003, April 10). Epidemics and economics. Available online at www.economist.com/PrinterFriendly.cfm?story_id=1698814

Forero, J. (2005, December 14). Bolivia regrets IMF experiment. *New York Times.* Available online at www.nytimes.com/2005/12/14/business/worldbusiness/14iht-water.html?pagewanted=all

Geary, T. G., & Thompson, D. P. (2003). Development of antiparasitic drugs in the 21st century. *Veterinary Parasitology, 115*(2), 167–184.

Hotez, P. J., Brooker, S., Bethony, J. M., Bottazzi, M. E., Loukas, A., & Xiao, S. (2004). Hookworm infection. *New England Journal of Medicine, 351*(8), 799.

Kuzman, M., Tomic, B., Stevanovic, R., Ljubicic, M., Katalinic, D., & Rodin, U. (1993). Fatalities in the war in Croatia, 1991 and 1992: Underlying and external causes of death. *JAMA, 270*(5), 626.

Lave, L. B., & Seskin, E. P. (1970). Air pollution and human health. *Science, 169*(3947), 723–733.

Mary Mallon (Typhoid Mary). (1939). *American Journal of Public Health and the Nation's Health, 29*(1), 66–68. doi: 10.2105/ajph.29.1.66.

Mascie-Taylor, C. G., & Karim, E. (2003). The burden of chronic disease. *Science, 302*(5652), 1921–1922.

McCornick, P., & Pasch, J. (2011). Water and health: Fragile sources. In R. Parker & M. Sumner (Eds.), *Routledge handbook of global public health.* New York: Routledge.

Molden, D., & de Fraiture, C. (2004). Investing in water for food, ecosystems and livelihoods. *Blue Paper.* Stockholm: Comprehensive Assessment of Water Management in Agriculture.

Muennig, P. (2009). The social costs of childhood lead exposure in the post-lead regulation era. *Archives of Pediatric and Adolescent Medicine, 163*(9), 844–849. doi: 163/9/844 [pii]10.1001/archpediatrics.2009.128.

Muennig, P., Pallin, D., Sell, R. L., & Chan, M. S. (1999). The cost effectiveness of strategies for the treatment of intestinal parasites in immigrants. *New England Journal of Medicine, 340*(10), 773–779.

Murray, C.J.L., King, G., Lopez, A. D., Tomijima, N., & Krug, E. G. (2002). Armed conflict as a public health problem. *BMJ, 324*(7333), 346.

Platt, O. S., Brambilla, D. J., Rosse, W. F., Milner, P. F., Castro, O., Steinberg, M. H., & Klug, P. P. (1994). Mortality in sickle cell disease: Life expectancy and risk factors for early death. *The New England Journal of Medicine, 330*(23), 1639–1644. doi: 10.1056/NEJM199406093302303.

Pope, C. A., III, Burnett, R. T., Thurston, G. D., Thun, M. J., Calle, E. E., Krewski, D., & Godleski, J. J. (2004). Cardiovascular mortality and long-term exposure to particulate air pollution: Epidemiological evidence of general pathophysiological pathways of disease. *Circulation, 109*(1), 71.

Prüss-Üstün, A., Bos, R., Gore, F., & Bartram, J. (2008). *Safer water, better health: Costs, benefits and sustainability of interventions to protect and promote health.* Geneva: WHO.

Sachs, J., & Malaney, P. (2002). The economic and social burden of malaria. *Nature, 415*(6872), 680–685. doi: 10.1038/415680a.

Sen, A. (1993). The economics of life and death. *Scientific American, 268*(5), 40–47.

Talman, A. M., Domarle, O., McKenzie, F. E., Ariey, F., & Robert, V. (2004). Gametocytogenesis: The puberty of Plasmodium falciparum. *Malaria Journal, 3,* 24. doi: 10.1186/1475-2875-3-24.

UN. (2010). *State of the world's cities 2010/2011—Cities for all: Bridging the urban divide.* Geneva: UN-HABITAT.

Wellems, T. E., Hayton, K., & Fairhurst, R. M. (2009). The impact of malaria parasitism: From corpuscles to communities. *The Journal of Clinical Investigation, 119*(9), 2496–2505. doi: 10.1172/JCI38307.

Wormser, G. P., & Steffen, R. (2010). *CDC health information for international travel 2010 (the yellow book)*, eds. Gary W. Brunette, Phyllis E. Kozarsky, Alan J. Magill, David R. Shlim, and Amanda D. Whatley. Atlanta, GA: Department of Health and Human Services, Public Health Service, 2009. *Clinical Infectious Diseases, 50*(4), 624. Available online at http://cid.oxfordjournals.org/content/50/4/624.full

CHAPTER 11

The Social Environment and Disease

KEY IDEAS

- Health outcomes are shaped not only by biology and the physical environment but by one's "social environment."

- Race, ethnicity, class, and gender play profound roles in shaping our health behaviors and the institutions we access.

- These social forces especially play a role in infectious diseases such as HIV/AIDS and tuberculosis and in chronic diseases such as obesity.

- Women's networks and social capital have received a lot of attention and support in global aid and global health in recent decades, especially in the areas of microfinance and children's development.

In chapter 10, we discussed some of the factors within the physical environment leading to disease. But the **social environment**—the people and institutions with whom one interacts most regularly—is also a very important determinant of how long people live. Our interpersonal interactions determine how much exercise we get, how well we eat, and not only whom we sleep with but how we sleep with them—with or without protection (whether condoms or mosquito nets), in close quarters with family or not.

The way that we build our communities and our social networks also has a profound influence on our social environment. Poor countries cannot afford to tackle the rising prevalence of chronic disease with medicine. This is forcing governments to become more creative in how they address problems such as diabetes and hypertension. For example, even some of the world's poorest countries are now working to reshape the way that people get to work, play, eat, drink, and interact to produce healthier communities. Countries such as China, Colombia, Chile, and even Ecuador are thinking more about how to design urban environments so that their dwellers move from cars to public transit systems, get on bicycles, and transition toward healthier foods.

In this chapter, we explicitly articulate some ways in which **social forces**—patterns in social organization that often help to shape human behavior—of race, class, and gender relate to global health, focusing especially on gender. Although we discuss these social forces in a separate section (toward the end of the book, no less), we hope that readers recognize that these social forces animate all disparities in global health as well as many of the analytical lenses and concerns we highlight throughout this textbook. Analyses of different policies' impact on different groups by race, class, and gender cannot be add-ons but rather important components of public health work, including the sorts of cost-effectiveness analyses discussed in chapter 3.

We select a few diseases to highlight how policies that shape the social environment also shape the health of communities and nations alike. We begin with HIV and tuberculosis, two intertwined diseases that arise from socially patterned human contact. We then discuss obesity as a condition that arises from a confluence of social interactions, national policies (including community design and food subsidies), and food industry policies. Finally, we discuss new urban planning policies that attempt to address how the physical and social environments work together to shape health outcomes.

THE ULTIMATE TRIFECTA: RACE, CLASS, AND GENDER

Academics often talk about race, class, and gender together because these socially constructed forces profoundly shape the identities of each and every one of us as well as the power inequalities among us. Although many people think of race and gender as biological constructions, many of the social assumptions about someone of a certain race or gender are **socially constructed**—that is, they are not based on genetic variations as much as mutable, changing, historically and geographically embedded conditions and shared perceptions.

For instance, it may surprise contemporary US parents to learn that until World War I, there were no color signifiers for boys' and girls' clothing. Baby pictures of future president Franklin D. Roosevelt showed him with well-combed, wavy long hair and wearing a white dress. White dresses and diapers were considered standard because they were practical and could be bleached. Between the two World Wars, clothing retailers began to advertise that the "generally accepted rule is pink for the boys, and blue for the girls. The reason is that pink, being a more decided and stronger color, is more suitable for the boy, while blue, which is more delicate and dainty, is prettier for the girl" (Frassanito & Pettorini, 2008). The current pattern of blue clothes with pictures of ball-playing bears and trucks for boys and angel-adorned pink clothes for girls did not proliferate until the 1980s, with the growth of prenatal gender testing (Paoletti, 2012).

Many other commonplace presumptions about appropriate behaviors, occupations, and "essential" natures for boys, girls, men, and women have turned topsy-turvy over time—secretaries and bank tellers were overwhelmingly male, for example, until the Civil War turned men to other pursuits. Further, when such occupations become "feminized," they tend to erode wages, be seen as "deskilled," and lose prestige. Historians have long questioned what precisely divides chefs from cooks, doctors from nurses, artists from craft makers, administrators from secretaries, professors and principals from teachers, and so on besides gendered representation and lobbying by professional accreditation organizations. It is impossible to speak of what characteristics appear to be "naturally" gendered without also speaking about power relationships. When we think about how these occupations come with different incomes and occupational hazards, we begin to see how these gender roles also shape gender health disparities.

Social Class

Of the three socially constructed forces, we have discussed permutations of class the most, especially in chapter 8 on poverty. **Social classes** are economic and cultural arrangements of groups in society, namely marked by income (and all of its complications in terms of purchasing power, as we discussed previously). Alongside income, wealth (such as inheritances, parents' homes, land, etc.), education, and occupation also serve as key markers of social class. (To get your own social class coordinates in the US context, go to www .nytimes.com/packages/html/national/20050515_CLASS_GRAPHIC/index _01.html.)

FORMS OF CAPITAL IN SOCIAL CLASS

The French sociologist and theorist Pierre Bourdieu emphasized that several **forms of capital** are important in the reproduction of social class (or, to more optimistic folks, in the potential for class mobility).

Economic capital, or command over financial resources, is familiar to most of us. Human capital, or the educational goods that can be commodified and bought and sold in the marketplace, largely consist of the skills and degrees we list on our resumés and curriculum vitae. For example, knowing how to program in a new computer programming language or speaking fluent Mandarin, Arabic, Spanish, and German (we wish) are two examples of valuable human capital. Over the past few decades, education policy around the world has increasingly emphasized human capital formation as a primary goal. Some argue that this has happened at the expense of other functions of a basic education, such as the development of social and active citizens and critical thinkers.

We talked a bit about social capital in chapter 2 and a number of times since then as the extent to which someone is connected with others around them. This was a simplification. Social capital is quite difficult to define. It has become quite a trendy concept in recent decades, and different theorists describe it in different ways (Woolcock, 1998). You have probably gathered by now that social capital has something to do with one's network of family, close friends (so-called strong ties), acquaintances and other friends (so-called weak ties or Facebook friends), colleagues, and others. Some researchers emphasize the positive aspects of social capital because emotional support networks, the sharing of resources, and active participation in civic associations are all essential to social cohesion and population well-being (Putnam, 2001; Sampson, 2002). Others, however, warn that policy makers should not romanticize social capital—after all, people can spread bad habits as well as good ones, exclude people as well as include them, or worse yet, combine these two patterns to engage in mob violence against a specific group of people. That is, in harnessing the social capital and rich sense of community among the less powerful, policies should not inadvertently exclude the *least* powerful or the hardest to reach. Some international development and global health researchers also warn that attention to social capital and civil society should not lead policy makers to overrely on nonprofits and voluntary organizations to do the job of governments.

Cultural capital consists of the knowledge, skills, and attitudes that promote social mobility. In lay terms, it consists of all the habits and knowledge one might possess to not be revealed as a wannabe or poseur in a given cultural milieu; this cultural capital might consist of knowing what fork to use in a fancy restaurant (and feeling a sense of entitlement and comfort in the setting), rattling off the latest underground hip-hop mix tapes among professional DJs, or discussing avant-garde Iranian films by Abbas Kiarostami at a dinner party with writers and artists. The phrases *streetwise* and *book smarts* refer to the fact that different sorts of cultural capital are most useful in different settings. Likewise, different racial and ethnic groups, immigrant groups, and other communities have different sets of skills that are valued and provide important survival mechanisms.

Unlike economic capital, human, social, and cultural capital tend to accrue value and authority with use. For public health workers, it is important to acknowledge the value of different social networks or sets of cultural capital so that breast cancer or safe drinking water programs might use different skill sets embedded in different communities, but it is also important to refrain from treating these different sets of cultural capital as if they were of *equal* value—after all, some of these communities do have much less power than others and their health outcomes reflect that fact. Finally, it is important not to essentialize any sets of norms as inevitable, as if this community of people will always act according to certain norms and values. After all, these sets of capital evolved over time in response to larger structural conditions, such as laws, conquest and violence, the physical environment, the doctrines of key leaders, and other factors.

Race

We know that there are more genetic variations between people of a single racial and ethnic group than there are between different racial and ethnic groups. Racial categories are not based on genetic variations per se as much as phenotypic characteristics or geographic ancestry, cultural traditions, and social class. They have often changed through time. *Mexican, Chinese,* and *Japanese* were at one point listed as different races on the US Census, before they became subsumed into *Latino ethnicity* and *Asian/Pacific Islander race.* There are countless books on the historical processes via which Italian, Irish, and Ashkenazi Jewish immigrants became white in the United States; as such, race is "an unstable and 'decentered' complex of social meanings constantly being transformed by political struggle" (Omi & Winant, 1994, p. 55). *Ethnicity* tends to be associated with an emphasis on political-historical characteristics, but race and ethnicity are contested terms and have often been used interchangeably (Oppenheimer, 2001). A Latino identity in the United States and the Panará indigenous group in the Amazon, for instance, are sometimes seen as ethnic identities and other times as racial ones. Despite its social construction, race remains an important factor in global health because the racialized experiences of different groups—and their very disparate health outcomes—remain real.

Just as there is no single pathway between social class and health, there is no single pathway between race and health, especially across societies. There are dramatic health disparities by race and ethnicity in most diverse societies, mostly because social class, education, occupational prestige, wealth, and so on tend to be unequally distributed along racial lines. It is difficult to disentangle all of these factors. The role of racism, race-based discrimination, and stereotyping, however, tends to truncate the class mobility of certain groups. Thus, low-income South African "colored" folks (mostly of South Asian descent) experienced apartheid differently than South African blacks and whites did, just as high-income Chinese Singaporeans face different daily experiences than high-income Malay Singaporeans do.

Typical pathways between social class and health outcomes can be altered not just by individual discrimination (such as doctors prescribing suboptimal prognoses to members of a minority racial group) but by **institutional racism** as well. In Sri Lanka, for example, some argue that university admissions may be facially neutral, but that the criteria used consistently and disproportionately grant admissions to certain racial groups.

GENDER AND SOCIAL CAPITAL

Despite the popular phrase of "old boys' networks," many international development policy makers tend to see social capital as women's capital. Thus, large NGOs such as Care, the Grameen Bank and other microfinance institutions, and grassroots peace organizations disproportionately work with women. These organizations build their work on the premise that women have less access to traditional economic capital but that they are also socialized to share resources, build networks of trust, and rely on collaboration rather than confrontation in adjudicating conflicts. In short, women are seen as more trustworthy. Ideally, these organizations will help women to better harness the forms of capital they do possess in order to earn higher incomes, earn greater decision-making power within their households, and slowly build other social and political capabilities.

Microfinance institutions' work with women's networks is controversial, and the majority of academic studies tend to be critical. They state that these networks rarely change larger gender roles or enhance other capabilities, with men often continuing to decide how newly generated income is spent, and that they often shift the focus of international development from social and political citizenship to "financial self-sustainability" (Mayoux, 2001; Rankin, 2002).

Gender and Health

Gender refers to a set of characteristics—biological, behavioral, social—differentiating men from women and masculine from feminine traits. In the context of global health, policy makers have paid increasing attention to women's health in particular (figure 11.1).

Public health officials have stated that addressing women's health issues demands a "social transformation" more than a medical one; the differential power between men and women in almost every society around the globe means that women's health is irrevocably tied to gender roles and inevitably involves men. In Bombay, one-fourth of all deaths of women between the ages of fifteen and twenty-four are caused by "accidental" burning. In Kenya, the headmaster of a boarding school states that the boys who raided a girls' dormitory, raping seventy-one and killing nineteen, "never meant any harm to the girls. They just wanted to rape." In the United States, up to 35 percent of all emergency room visits consist of women victims of battering and domestic violence (Holloway, 1994). In some years, almost half of all women killed in New York City were murdered by their intimate partners (Stayton et al., 2008). The **feminization** (whereby a phenomenon that mostly involved males before now mostly affects females) of the AIDS crisis in sub-Saharan Africa and the feminization of poverty and low-skilled work in the United States are in most ways distinct phenomena. Nevertheless, they are correlated with the fact that men tend to enjoy greater economic and social freedoms than women do, and that unequal codes of conduct, violence, and access are often not just condoned but encouraged (Lewis, 2006). Gendered social determinants lead to health disparities through multiple pathways, including (1) discriminatory practices and norms, (2) differential exposures to disease and injuries, (3) biases in health systems, and (4) biased health research (Sen, Östlin, & George, 2007).

Assumptions about men and women's tendencies and natural roles in society shape mass health risk behaviors and public policies meant to control or address risk behaviors. Questions extend beyond whether explicitly health-oriented policies such as family planning are sanctioned and provided, whether diseases that disproportionately affect one gender are given research and implementation funds, and whether doctors treat each patient according to his or her specific needs. (Until recently, for example, overwhelmingly male doctors tended to tell older women with breast cancer that they should undergo mastectomies and younger women that they should undergo chemotherapy. These prognoses did not always correlate with the specific cancer cases as much as the doctors' assumptions that younger women wanted to hold onto their breasts no matter what, whereas older women were no longer sexualized beings [Holloway, 1994; Lewis, 2006; Love & Lindsey, 2010; Sen et al., 2007; Stayton et al., 2008]).

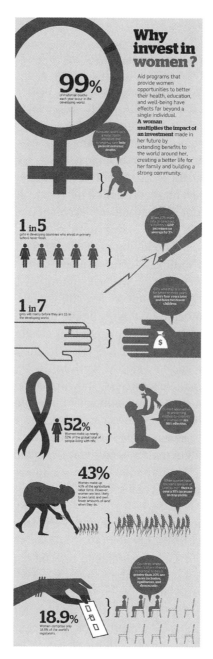

Figure 11.1. From a purely economic perspective, it makes more sense to invest scarce aid dollars in women rather than men because women are more likely to comply with interventions, pass on information to their children, and are less likely to squander income on alcohol or other drugs than are men.

Source: USAID.

THE MISSING WOMEN PHENOMENON

It is estimated that there are more than one hundred million girls and women missing worldwide—they were never born because of sex selection bias, they were victims of infanticide, or they died premature deaths from severe malnutrition, physical abuse, or other factors that tend to disproportionately affect females. Namely, because boys tend to be valued more than women in many societies. They tend to earn higher wages and are thus better able to provide for their families in the future and bring prestige, whereas girls come with much higher costs, especially in terms of dowries, and lower returns, especially in terms of future wages. Such tragic calculations are especially consequential in contexts where infant mortality is high, where there is not enough food to feed multiple children, where there is not enough money to send multiple children to school, and where governments pressure families to have only one or two children, as in China.

This phenomenon was first extensively analyzed and brought to widespread attention by Amartya Sen, a Nobel Prize–winning economist who noticed that some nations had considerably more males than females, despite the fact that women tend to live longer than men (figure 11.2). Although it is true that one hundred boys are born to every ninety-five girls in most of the world, women tend to outnumber men by age thirty-five. (Whether by war, violence, drunk driving, disease, heart attack, or other means, the mortality ratios for young men are usually higher than those for young women.) Yet, in northern India, there are roughly eighty to eighty-five girls per one hundred boys. This contrasts even with ratios in southern India, where there are between ninety-five or ninety-six girls per one hundred boys (Sen, 1999) (see figure 11.2). Male-to-female ratios are therefore a powerful measure of the status of women in society. Countries that have high proportions of males relative to females tend to have high numbers of poorly educated women, to deprive females of food or medical care in times of scarcity, to perform infanticide, or to perform sex-selective abortions. Some examples of nations with disproportionate numbers of males include India, China, Afghanistan, and Pakistan.

What should be done in response? Sen points out differences in natality bias are not fully explained by the availability of medical resources, predominant religious background, income, or economic growth of specific contexts. Thus, it is imperative to not only address the *well-being* of women but also the *agency* of women. It is different to help

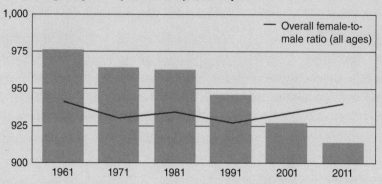

Falling number of girls aged 0–6 years in India since 1961

Number of girls aged 0–6 years for every 1,000 boys

Figure 11.2. The missing women phenomenon. Some nations have many more boys than would be expected by natural sex ratios at birth.

Source: Census of India, 2011.

a friend adopt healthy habits as an equal than it is to tell a patient what to do in well-meaning ways. He thus advocates that women's capabilities be expanded via support-led policies such as those in Kerala. These capabilities might include the ability to earn an independent income and find employment outside the home, have ownership rights, be literate and educated, and participate in decision making inside and outside the family. Enhancing capabilities, then, is fundamentally different from raising money for a large dowry or an expensive engagement ring, without addressing the daughter's lack of empowerment, in an attempt to ensure her well-being.

Sen's emphasis on agency and informed decision making becomes more acute in his comparisons of Kerala, northern Indian states, and China. How does Kerala maintain a much higher female-to-male ratio than most Indian states when its birth rate is much lower, at 1.7 instead of the 3.0 Indian average? And how does the state maintain birth rates comparable to China's—and female-to-male ratios much more favorable than China's—without coercion? To adherents of the capability approach, as described in chapter 5, Kerala's approach is commendable because of its combination of support-led policies and democratic governance; ideally, under such circumstances, the people themselves help to address extreme gender inequalities.

A recent book—with the updated estimate of 160 million missing women—has reignited public debates on what policies might best address this issue (Hvistendah, 2011). Social conservatives have argued that the issue of missing women must be addressed by banning not just sex-selective abortions but abortions altogether. Others, including Hvistendah, have retorted that the biggest group of victims are not fetuses but women, and that the practice of sex selection should not justify curtailing women's rights to family planning. Further, she argues that the high prevalence of sex-selective abortions and forced sterilization in Asia stems partly from mandated policies by foreign governments to introduce abortions as a means of population control rather than as women's family planning options. Other more socially accepted practices (currently used primarily by wealthier households in industrialized countries), such as gender selection in the process of in vitro fertilization, suggest that abortions are hardly the only means of sex selection.

In the meantime, the skewed gender ratios have significant implications for social stability, and sex trafficking, sex work, and child trafficking networks have proliferated as a result. As many as 90 percent of Burmese women in China enter forced marriages (Hvistendah, 2011). In some cases, local Chinese governmental officials are charging families between US$1,000, five times a household's annual income, and US$5,000 for the families to be able to keep their children. In such circumstances, officials seized dozens, if not hundreds, of children whose parents did have proper marriage papers or permits for additional children, selling these babies to orphanages that catered to foreign adoptions (LaFraniere, 2011). It speaks to the power of parental love that even under such circumstances, many parents continued to look for their daughters, hoping to find them in orphanages, years after the illegal seizures.

Social class, race, and gender often intersect in patterned ways. As policy makers in Quito, Ecuador, design a new public health food program, then, they might keep in mind that low-income mestizo women will probably respond differently than upper-class mestizo women, low-income mestizo men, or indigenous Quechua women. These **intersectionalities,** or intersections among gender, race, age, and social class, also inform how diseases such as HIV, tuberculosis, and obesity tend to affect and wreak havoc on some subpopulations more than others.

THE HUMAN IMMUNODEFICIENCY VIRUS (HIV)

About thirty to thirty-five million people were living with HIV worldwide in 2011, about two-thirds of whom live in sub-Saharan Africa (UN, 2010). This amounts to about five out of every one hundred people living there. The prevalence is below 0.5 percent in other regions of the world. In absolute terms, the second largest population of HIV-infected people reside in South and Southeast Asia (about four million) but this only represents 0.3 percent of the population. The number of new infections has reached a plateau and may be declining by the time you read this.

HIV/AIDS has wreaked devastating effects in South Africa. The country had a life expectancy of sixty-one in 1992, and it has reported a steady life expectancy of fifty-two since 2003. Although health outcomes have not worsened in the past decade, most other countries with similar GDPs hover far above South Africa on the graph.

HIV infection is most often transmitted through unprotected sex and injecting drug use. It can also be spread from mother to infant during birth or during breast-feeding. Thus, prevention efforts involve encouraging condom use, using medicines to reduce transmission of the virus from the mother to the infant during birth, and changing breast-feeding practices among HIV-positive women. To reduce sexual transmission, one widely promoted preventive campaign is ABC, an acronym for Abstinence, Being faithful, and, failing that, Condom use. The primary preventive modality for injecting drug users is providing clean needles, often referred to as *needle exchange,* because it involves swapping used needles with clean ones. This is known as a "harm reduction" policy because it does not focus solely on changing behaviors or punishing drug users as much as reducing the social and personal harm they unleash via their drug use. Finally, efforts to reduce transmission from mother to infant involve screening pregnant women for HIV in high-risk settings and providing treatment with powerful antiviral drugs prior to delivery.

Policy makers tend to think of HIV and the acquired immunodeficiency syndrome (AIDS) as one entity, so much so, in fact, that most publications simply refer to the two as HIV/AIDS. Still, HIV and AIDS should probably be discussed as separate phenomena, especially when thinking about them from a policy-making perspective.

HIV refers to a virus that ultimately leads to a disease called AIDS. AIDS attacks the immune system, particularly a type of cell called a T-cell, and causes a slow deterioration in one's ability to fight off disease. People who are infected with HIV can be healthy for at least six months, or even decades, before they become sick and severely compromised. The length of this interval partly depends on one's genetic makeup. Mostly, it depends on whether the person is otherwise healthy, well-nourished, living in a healthy environment, and receiving medical care.

Even without treatment, those who are quite healthy can live with HIV for longer than a decade before they develop any symptoms. This time frame is greatly shortened when the immune system is further stressed by malnutrition, exposure to other infectious diseases, or exposure to harsh living circumstances. For these reasons, the time from HIV infection to AIDS tends to be much shorter in poor countries than in rich ones (Wegbreit, Bertozzi, DeMaria, & Padian, 2006). When treated, HIV can become a chronic disease, and those who are infected may be much more likely to die of something else before they develop AIDS. In short, there is no reason for the average person with HIV to develop AIDS. But preventing AIDS is not as easy or as straightforward as it seems.

HIV—A Brief History

HIV was thought to exist in nonhuman primates long before it made its leap to humans in central-west Africa sometime in the nineteenth or twentieth century (Korber et al., 2000; Worobey et al., 2008). The most common type, HIV-1, has been tracked back to Cameroon. There, people who prepare chimpanzee meat tend to chop the meat with bare hands using a cleaver. This process is quite bloody and bone fragments can penetrate the skin. These people probably had a very high prevalence of simian immunodeficiency virus, a virus that does not typically cause severe disease in humans. At some point, though, this virus adapted to the human host and became HIV.

HIV was then probably slowly spread through IV drug use, prostitution, and polyamorous relationships over a period of time until it reached a critical mass. Some epidemiological accounts in the 1980s emphasized the role of a handsome flight attendant who was quite lucky at love. (Activists, especially in the gay community, protest popular media portrayals of "Patient Zero" as somehow culpable or responsible for the epidemic.) Eventually, whether via straight sex, gay sex, or injecting drug use, the virus made its way all over the world.

Why Some Countries Have Little HIV and Others Have a Lot

The virus is most infectious when someone is very recently infected. During this time—usually around the first few months after contracting the disease—the body's immune system has not had a chance to fully tackle the new invader. For this reason, the virus causes a flu-like illness and the viral count is very high. After a while, the body gets a handle on the virus. Although it does not get rid of it completely, the body does reduce the number of viruses in the blood to very low levels. After a while, the virus slowly wears out the immune system to the point that it can once again reach high levels in the blood. At this point, the infected person develops AIDS and usually passes away in less than a year.

Because levels in the blood are low after the initial infection, the virus is not easy to transmit. For instance, even before the availability of modern drugs, HIV-negative people partnered with HIV-positive people could go for years without ever becoming infected (Gray et al., 2001). This is true even when they are less than perfectly careful about protection. But if one partner becomes infected during the relationship, the other is very likely to become HIV-positive because they will have unprotected sex when the viral load is quite high. The HIV virus therefore does best when spread through a social network that shares bodily fluids in one form or another on a frequent basis. In 2011, the primary modes of transmission were via sexual networks, prostitution, and intravenous drug use.

Sexual networks are by far the most common means of transmission. They typically work like this: Fred has a wife with whom he lives, but he also sees Brenda, whom he visits when he travels, which is once every week. On occasion, his business takes him farther to another town, in which he sees Suzy. Brenda and Suzy do not get much from Fred other than occasional company, so they keep a few additional lovers themselves. These lovers, in turn, keep a few others, creating a large web of people who are sexually intertwined. When the virus is introduced into this network, everyone ends up having sex with a recently infected person—the time when the virus is most easily spread. As a result, the virus moves through the network very efficiently. Because Fred's network overlaps with other networks throughout the country, the virus spreads rapidly over a wide geographic swath. In some locales, the percentage of HIV-infected people has far exceeded 50 percent.

Therefore, local sexual practices are primary determinants of whether HIV meets a dead end (e.g., the nonadulterous spouse of a sex worker's client) or continues on from person to person. For this reason, some societies see explosions of HIV, whereas others are relatively unaffected. The virus has not taken hold in places where most people tend to have fewer partners or when people tend to be serial monogamists; when the number of recently infected people is small and each new infection is a relative dead end, the prevalence will be quite low.

Similarly, with prostitution, the sex worker must be recently infected to transmit the virus to a client. Rather than work in social networks, prostitutes tend to work serially with clients. If a sex worker has a dedicated base of not-so-lucky-in-love clients, it remains rather difficult for HIV to break into the larger population; even if such a sex worker becomes infected, and all of his or her clients become infected, the infection is unlikely to spread rapidly through the larger population.

However, if the sex worker has a fairly high volume of clients, and the clients visit multiple sex workers, an explosion of HIV will occur. Even in this setting, it is possible to reduce the spread of the virus by ensuring that condoms are used with most sexual encounters. The average volume of clients a sex worker has can vary greatly by region. For instance, for some, sex work is a side business to supplement income. In this model, the prevalence of HIV can remain quite low.

The explosion of HIV in Thailand in the 1990s was almost certainly related to that nation's reputation as a tourist destination for clients of sex workers (Weniger et al., 1991). These people typically visited multiple sex workers, and the sex workers typically had many clients per day. As might be predicted by what we now know about transmission of HIV, the introduction of condom use campaigns stemmed the epidemic. Today, paid sex is probably as prevalent as ever in Thailand, but HIV is declining rapidly simply because more people are using condoms (Nelson et al., 1996). In sub-Saharan Africa, relatively small changes in social sexual practices have led to significant drops in new infections (Cohen, 2010a, 2010b). This gives great hope that prevention campaigns will reverse the tide of HIV. Indeed, though some places are still seeing increases, it already looks like the number of new infections worldwide will soon begin to decline.

HIV as a Chronic Disease

In the chapter on aid, we saw that AIDS in Africa led in part due to the large increase in aid to poor countries. Much of that aid went to testing people for HIV and then treating those who tested positive. This is a relatively inefficient way of tackling the crisis. Treating people does reduce the number of viruses in the blood to the point that is almost impossible to transmit the disease, but it does nothing to reduce the viral load when people are most infectious—in the interval immediately following initial infection. Not only is it less common that people get tested immediately following exposure but the test used as this textbook goes to press cannot reliably detect the disease until people develop antibodies. Once someone develops antibodies (usually six weeks to six months after infection), the viral load drops and the person is less infectious. One alternative test, viral RNA, can detect the disease as early as nine days postexposure and may serve as a more reliable way of controlling new infections.

Regardless, it is much easier to reduce the prevalence of disease by preventing infection in the first place. This involves changing the nature of sexual networks and increasing condom use. Nevertheless, this global push to treat people who are HIV positive has had a profound effect on drug pricing, global aid, and deaths due to AIDS. It has also had spillover effects, with prevention programs going into full swing. As a result, HIV/AIDS has become much less of a problem than experts once feared, despite the fact that any reasonable cost-effectiveness analysis suggested that funds be diverted to prevention. The case of HIV aid just goes to show that the most scientifically logical approach is not always the best approach. In this case, HIV and AIDS cases prompted a whole new era of global aid, with massive spillover effects that benefited public health overall.

Prevention and Treatment

Effective modes of prevention of HIV vary greatly from place to place. In Africa, preventive campaigns have proven to be very effective at reducing the prevalence of disease. These focus simply on increasing condom use and reducing the total number of partners one has in his or her social network.

In the United States, HIV is a disease of the poor. Reducing drug use and organized drug crime can go a long way toward addressing HIV infection. Needle exchange appears to be a cost-effective means of reducing HIV prevalence among intravenous drug users (Belani & Muennig, 2008). Public health departments also need to be vigilant and to intervene in social networks when needed. For instance, a spike in HIV occurred among young gay males in the early 2000s in the United States as a result of HIV fatalism and risky behaviors such as *bugchasing*, a form of *self-harm*. This partly occurred because the advent of more effective treatments meant that few young gay males had personally known someone who died of the disease. It was ultimately stemmed with aggressive social marketing campaigns on the part of local health departments, but health education campaigns probably could have caught and prevented the spike in HIV infections sooner.

TUBERCULOSIS

Tuberculosis, nicknamed TB, is a very common disease. About one in three people worldwide are infected with TB (Donald & van Helden, 2009; Dye, Scheele, Dolin, Pathania, & Raviglione, 1999). Usually, those who are infected do not develop symptoms or easily transmit the disease until their immune system becomes compromised. Most infected people therefore die of something else before the disease becomes "active." Of every person infected, only a fraction (about 10 percent on average) actually develops active disease. Inactive infection is diagnosed with a simple screening test that many readers are familiar with. In this test, a small amount of dead TB particles are injected into the skin, making a tiny bubble. If the immune system recognizes the dead TB, it will attack it, leaving a red, hard, and inflamed bump where the injection was. If the immune system has not encountered TB before, the tiny bubble will just disappear.

This detail regarding the immune response to TB is important for understanding why TB is such a problem worldwide. In most people, the TB bacillus (the particle that causes infection) does a pretty good job of staying alive while under attack by the immune system. It builds a protective barrier around itself in the body and it lives there for decades, happily sheltered from attack by the body's immune system. The TB bacilli like to make their little immune igloo in the lungs where they can get plenty of oxygen. Although TB can also live in other tissues, such as bone, such infections are less common than lung infections, probably because of the fact that their lung igloos come with central air. Over time, the person hosting the TB might weaken with old age or develop other immunological problems, such as AIDS. When this happens, the TB leaves its little house, multiplies, and spreads to other parts of the lung or body, forming **active tuberculosis** (Davies, 2005).

In active tuberculosis, people develop symptoms (e.g., chest pain, coughing up blood, or night sweats) because the TB has broken out of its shell. In this stage, the disease can be highly infectious, and if untreated, lethal (about 50 percent will die). People with active TB cough and sneeze out live TB into the air, causing others to inhale the bacilli (which are usually then walled off in the lungs of their new hosts, awaiting their big redebuts).

The AIDS epidemic caused an explosion of active tuberculosis cases worldwide. In fact, TB is the leading cause of death among people who develop AIDS. In addition to those with AIDS, people who are undernourished are especially susceptible to tuberculosis, which is one reason why it tends to be more common in poor countries. Although normal human aging is also a major risk factor that can bring out the infection (and rich countries have many more elderly people than poor countries), most of the latent cases in wealthy nations have either never been exposed to TB or have already been screened and treated for latent infection.

Whether latent or active, treatment of tuberculosis can be tricky, requiring a long course of antibiotics. Even trickier, many cases have become resistant to the standard therapy. Resistance varies worldwide, leading to different recommendations for asymptomatic people who live or contracted the infection in different places (Khan, Muennig, Behta, & Zivin, 2002). In fact, tuberculosis is one of the **superbugs.** A superbug is a colloquial term for an organism that has evolved to develop resistance to drugs that previously effectively killed them.

In the case of tuberculosis, there are strains that are resistant to most known therapies. This resistance likely developed because therapy takes a very long time to complete. Most people tend to forget to complete a course of antibiotics for six days, let alone six months. When people take only a partial course of antibiotics, they require retreatment. Unfortunately, this process of treatment and retreatment allows bacteria to evolve. When you knock out the weakest bugs with a partial round of antibiotics, only the most antibiotic-resistant bacteria survive. These stronger bugs multiply, carrying their hardy genes with them. These are more prepared for the next round of therapy, and a higher than normal dose of drug is needed to kill them. The weakest of those strong bugs get knocked down, and so on, until one is left with superbugs. Superbugs can be almost impossible to effectively treat and can spread to other people (Gandhi et al., 2006).

Because treatment goes on for so long, an important component of treatment is "directly observed therapy," in which the patient is required to come to a particular place to take his or her medication. If the patient fails to show, health officials can track him or her down to make sure the therapy is reinitiated.

OVERUSE OF ANTIBIOTICS

The term *superbug* refers to bacteria, parasites, or viruses that have become resistant to standard therapies. Bacteria become resistant to antibiotics (and viruses to antiviral medications, etc.) when they are used widely. Some of these uses are appropriate treatments for dangerous infections, but oftentimes the drug was never called for in the first place. For instance, despite the fact that the common cold has no cure, and, besides that, it is a virus and not a bacteria, some doctors prescribe antibiotics for a cold. (Why? In a health care system driven by demand, some doctors keep the appointment short rather than explaining the situation to their patients, giving patients something tangible—drugs—instead.) This inappropriate overuse of the drug means that there are more drugs in the general population, leading to drug resistance.

Other common misuses include prescribing antibiotics for conditions that do not call for them, such as diarrhea or ear infections that are not accompanied by a fever. In these cases, the harmful bacteria usually would have been attacked by the immune system, and the patient would have recovered anyway. Instead, the bacteria were exposed to antibiotics and given the chance to evolve.

Inappropriate use can also occur when people do not take their entire course of the medication. Many people feel better once the number of harmful bacteria in their body begins to fall. But the harmful bacteria are often still there if the treatment is stopped early, and they can then grow back.

A more troubling, avoidable, inappropriate use of antibiotics occurs when livestock is placed in unsanitary and overcrowded conditions so that farms can maximize profits. Under these circumstances, farm animals are usually given "preventive" antibiotics or antiparasitic medications in their feed.

Prevention and Treatment

The prevention of TB requires ensuring that people do not live in overcrowded housing, have access to adequate medical care, and that social rates of new HIV infections are brought under control. In middle- and high-income countries, **extended contact investigation** is often used. This involves contacting people who were exposed to those with the most infectious forms of TB, testing them, and providing long-term treatment as needed.

The Bacillus Calmette-Guérin (BCG) vaccine has been developed to reduce the prevalence of TB, but it is not 100 percent effective. It is used in many low-income countries with mixed results. The vaccine is thought to be reasonably effective at treating childhood forms of tuberculosis. It may also help prevent pulmonary tuberculosis in adulthood but, despite its widespread use worldwide, this has yet to be proven beyond doubt.

SOCIAL NETWORKS AND CHRONIC DISEASE

Christakis and Fowler (2007) shocked the world (or at least many social scientists and public health nerds) when they fairly convincingly argued that obesity is a contagious disease. They showed that when one person gains weight within a social network, other people tend to gain weight as well. What was so very surprising about this is that the people who gained weight did not have to be in proximity to one another. They could be all the way across the country. We are used to thinking of the common cold as a contagion, and thinking of HIV and AIDS as socially constructed diseases that appear disproportionately in certain subpopulations, even though they are not transmitted differently in different subpopulations . . . but obesity?

What is less surprising is that risky health behaviors tend to spread through social networks as well. After all, your friends are the ones who typically start you smoking or encourage you to stop. The same goes for drinking, for safe or unsafe sex, or for drugs. In fact, the advertising industry has long understood that social networks provide a powerful means to get people to do something that they want them to do, such as buying a product. Public health practitioners can use these techniques to encourage people to become healthier, too.

Public Health Advertising

To get someone (the "target audience") to buy a product, the target audience not only needs to be aware of the product but also must desire it. The most desired products tend to be in the hands of the most popular members of popular groups ("thought leaders"). The objective, then, is to compel such thought leaders to use the product. Once the specific preferences for such people have been studied, they are specifically targeted with a well-honed message ("the communication"). In selling its iPod, Apple's advertising partner targeted young urbanites with images of multicultural silhouettes dancing while wearing the trademark white earphones. Multiculturalism captures one essence of the cosmopolitan life, as does going out and dancing. According to marketing research, this created a feeling or emotion around the product that was perfectly in line with the values, lifestyle, hopes, and desires of the target audience. Once the thought leader group adopted the technology, the iPod became the must-have electronic for young suburban kids, then thirty-somethings. It worked. It was so desired that classified ads online could be found in which people were willing to trade sex for an iPod. After just a few years on the market, grandmothers could be seen using the device in the New York subway. The product's name ultimately overtook the generic MP3 player description and became the standard electronic for listening to music. (Like Band-Aid or Google, the thought leader's name became a verb, so that few people ask for "an adhesive bandage," command you to "enter the keyword in a search engine," or talk about "MP3 player mixes.")

Similarly, the New York City Department of Health and Mental Hygiene targeted young groups in its advertising. One objective was to increase condom use. So, special condoms were purchased with the subway logo on them (another supposed signifier of "hip" urban life) and distributed in trendy bars and restaurants. The simple association of condoms with urban life may have done a lot to increase the uptake of their use. Once that happens, the behavior is more likely to become normalized, and the hope is that eventually both men and women purchase condoms without a second thought before going out or going on a hot date. The same department's campaign to increase tap water consumption over bottled sugary drinks relied not only on the notion of environmental conservation (no plastic bottles) but fear of fat. One subway advertisement showed a drink being poured into a glass from a bottle, but in place of liquid, the drink contained what looked like human fat (see figure 11.3).

However, much more sophisticated advertisements are needed. Madison Avenue firms in New York City study human psychology to improve the effectiveness of their advertising campaigns. In response to what some see as too much advertising and consumption (particularly for products that damage health or damage the environment) *culture jamming* has risen in response. This is the process of modifying existing advertisements or creating new advertisements in ways intended to counter the harmful effects of conventional corporate ads (see figure 11.4).

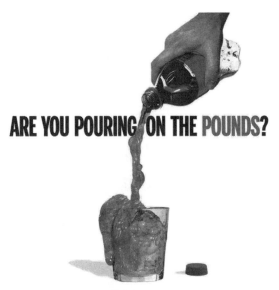

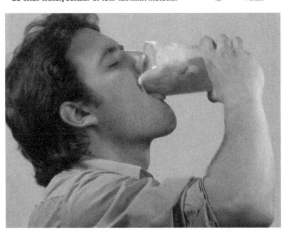

Figure 11.3. A public communications campaign from the New York City Department of Health and Mental Hygiene. Top panel: An advertisement frequently seen on the subway. Bottom panel: Still from an accompanying YouTube video.

Source: New York City Department of Health and Mental Hygiene.

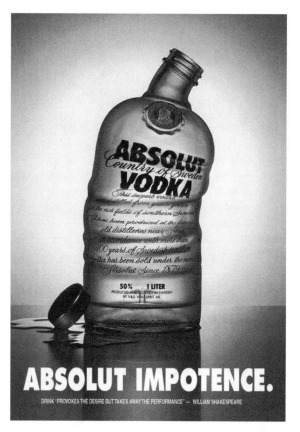

Figure 11.4. Adbusters is an organization stocked with disenfranchised advertisers that seeks in part to counter the harmful effects of consumer advertising in a process called *culture jamming*. This ad attempts to delink male virility and alcohol. It might be particularly effective at reducing alcohol consumption because most men know what alcohol can do when they actually do get lucky with their bar date.

Source: Adbusters.org. Available online at www.adbusters.org/content/absolut-impotence.

INDIVIDUAL RISK BEHAVIORS, URBAN PLANNING, AND HEALTH

Public health departments have long attempted to facilitate these healthy social norms by targeting advertisements to supposed thought leaders, much the same way that branded Apple targeted certain demographic groups—urban graphic designers—in making the relatively more expensive iPod the socially acceptable standard for owning an MP3 player. Governments tend to have more limited advertising budgets, and such campaigns can look quite pitiful, with very low production values. Still, governments have a number of advantages over private agencies. For one, given the resources and political will, they can better shape behaviors not only through advertising but also by transforming the communities in which people work, live, and play.

Exercise campaigns can be coupled with the installation of parks, bike lanes, and public transit systems. Sugar taxes can be combined with cleaner public water systems and campaigns promoting personal water bottle use. (This has the benefit of substituting water for unhealthy drinks and reducing the pollution produced by transporting bottled beverages and disposing of the plastic.) In both of these cases, normalization of healthy behaviors can be facilitated not only by changing thought leaders' preferences, but also by shaping the physical and policy environment to usher in those behaviors.

Still, campaigns that focus on changing individual behaviors via incentives and marketing are unlikely to be sufficient on their own. They must also provide resources (so that it becomes easier for individuals not just to recognize but also to realistically choose the healthier alternative) and begin to address structural inequalities. One of the most successful campaigns in New York, for example, helped more than 14 percent of smokers in the city quit in just two years, an impressive outcome. The campaign involved more than public information and scare tactic posters, however. The city also gave away over ninety thousand nicotine patch and smoking cessation kits in 2003 and 2005 alone, primarily to nonwhite and poor residents. Between 2002 and 2006, the percentage of smokers in the city decreased by almost 20 percent (Colgrove, 2011). In other words, before attempting to convince folks that something is good or trendy, governments need to make sure that it is also possible or at least not a lot of work, expensive, or a total drag (no pun intended).

For instance, with regard to bicycling, New York City embarked on a multipronged approach of giving away free gear (lights, helmets, and maps), promoting bicycling through advertising, and building (or painting green) 390 miles of new bicycle lanes between 2002 and 2010. By 2011, the number of commuter bicyclists in New York City had risen by 62 percent since 2008 and 262 percent since 2000 (O'Grady, 2011).

Some specific bicycle lanes were painted in neighborhoods without local community input, and the response was so furious that the bike lanes were turned back into car lanes. That said, the overwhelming majority of new bicycle lanes in New York City have been a resounding success, and they have made it much easier for nondaredevils to safely ride the streets. It also helps that the city distributes free bicycle maps at most subway stations, that there are no restrictions on bringing bicycles onto subway cars (as there are in other metropolitan cities in the United States), and that Google maps helps one find not just the best walking and driving routes from point A to point B but the best public transit and bicycling routes as well. The city has also mandated that employers allow workers to bring their bicycles inside but this has not yet been enforced well.

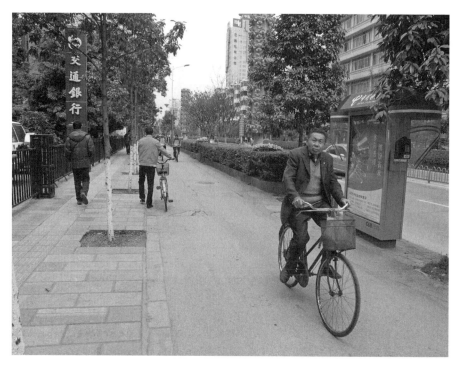

Figure 11.5. A bike lane in Kunming, China. Sophisticated bike lanes are a regular feature of mainstream Chinese urban planning.

Source: Michael Kodransky. Available online at www.flickr.com/photos/itdp/5667737574/.

Nevertheless, the United States overall is way behind cities such as Barcelona, Spain; Paris, France; London, England; and for that matter, Curitiba, Brazil, and Guangzhou, China (see figure 11.5). In those cities, folks who cannot afford to buy a bicycle (or worry constantly about it getting stolen) can still cheaply rent bicycles at stations conveniently located at public transit stations, and congestion pricing in the cities heavily taxes cars—providing yet another (dis)incentive for folks to drive into town. Years after Bangkok, Hangzhou, and many other major cities, New York City was just getting its first bike share program at the time of press. Without the snazzy bicycles and streetcars, Londoners would just complain that the politicians' congestion tax made their commutes too expensive and vote them out of office. The combination of citywide changes and individual-based incentive programs helps Londoners instead to brag that they lost six pounds (or, as they would say, about half a stone) in just a couple of months by cycling to work without spending money or time at a gym. Both citywide changes, especially in zoning and the promotion of mixed-use and dense areas, and individual-based incentive programs appear to be essential in encouraging population-wide lifestyle changes (Appleyard et al., 2007; Goldman & Gorham, 2006).

Unfortunate disconnects arise when governments spend money trying to convince low-income families to "value" or take advantage of opportunities that do not meaningfully exist. It is difficult for poor people to "simply" stop eating junk food when they do not have access to fresh produce in their local bodegas or their neighborhoods, when such fresh produce tends to exist at the Whole Foods Market on the other side of town and cost half their paycheck, and when they do not receive a good education on how to make budgetary choices. (That said, many well-educated folks and Congress need help learning to budget as well.) For example, New York City offered US$1,000 to low-income African American and Latino high schoolers who scored perfect fives on Advanced Placement (AP) exams, but several student-led community organizing groups held protests at City Hall demanding that their schools even *offer* AP classes and college-preparatory course work (Alonso, Anderson, Su, & Theoharis, 2009).

So-called market-oriented incentive programs can play an important role in health policy making, but they must be well-designed to fit the local context's cultural norms, infrastructure, and resources. Real-life public health policies aiming at comprehensive reform must be multipronged, and they end up being quite complex. For example, in 2004, New York City's Department of Health launched "Take Care New York," which focused on biomedical interventions such as cancer screenings and clinical guidelines for cholesterol control. Thomas Friedan, the city's health commissioner and later the head of the Centers for Disease Control in the Obama administration, stated that the campaign's "success depends greatly on the power of clinical setting and on the influence of physicians and other providers" (quoted in Corburn, 2009, p. 120).

Attempts at More Comprehensive Approaches

In the end, the ten leading risk factors (smoking, obesity, high blood pressure, illicit drug use, unsafe sex, etc.) cumulatively account for only 30 percent of disease among men in the United States (Murray et al., 2006). An increasing number of city planners thus see that they need to tackle individual risk behaviors and larger social environmental structures in more comprehensive ways. Many are evaluating public transit, housing, economic development legislation, zoning, and other aspects of the built environment to help to determine how, and how long, residents live.

In the same year as the Take Care New York campaign, the San Francisco Department of Public Health's Strategic Plan tackled not only unhealthy eating, smoking, and other individual risk behaviors but also the four priority social determinants of (1) low socioeconomic status, (2) social isolation and connectedness, (3) institutional racism (including racial disparities in where sewage treatment plants, hazardous lots, amenities such as public parks and well-funded schools, and well-stocked produce suppliers were located), and (4) transportation. By 2007, they had developed the healthy development measurement tool (HDMT, www.thehdmt.org), a comprehensive evaluation metric for all cities and neighborhoods to use themselves in considering health needs in urban development. The measurement tool includes 6 key elements, 28 objectives, and 125 indicators. For example, the "Healthy Economy" key element has four objectives, such as "increase high-quality employment opportunities for local residents." This particular objective has four indicators, including "jobs paying wages greater than or equal to the self-sufficiency wage" and "proportion of estimated entry-level jobs accessible to individuals with a GED or high school diploma." Each of these indicators then comes with a table on the exact local "self-sufficiency wages," as well as how they were calculated, so that another city can calculate its own.

In sharp contrast to the Take Care New York indicators, most of the HDMT indexes focus on environmental factors such as neighborhood violent crime rates, clean air quality, affordable and high-quality child care and schooling, proportion of residents within a half mile from a bank or credit union, and so on. HDMT tracks health outcomes such as diabetes hospitalization rates per thousand residents, but mainly as part of its baseline and impact assessments.

In 2006, San Francisco also launched the Healthy San Francisco program to subsidize medical and dental care to uninsured residents. San Francisco residents who make less than 500 percent of the federal poverty line (in 2011, that was US$54,480 for a household of one) are eligible for the program. (See www.healthysanfrancisco.org for more information.)

In 2009, Take Care New York initiated a revamped campaign. When compared to the 2004 version, the 2009 Take Care New York objectives pay much greater attention to environmental and social factors outside the clinical setting, especially in the "make all neighborhoods healthy places" section. The "promote physical activity and healthy eating" section, for instance, emphasized new restaurant bans against transfat and attempted reforms regarding soda and salt, alongside clinical recommendations. Likewise, the "reduce risky alcohol use and drug dependence" section advises policy makers to "promote alternatives to incarcerating for low-level drug offenses" and develop counter-alcohol advertising campaigns alongside "increasing the use of buprenorphine for opioid dependence."

As compared to the San Francisco Health Department's indicators, however, Take Care New York 2012 continues to focus on individuals as units of analysis and biomedical models. This is especially pronounced in the "raise healthy children" section, which is fairly narrowly confined to promoting breast-feeding and immunization, screening for developmental disorders, and other medical interventions.

Although these practices are evidence based and important, they do not integrate with urban planning and other social determinant–oriented social policies to the same degree as San Francisco's model. Take Care New York's framework notably sidelines discussions of civic engagement, social cohesion, and governance. Frieden stated as much when he said that "the sanitary measures adopted are sometimes autocratic, and the functions performed by sanitary authorities paternal in character." At the same time, Mary Bassett, who worked as deputy director of health promotion and disease prevention with Frieden, noted that "health never improves without the engagement of the community . . . You have to change the policy environment, but health never improves through engineering alone" (quoted in Colgrove, 2011, pp. 255–256).

SUMMARY

The social environment is thought to be one of the biggest drivers of health from childhood through adulthood. Harsh living conditions place psychological stress on the family. This can affect adult health behaviors, and health more generally, in adulthood, but it can also affect children for the remainder of their lives, even if conditions improve. Race, class, and gender are all factors that can affect one's social environment, with low-income people, ethnic minorities, and women sometimes relegated to lower-paying jobs and professions. In low-income countries, discrimination against these groups is sometimes even sanctioned by the government. Girls, minorities, and the very poor are sometimes unable to attend school altogether. When faced with an economic choice between educating boys or girls, many families will choose to educate boys, for instance. Wealthy countries often attempt to improve the social environment through education, health, employment, and urban planning policies. There is a strong global movement currently under way to improve living conditions in urban areas by building projects such as parks and bike lanes in the hope that improvement in conditions will improve the social environment and health.

KEY TERMS

active tuberculosis	*forms of capital*	*social classes*
cultural capital	*gender*	*social environment*
economic capital	*institutional racism*	*social forces*
extended contact	*intersectionalities*	*socially constructed*
investigation	*missing women*	*superbugs*
feminization	*phenomenon*	

DISCUSSION QUESTIONS

1. What are the five most common diseases in the country where you live? In what ways may these diseases be socially constructed? Are they evenly distributed through the national population?

2. If men and women have very different life expectancies but do not tend to die from diseases biologically tied to a single sex (such as testicular cancer or ovarian cancer), what are some of the key ways in which gender shapes health outcomes?

3. You have been appointed the new food policy chief in a city in Pakistan. You would like to change the diets of the local populace and especially help young girls eat more and healthier. What issues would you consider in designing your program, outside of budget limitations? Does the local social environment shape your policy proposals? How so?

FURTHER READING

Alcabes, P. (2010). *Dread: How fear and fantasy have fueled epidemics from the Black Death to the avian flu.* New York: PublicAffairs.

Game changer: Janette Sadik-Khan, road ruler. Time Video. Available online at www.time.com/time/video/player/0,32068,1155928905001_2093105,00.html

Man drinking fat. NYC health anti-soda ad. Are you pouring on the pounds? (2009). [Advertisement from the New York City Department of Health and Mental Hygiene.] Available online at www.youtube.com/watch?v=-F4t8zL6F0c

REFERENCES

Alonso, G., Anderson, N., Su, C., & Theoharis, J. (2009). *Our schools suck: Students talk back to a segregated nation on the failures of urban education.* New York: New York University Press.

Appleyard, B., Zheng, Y., Watson, R., Bruce, L., Sohmer, R., Li, X., & Qian, J. (2007). *Smart cities: Solutions for China's rapid urbanization.* New York: National Resources Defense Council.

Belani, H. K., & Muennig, P. A. (2008). Cost-effectiveness of needle and syringe exchange for the prevention of HIV in New York City. *Journal of HIV/AIDS & Social Services, 7*(3), 229–240.

Christakis, N. A., & Fowler, J. H. (2007). The spread of obesity in a large social network over 32 years. *New England Journal of Medicine, 357*, 370–379. doi: 10.1056/NEJMsa066082.

Cohen, J. (2010a). The ins and outs of HIV. *Science, 327*(5970), 1196.

Cohen, J. (2010b). New HIV infections drop, but treatment demands rise. *Science*, *330*(6009), 1301.

Colgrove, J. (2011). *Epidemic city: The politics of public health in New York*. New York: Russell Sage Foundation.

Corburn, J. (2009). *Toward the healthy city: People, places, and the politics of urban planning*. Cambridge, MA: MIT Press.

Davies, P. D. (2005). Risk factors for tuberculosis. *Monaldi Archives for Chest Disease*, *63*(1), 37–46.

Donald, P. R., & van Helden, P. D. (2009). The global burden of tuberculosis—combatting drug resistance in difficult times. *New England Journal of Medicine*, *360*(23), 2393.

Dye, C., Scheele, S., Dolin, P., Pathania, V., & Raviglione, M. C. (1999). Global burden of tuberculosis: Estimated incidence, prevalence, and mortality by country. *JAMA*, *282*(7), 677.

Frassanito, P., & Pettorini, B. (2008). Pink and blue: The color of gender. *Child's Nervous System*, *24*(8), 881–882.

Gandhi, N. R., Moll, A., Sturm, A. W., Pawinski, R., Govender, T., Lalloo, U., et al. (2006). Extensively drug-resistant tuberculosis as a cause of death in patients co-infected with tuberculosis and HIV in a rural area of South Africa. *Lancet*, *368*(9547), 1575–1580.

Goldman, T., & Gorham, R. (2006). Sustainable urban transport: Four innovative directions. *Technology in Society*, *28*(1–2), 261–273.

Gray, R. H., Wawer, M. J., Brookmeyer, R., Sewankambo, N. K., Serwadda, D., Wabwire-Mangen, F., et al. (2001). Probability of HIV-1 transmission per coital act in monogamous, heterosexual, HIV-1-discordant couples in Rakai, Uganda. *Lancet*, *357*(9263), 1149–1153.

Holloway, M. (1994). Trends in women's health: A global view. *Scientific American*, *271*(2), 66–73.

Hvistendah, M. (2011). *Unnatural selection: Choosing boys over girls, and the consequences of a world full of men*. New York: Public Affairs.

Khan, K., Muennig, P., Behta, M., & Zivin, J. G. (2002). Global drug-resistance patterns and the management of latent tuberculosis infection in immigrants to the United States. *New England Journal of Medicine*, *347*(23), 1850–1859.

Korber, B., Muldoon, M., Theiler, J., Gao, F., Gupta, R., Lapedes, A., et al. (2000). Timing the ancestor of the HIV-1 pandemic strains. *Science*, *288*(5472), 1789.

LaFraniere, S. (2011, August 4). Chinese officials seized and sold babies, parents say. *New York Times*. Available online at www.nytimes.com/2011/08/05/world/asia/05kidnapping.html

Lewis, S. (2006). *Race against time: Searching for hope in AIDS-ravaged Africa*. Toronto: House of Anansi Press.

Love, S. M., & Lindsey, K. (2010). *Dr. Susan Love's breast book*. Cambridge, MA: Da Capo Lifelong Books.

Mayoux, L. (2001). Tackling the down side: Social capital, women's empowerment and micro finance in Cameroon. *Development and Change, 32*(3), 435–464.

Murray, C.J.L., Kulkarni, S. C., Michaud, C., Tomijima, N., Bulzacchelli, M. T., Iandiorio, T. J., & Ezzati, M. (2006). Eight Americas: Investigating mortality disparities across races, counties, and race-counties in the United States. *PLoS Medicine, 3*(9), 1513–1524.

Nelson, K. E., Celentano, D. D., Eiumtrakol, S., Hoover, D. R., Beyrer, C., Suprasert, S., et al. (1996). Changes in sexual behavior and a decline in HIV infection among young men in Thailand. *New England Journal of Medicine, 335*(5), 297.

O'Grady, J. (2011, 29 April). *Biking on the rise in the city, DOT Says*. National Public Radio. Available online at www.wnyc.org/articles/wnyc-news/2011/apr/29/department-transportation-says-streets-aresafer-biking

Omi, M., & Winant, H. (1994). *Racial formation in the United States: From the 1960s to the 1990s*. New York: Routledge.

Oppenheimer, G. (2001). Paradigm lost: Race, ethnicity, and the search for a new population taxonomy. *American Journal of Public Health, 91*, 1049–1055.

Paoletti, J. (2012). *Pink and blue: Telling the girls from the boys in America*. Bloomington: Indiana University Press.

Putnam, R. D. (2001). *Bowling alone: The collapse and revival of American community*. New York: Simon & Schuster.

Rankin, K. N. (2002). Social capital, microfinance, and the politics of development. *Feminist Economics, 8*(1), 1–24.

Sampson, R. J. (2002). Crime and public safety: Insights from community-level perspectives on social capital. In S. T. Saegert, J. Phillip, & M. R. Warren (Eds.), *Social capital and poor communities* (pp. 89–114). New York: Russell Sage Foundation.

Sen, A. (1999). *Development as freedom*. New York: Knopf.

Sen, G., Östlin, P., & George, A. (2007). Unequal, unfair, ineffective and inefficient. Gender inequity in health: Why it exists and how we can change it. *Final Report to the WHO Commission on Social Determinants of Health*. Available online at www.who.int/social_determinants/resources/csdh_media/wgekn_final_report_07.pdf

Stayton, C., Olson, C., Thorpe, L., Kerker, B., Henning, K., & Wilt, S. (2008). *Intimate partner violence against women in New York City*. New York: New York City Department of Health and Mental Hygiene.

UN. (2010, January 7). *The Joint United Nations Program on HIV/AIDS*. Available online at www.unaids.org/en

Wegbreit, J., Bertozzi, S., DeMaria, L. M., & Padian, N. S. (2006). Effectiveness of HIV prevention strategies in resource-poor countries: Tailoring the intervention to the context. *AIDS, 20*(9), 1217.

Weniger, B. G., Limpakarnjanarat, K., Ungchusak, K., Thanprasertsuk, S., Choopanya, K., Vanichseni, S., et al. (1991). The epidemiology of HIV infection and AIDS in Thailand. *AIDS*, *5*, 71.

Woolcock, M. (1998). Social capital and economic development: Toward a theoretical synthesis and policy framework. *Theory and Society*, *27*, 151–208.

Worobey, M., Gemmel, M., Teuwen, D. E., Haselkorn, T., Kunstman, K., Bunce, M., et al. (2008). Direct evidence of extensive diversity of HIV-1 in Kinshasa by 1960. *Nature*, *455*(7213), 661–664.

CHAPTER 12

Globalization, Internal Conflict, and the Resource Curse

KEY IDEAS

- Globalization promises to bring amazing advances in health, technology, and global peace, but it also presents challenges for public health. In nations with weak governance, increased income—whether in the form of trade, aid, or natural resources—can lead to civil war when different groups vie for power and wealth.

- The most contentious working definition of globalization is that of trade liberalization, often imposed by intergovernmental institutions such as the WTO.

- Poor governance exacerbates the potential for so-called resource curses and civil conflict, whereby the presence of rich natural resources brings about inequality and strife rather than a higher quality of life.

GLOBALIZATION AND HEALTH

Globalization takes many forms: mass migration, ease of travel, social networking via websites and applications such as Facebook and Twitter, diffusion and mixing of musical genres such hip-hop and bhangra, and racial blending. Who would argue that the blending of people, cultures, and ideas is a bad thing? As it turns out, some do complain about globalization but not technological advances, cultural exchange, or attempts to create a socially just "global village." Rather, the so-called antiglobalization groups are protesting a more narrowly defined version of globalization, especially trade liberalization. The

antiglobalization groups are a diffuse and varied bunch that include the traveling South Korean farmers protesting subsidized beef from the United States, the residents of the disappearing Tuvalu islands pleading for help in stemming climate change, and collectives of anarchists. They are advocating for stronger international regulations on free trade, and many of them are doing so for health reasons.

Globalization, including the free trade of goods across borders, is undoubtedly a positive development overall. But like many good things, it carries with it unintended side effects. These include the ability of diseases to spread rapidly across borders, damage to local economies, and incentives for bad people to dominate weakly governed but resource-rich nations for their own benefit. Other conflicts arise, too. For instance, how do we balance the incentives for drug companies to innovate against the need for poor nations to use their innovations to combat HIV/AIDS, heart disease, and cancer? In this chapter, we focus on free trade and the resource curse.

WHAT IS SO WONDERFUL AND TERRIBLE ABOUT FREE TRADE?

Free trade is great in theory. Currently, nations place taxes or other regulations on goods from other countries that enter their borders. This requires substantial layers of bureaucracy and costs on a good thing—inexpensive goods and services from abroad. After all, if we have free trade across borders, the consumer can simply pick those goods that are the highest quality for the price. Some of these goods and services, such as pharmaceuticals, can directly improve health. Cheaper goods and services, coupled with less bureaucracy involved in procuring them, can indirectly improve the health of very poor nations by growing the economy and thereby lifting very poor people out of poverty. Free trade also challenges the very notion of borders, offering the hope of less armed conflict.

Of course, transactions in the real world are never so simple. Many nations' internal markets are fragile, and floods of cheap goods can lead to increased unemployment and thereby worsen poverty. Moreover, some goods, particularly agricultural products, are subsidized by foreign governments. This makes for unfair competition for nations that cannot afford to subsidize the goods that they produce.

There are many other reasons for regulating the flow of goods across borders as well. Some nations produce lead-tainted toys or medicines laced with radiator fluid. Without proper border checks, a country that otherwise produces goods with high consumer safety standards risks harming its people by importing unsafe goods. This threat was illustrated by the case of Panama, a nation that produces high-quality, low-cost medicines for its people. Panama ended up poisoning its people with fake glycerin, a common inert ingredient in medications. The government believed that it was purchasing quality glycerin from Spain. Instead, it was purchasing radiator fluid from an unscrupulous, unregulated company in China that had been passed through to Panama via Spain.

Since the 1960s, the world has rapidly industrialized, thanks in part to multinational corporations that cross borders. Many of these multinational corporations have economies larger than those of entire countries. Although many bring unimaginable benefits to the global economy—cures for diseases, four-pound computers that perform more calculations than a computer the size of a room did ten years ago, trains that run more than two hundred miles an hour—others, such as cigarette companies and fast food chains, bring harm. The profit motive of corporations, good or bad, incentivizes them to constantly move to nations where environmental regulations are weak, obviating the benefits of environmental regulations in wealthier nations. With a global standard for environmental and health regulations, it would be possible to reap many of the benefits of multinationals without realizing as many of the harms. But, as we have pointed out many times previously, global governance on such matters is nearly nonexistent.

GLOBALIZATION IS NOT EXACTLY A NEW PHENOMENON

In the mid-nineteenth century, US bullet cartridges were coated in lard (pork fat) and tallow (beef fat) (Hibbert, 1980). To use these, one was required to "bite the bullet" before it was put in the rifle and fired. Many rifles were made in England, and the English rifles were used by Indians under British rule. But many of the bullet cartridges were made in the northeastern United States and sold to the United Kingdom. Consuming pork fat is seen as sacrilegious by Muslims, just as consuming cow fat is by Hindus. When it became known that Muslims and Hindus had been inadvertently sinning at the hands of the British, they were none too happy. Little did the New Englanders making these cartridges know that their run-of-the-mill bullet coatings would spark a major rebellion. When the Hindus and Muslims discovered what they were biting, they rose up and the mutiny eventually contributed to the campaign for Indian independence.

Today, trade flows, the global repercussions of local events, and traveling phenomena are ever-more complex. The earthquake, tsunamis, nuclear fallout, and rolling blackouts in Japan in 2011 immediately shut down car factories in the United States and Apple electronics factories in China; transcontinental supply chains are much more integrated now. On the upside, this dimension of globalization also compels South Koreans to care about cotan (a mineral that is used in cell phone manufacturing plants) reserves in rainforests in Congo, the Chinese to care about Australia, and Africans to care about trade agreements in Europe. Moreover, as we become an economically globalized world, perhaps the cost of war has become more tangible now than people dying in remote battlefields were decades ago.

Not only would effective global governance help stem the spread of disease via monitoring and containment, it could also help to prevent outbreaks from ever happening in the first place. For instance, multidrug-resistant organisms arise from overuse. In many places, it is possible to simply buy antibiotics over the counter, and these are often sold to people who do not understand how to use them. Often, people take them for inappropriate infections or use inappropriate dosing, providing an opportunity for organisms to mutate. This also occurs when agriculture is not regulated; it is more profitable to raise livestock in overcrowded conditions and to stem infections with antibiotics than it is to run a smaller farm.

The labor, environmental, social, and health spillover effects of trade policies may be contained as technology advances. EMRs can stem drug resistance by ensuring that medical providers are administering the correct antibiotic given the patients' diagnosis, for instance. Middle-income nations can sometimes leapfrog over problems associated with industrialization by using modern technologies to protect the environment and workers.

But technology is also creating many of the problems. Epidemics such as SARS spread much more rapidly than they did before leisure flight travel was so commonplace. A boat containing a SARS patient would probably be detected well in advance of landing in a trans-Atlantic trip.

Our global governance institutions have not caught up with the ways global public health problems currently unfold. For example, only one in four people sick with tuberculosis has access to life-saving drugs that cost just US$16 for a full course of treatment, and some of these folks are not getting full-strength medications (Dye, Scheele, Dolin, Pathania, & Raviglione, 1999). Some drug manufacturers place only small quantities of drug in their pills so that the pills can pass basic inspections by regulators. Sometimes, antibiotic resistance arises when unscrupulous drug companies place too little medication in the drugs they sell. Multidrug resistant tuberculosis (MDRTB) affects roughly half a million people each year (Farmer, 2004; Frieden et al., 1993; Garrett, 2000). Of those who contract MDRTB, most die from it. More than one-third of countries around the world report MDRTB rates higher than 2 percent (Khan, Muennig, Behta, & Zivin, 2002). In the United States, there are high rates of MDRTB in states with high prison populations, such as California, New York, and Texas. These drugs must be taken for a long time, so it provides an opportunity for the TB to slowly adapt to having the medications in its environment. It is conceivable that MDRTB will one day be as common as regular tuberculosis, a disease that kills two million people a year, five thousand a day, two hundred people an hour. In the meantime, coordinated and well-allocated resources could go a long way in stemming the spread of MDRTB.

Because the WTO is a global governance institution, we would expect that it would help provide such protections. But as we discussed in chapter 8, it does not. Decisions are made in backroom deliberations rather than via public votes, and these decisions tend to focus on maximizing trade profits with little consideration given to saving lives.

SPILLOVER EFFECTS OF POOR GLOBAL GOVERNANCE

Without an effective global government, it is difficult to tackle global pandemics, to prevent war, to stem plagues, to address antibiotic resistance, or even to build international roads. Rivers that start in one country can be completely depleted or polluted by the time they flow into the next.

In the next section of this chapter, we look at one example of one problem associated with a lack of global governance, **civil conflict.** This is meant to illustrate the scale and scope of the problems we face when governments cannot coordinate to act in the interests of the world's people. We start off by introducing civil conflict as a public health problem. We then discuss how civil conflict can be paradoxically fostered by a nation's natural resource wealth.

CIVIL CONFLICT AS A PUBLIC HEALTH PROBLEM

Before we can understand the resource curse—a phenomenon driven by global markets—we must take a step back and understand civil conflict as a public health problem. Despite their name, civil conflicts transcend borders; they are a major problem in global governance. Even if the actual fighting is happening within a country, the conditions that led to or exacerbate the violent conflict can involve volatile global commodity markets, corrupt politicians, a weak set of international regulatory or peacekeeping institutions, and unscrupulous business and trade partners (such as certain gun suppliers, diamond buyers, or oil companies).

If a California governor began killing off people in Los Angeles because they were overrepresenting an opposition party, the US government would quickly send in the national army. But there is no clear way of stopping this from happening within Rwanda or Somalia. At least not really. A dictator (almost always a man) has so poorly governed a country that he stirs up ethnic hatred or starts a war with a neighbor in order to stay in power. Often, the dictator is funded by national riches, such as oil and diamonds, as well as the production of illicit commodities, such as opium and cocaine. So, one could tackle the problem by closing bank accounts, banning exports of oil, or moving in with a military force.

But who might take action? The UN might pass a Security Council resolution. Regional governance organizations such as the Arab League might go at it alone if the UN fails to act. Certainly, NGOs and civil society groups would become involved in delivering humanitarian assistance to the groups that were most affected. But the ultimate action taken depends on the collective political will to act, the players involved, and the resources at stake. For instance, public policies in Burma (Myanmar) continue to effectively commit genocide against one of its ethnic minorities, the Rohingya. This is happening even as the country moves to a more democratic model of governance. Though it has significant mineral resources that many nations want, these are mostly currently controlled by Thailand and China (though other nations such as the United States were moving in at the time of press). Any change in the status quo would mean huge losses for China's companies. But the remaining Rohingya population is small, and as a poor Muslim minority group, it has little international voice.

It is incredibly difficult to estimate the collective numbers of casualties in contemporary conflicts such as the killing off of the Rohingya. One week prior to the time of writing this section, there was a conflict between Rohingya and non-Rongya Burmans in Arakan state, and it was estimated that ten thousand Rohingya were displaced from their homes. However, this estimate was almost entirely subjective because there was no way to measure who was moving where.

However they are derived, it is likely that the numbers are large. One estimate suggests that the twenty-five largest instances of violent conflict in the last century led to approximately 191 million deaths, with civilians suffering most of the casualties (Thoms & Ron, 2007; WHO, 2002). This is more than the size of the entire population of Japan. Each year, almost two million people die because of violence, including interstate or civil conflicts (Iqbal, 2006). In Iraq, where more reliable numbers are possible, it was estimated that 650,000 Iraqis died in the first three years after the 2003 post-invasion insurgency alone (Burnham, Lafta, Doocy, & Roberts, 2006). In the Sudan, more than two million people were killed since 1983, and over four million people were internally displaced. Imagine four million people without shelter or latrines and you will get a sense of the public health problems associated with these conflicts. The WHO sets emergency levels at one death per ten thousand people per day, but some villages in the Sudan experienced death rates of five times that (Zwi, 2004).

By now you probably will have guessed that the most devastating, long-ranging, and pervasive effects are not of bullets or doctors who treat wounds but from displacement of people from their ecological niche, disruption of food supplies, and loss of economic opportunity among the innocent bystanders of conflict.

In conflict, of course people die from wounds from weapons, but heightened rates of infectious diseases such as malaria, cholera, and typhoid fever tend to take many more lives. Sexual violence also tends to increase, along with increased numbers of HIV/AIDS infections (too often from rape). Food insecurity and rape are often not just by-products of war, but are also sanctioned by despotic governments who wish to eliminate or psychologically terrorize segments of their population. Skyrocketing rates of acute and chronic malnutrition and mental illness compound these challenges (Zwi, 2004).

Just as physical and mental disease rates skyrocket, the ability to address them crumbles in conflict situations. An unstable political environment makes any public policy difficult to legislate and implement. But areas of conflict are almost always lacking in these basic services to begin with. The states' inability to provide for their constituencies, especially in an equitable, relatively transparent or democratic manner, is also the root cause of many instances of violent conflict as frustration with ineffective, thieving governments rises.

When Liberia experienced conflict at the end of the twentieth century, there were points when only roughly 30 percent of Liberians could access clean water or latrines (Iqbal, 2006). In Sudan, violent conflict prevented children from attending schools, becoming immunized, or receiving adequate nutrition or infant care. A girl born in southern Sudan in the heart of the conflict had a greater chance of dying than completing primary school (Zwi, 2004).

What can be done to address the aftermath of conflict in the absence of a global governance structure? There are humanitarian efforts, such as those by the group Doctors Without Borders. There are development aid efforts, such as those described in chapter 4, for the reconstruction periods after conflict. But the lag in international aid, coordination, and interventions is a consistent problem in addressing the public health implications of violent conflict (Canavan, Vergeer, & Bornemisza, 2008). Regardless, such efforts are merely superficial bandages. Unless policy makers can address the root causes of the conflicts, and unless intergovernmental institutions, national governments, and NGOs can together build the social, economic, and political institutions needed to provide entire populations with human security, conflict will remain a major public health problem.

RESOURCE CURSES AND CIVIL CONFLICT

In 1975, most Venezuelans were optimistic about their country's rich natural resources, economic growth, and a corresponding rise in their quality of life in the coming decades. But Juan Pablo Pérez Alfonzo, a Venezuelan former oil minister and founder of OPEC, declared, "I call petroleum the devil's excrement. It brings trouble . . . Look at this *locura*—waste, corruption, consumption, our public services falling apart. And debt, debt we shall have for years" (quoted in *Economist,* 2003, p. 78).

The so-called resource curse, a **paradox of plenty,** is an overall umbrella term for the ailments plaguing countries that boast of great natural wealth such as diamonds and crude oil but surprisingly do worse, not better, in terms of economic, social, and human development. Endemic governmental corruption, insufficient taxation, excessive spending, lack of diversification, and lack of social investments are the most common symptoms of a resource curse (Humphreys, Sachs, & Stiglitz, 2007).

Combine these patterns with revenue volatility, and it becomes clearer why countries with precious commodities are often fragile states. The prices of commodities such as oil can also fluctuate wildly. When a nation teeters along dependent on revenue from oil or minerals, and the price of that commodity falls on international markets, the nation finds itself unable to finance basic, day-to-day operations. So countries that rely on oil cash leave their schools and roads half built until oil prices again increase. For some of the countries struggling with this paradox of plenty, revenues from oil and diamonds constitute the bulk of their GDP.

CHINA IN AFRICA

China has received heaps of attention in the popular press, mostly negative, for supporting dictators and human rights–abusing regimes in Africa with its economic aid. It also has been criticized for exporting Chinese workers for major African infrastructure projects without regard to local laborers or environmental consequences and for sidelining local industries (Alden, 2007). China received the bulk of international attention for selling arms to the Sudan, for instance. A closer look yields a more complicated picture, however.

China has been important for economic development in Africa since the 1960s. Its presence certainly has become more notable in the past two decades as its economic might has grown. The aid packages on offer by China tend to be loans with market-rate interest deals, so they look much more like business transactions than aid. However, these deals also tend to have much friendlier terms for African nations than their Western firm counterparts. Moreover, many Chinese-sponsored projects actually use local Africans for more than 90 percent of their labor. Finally, China also generally disburses oil-backed loans directly to Chinese companies rather than to corrupt governments (Brautigam, 2010).

Despite being called a *new colonialist,* Chinese arms transfers to African democracies have exceeded those of the United States. The United States, by contrast, has historically sent more arms to autocratic states than democratic ones (Midford & de Soysa, 2010). In fact, the Ukraine and Russia have exported many more arms to Africa, including to the Sudan and Zimbabwe, than China has. And regardless of whether it is exporting arms or is a new colonist in Africa, its activities remain somewhat small compared to those of the United States and Europe. Before the Libyan revolution, China imported an average of 150,000 barrels of oil per day from Libya, for instance. But Italy and France imported 581,000 barrels per day from that nation. China's development aid budget overall remains small, compared to the US one. Nevertheless, China has more of its stakes in Africa. In 2011, more than 44 percent of its aid was directed to this continent in comparison to roughly 1 percent of US aid (Midford & de Soysa, 2010).

As of 2011, China was also in the process of setting up six economic cooperation zones (see figure 12.1). Recall that these are the sorts of special "enterprise" zones that turned Shenzhen and other cities in China into economic powerhouses. China wants to replace its bottom-rung jobs

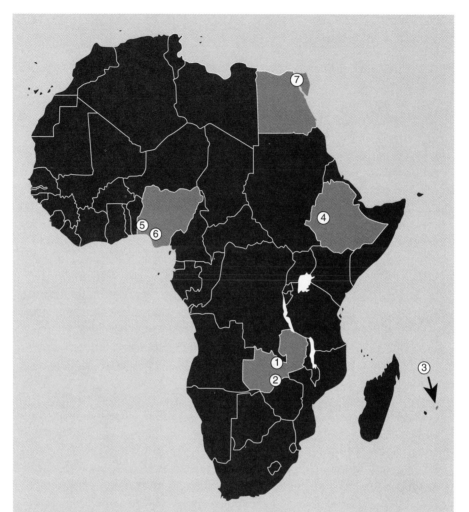

Figure 12.1. This map shows six special economic zones set up by the Chinese government in areas of Africa.

Source: Image ReferencePAR52903(RIO1985004K026) © Miguel Rio Branco/ Magnum Photos.

with better ones, so that "made in China" is not the pejorative, cheap signifier it currently is. This means that, if successful, these economic cooperation zones may bring the deplorable labor conditions and environmental consequences that China has suffered through since the 1990s to Africa. But they may also bring the infrastructural and technological advances that Africa needs to flourish.

This is not at all to excuse China; indeed, the situation beckons intergovernmental institutions such as the WHO and the UN as well as the European Union and the United States to hold *everyone* to the same standard. To address public health issues, global governance institutions must regulate arms sales to questionable autocratic regimes, set up some trade protections or subsidies for infant industries such as renewable wind energy for households, and set up guidelines regarding the percentage of local workers and local participation required in loan economic development projects as well as aid ones.

Venezuela's GDP has risen dramatically, so this one is a harder argument to make. Angola, Burma, Iraq, and Nigeria are all examples of countries that should be rich because they have a lot of oil but are poor because they are poorly governed. From 1965 to 1998, average GNP per capita decreased in OPEC countries, even as it increased in other low-income nations (Gylfason, 2001). There are, of course, exceptions such as Norway as well as more tempered cases such as Kuwait or Botswana. But how do we make these exceptional cases the norm? Burma, also known officially as Myanmar, appeared to be emerging from the resource curse at the time of writing but its future was still unclear.

There are some aspects of the resource curse that appear to be harder to escape. For example, a sudden increase in national revenues from the oil or other resource exports can cause inflation. This makes many other aspects of the national economy—such as health or education—more expensive because workers demand higher wages as their cost of living increases.

Finally, and most important, there is often governmental collusion with, rather than accountability of, industries in many resource-rich countries. Payments by oil companies too often line the pockets of individual politicians, who then allow the companies to drill for petroleum even where it is environmentally unsound or unsafe for health reasons. This is also true when the work has high social costs (such as mass displacement of people) or brings about unequal benefits (such as riches to one specific region or ethnic group, whereas others get no benefits from private companies *or* basics from government).

Alas, the answer is not a simple order of "democracy." The relationship between democracy and peace (or its flip side, violent conflict) is far from straightforward. Between democracy and civil conflict, some researchers argue that regimes that are neither total dictatorships nor democracies experience more violent conflict than either democracies or dictatorships (Hegre, Ellingsen, Gates, & Gleditsch, 2001). Still, although corruption certainly occurs in democracies, corruption is especially destructive (in terms of the health consequences) in low-income and autocratic settings because it is impossible to kick scoundrels out of office (Drury, Krieckhaus, & Lusztig, 2006). Some have recommended direct transfers of revenues—universal, transparent, and regular payments to individuals—that are then taxed by the government (Moss, 2011). Ideally, this sort of policy can kick-start new cycles of accountability for public fiscal coffers.

It is important to remember that resource-rich countries do not have to succumb to the resource curse. Botswana, for example, has been able to not only avert violent conflict but also build the sort of social democratic political economy—the sort of economic *and* political structures—that lead to prosperity and good health outcomes. Alongside Mauritius, it is the only African country that has held regular elections for more than forty years, since independence from colonial powers.

There is no single factor that differentiates these countries from the rest of the continent; Botswana and Nigeria inherited precolonial political institutions, but Nigeria has been plagued with its resource curse and Botswana has not. Some might say that Botswana has an easier time because it boasts of a relatively ethnically homogenous population (Sandbrook, Edelman, Heller, & Teichman, 2007). Research shows that even seemingly homogenous populations can splinter under economic duress, especially along class or religious lines. It makes a difference that Botswana's ruling governments have shared the benefits of growth so that they might survive and be reelected.

In Botswana, free public education and decent university systems have helped citizens to expand from hard labor–intensive jobs into more human capital–intensive jobs, such as tourism (McFerson, 2009; Sandbrook et al., 2007). Public health facilities are widely distributed across the countries and serve all subpopulations. Botswana provides antiretroviral therapy to the one hundred thousand or so HIV-positive citizens. When it and its neighboring countries experienced food shortages in 1983 and 1984, Botswana did not experience a famine partly because its government responded by creating jobs within its public programs; by contrast, Ethiopia and Sudan experienced famines even though their food decline had been smaller than Botswana's (Dreze & Sen, 1989). Botswana's experience suggests that good governance leads to good social policies, and in turn, good social policies lead to better health outcomes.

The Case of the Niger Delta

The Niger Delta, in the south of Nigeria, serves as a good case study of the complex interplay between domestic and international interests, ethnicity, unequal economic benefits, and violent conflict in an oil-rich area. Companies have been extracting oil from the area since the 1940s, and the national economy quickly became dependent on it. Oil constituted 25 percent of the national GDP in the 1980s and more than 60 percent by the late 2000s. With flares of civil conflict and general poor governance, other parts of the economy (such as groundnuts, rubber, and cocoa) shrank in absolute terms by as much as 65 percent (Okonta & Douglas, 2001). Large portions of the national population moved to the hub of oil production, the Niger Delta. As a result, the area quickly urbanized without much by way of social infrastructure or sufficient jobs.

Two main sets of violent tensions grew since the 1990s: first, the primarily Ogoni people of Ogoniland, a part of the Niger Delta, protested that Royal Dutch Shell, Chevron, and the Nigerian government forcibly appropriated their land without consultation or proper compensation in the 1950s. After attempting to gain compensation for more than three decades, an Ogoni group demanded in 1992 that oil companies pay them US$10 billion in compensation, that oil companies change their drilling procedures to prevent further environmental damage, and that citizens be involved in future decision making about local oil drilling. The Nigerian government banned freedom of assembly and declared that interrupting oil production was an act of treason. Military repression in 1994 led to the deaths of more than two thousand civilians and displacement of one hundred thousand villagers. Nine of the Ogoni leaders were found guilty of "incitement" and hanged without due process.

Complicating matters, long-simmering tensions between the Ijaw, the Itsekiri, and the Urhobo ethnic groups erupted over control of the resource-rich Warri region of the Niger Delta. In December 1998, the Nigerian military clamped down on Ijaw villages and killed hundreds of civilians. Although Nigeria became democratic in 1999, the root causes of the conflicts—namely, pervasive unemployment for young men, deep economic inequalities that leave the largest Ijaw group especially disenfranchised, a massive inflow of weapons, lack of participatory decision making on oil drilling, environmental degradation, and lack of compensation for past displacement and land appropriation—remain largely unaddressed. Thus, armed groups in the Niger Delta have grown markedly in the past decade, and conflict continues to this day, despite numerous governmental clampdowns and major attempts at amnesty for the armed rebel groups, offering training and rehabilitation in exchange for rocket-propelled grenades, explosives, and gunboats. In 2005, a US intelligence agency declared that Nigeria was on its way to becoming a failed state (*Economist*, 2009).

TRANSPARENCY IN THE NIGER DELTA?

Some of the governors in the Niger Delta are in charge of budgets that are bigger than those of entire African nations. But after they have lavished themselves with "Gloryland" mansions replete with miniature governments containing fleets of air transit, medical and educational infrastructure, and other forms of opulence, there is little left over for their constituents. In fact, one governor of the wealthy Niger Delta Bayelsa state escaped British authorities after being arrested for money laundering by dressing as a woman.

The corrupt governor Diepreye Alamieyeseigha, of Bayelsa state in the Niger Delta, was soon followed by another, Timipre Sylva, who, styling his bowler hat, took a different approach. Noting that "transparency has a direct link to development," he requested a complete audit of his state's finances. This audit included a look at the records of the local government authorities, which are responsible for funding the everyday citizens living in abject poverty in the Niger Delta. Not far into the audit process, it found that about 20 percent of the state budget was going to nonexistent workers. Many were shocked that the numbers were so low. But the audit process had an impressive side effect. Many of the militants who had been fighting in the name of ending corruption actually put down their arms, and the main militant group declared a cease-fire.

NATURAL RESOURCES AND CIVIL WAR

An especially gruesome and controversial corollary to the resource curse is civil war. As exploration technology advances and global demand for commodities increases, more nations garner access to natural resources. This may explain why civil war is more prevalent today than before 1960 (Ross, 2006).

This section focuses on oil and diamonds, but any natural resources can render countries vulnerable to the resource curse or to civil war. These include timber, gemstones, coffee, opium, and narcotics. In Mexico, narcotics constitute as much as 4 percent of GDP, around US$30 billion per year, employing half a million people. The world's largest drug market lies just to its north. In the four years after former President Felipe Calderón declared a clampdown on the trade, more than twenty-eight thousand people died in drug-related violent conflicts. In the drug-infested border town of Ciudad Juárez, the murder rate was 189 per 100,000 in 2010, many times higher than the already high 14 per 100,000 for the nation as a whole (Guillermoprieto, 2010). As the world's leading supplier of weapons, the United States reports that more than 10 percent of its gun dealers operate at the Mexican border (Shirk, 2011).

Mexico's resource curse situation cannot be remedied by the Mexican government alone in part because its gangs extend into the United States. Organized crime syndicates, politicians, multinational corporations, and innocent civilians are all migrating across borders. Development aid (to help avoid recruitment of corrupt police officers and young people into organized crime), judicial reform, transparency in gun and weapons sales, enhancements to the North American Free Trade Agreement (NAFTA) and other trade agreements, and immigration reform are all needed, alongside better drug policies. This all requires a good deal of international coordination.

Most scholars link natural resources to civil war through the same causal mechanisms described in the resource curse section, that is, that resource wealth weakens the state's ability to handle the economy (especially with a small tax base) and resolve social conflicts (Ross, 2006). Overall, the most prominent arguments include the claim that civil war is ignited or prolonged in conditions that highlight economic grievances (on top of more common political ones) (Collier, 2000; Collier et al., 2003; Collier & Hoeffler, 1998), as well as those of weak central governments (Fearon & Laitin, 2003). For example, resource wealth might increase the value of the state as a target so that insurgent groups can share in the riches as well. To avoid civil conflict, governments need to regulate how firms draw on natural resources and how the proceeds are distributed (see figure 12.2).

Still, as with the link between violent conflict and failed state governance, it is difficult to disentangle directions of causality in the link between violent conflict and natural, nonrenewable riches such as oil or diamonds. Income shocks, weak state institutions, mountainous terrain, and lack of population density are all correlated with civil war. Nevertheless, researchers continue to search for definitive and causal factors. More important, what sorts of policies should be implemented to avert conflict or to minimize damage and promote recovery remain fuzzy (Blattman & Miguel, 2010).

For instance, economic grievances and natural wealth might fuel civil war because there are then greater riches for different groups to fight over as well as more contraband materials to sell and fund insurgencies. Yet, it appears that civil conflict prompted the economy to become *more* dependent on resource exports in Angola. Further, gems, narcotics, and oil all seem to operate differently. In Burma, Colombia, Peru, and Afghanistan, for instance, rebel groups had no role in the drug trade when wars began (Ross, 2004). There are also lots of contradictory data on whether agricultural products, unlike opium or crude oil, are related to civil war (Ross, 2006).

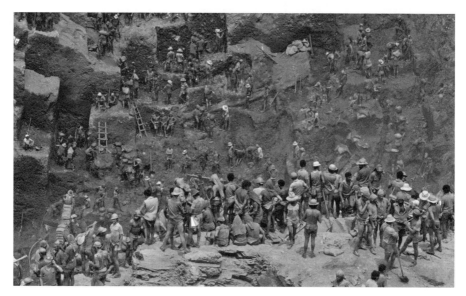

Figure 12.2. Natural resources in poorly governed nations not only encourage dangerous mining conditions, but also can lead to civil war.

Source: Magnum Photos/Miguel Rio Branco, 1985.

Similar reservations exist for analyses on the roles of national income and race and ethnicity in civil war. Is it really just low income and resource wealth that drive violent conflict or more precisely the number of unemployed young men trying to escape abject poverty? Are racial and ethnic divisions the cause of war or do military groups exploit and exacerbate these divisions in recruiting young men and child soldiers? Is it really the poorest who fight in rebel groups? Although social divisions, political grievances, resource abundance, and material incentives are all factors in civil wars, research shows material incentives to be most consistent, and for poverty measures (such as living in mud housing) to be more robust than political party affiliation (Blattman & Miguel, 2010).

In Mexico, the Zapatistas (a group that is variously armed and fights in the name of social justice) calls for distributive justice and the "suspens[ion of] the robbery of our natural resources" (Ross, 2010, p. 19). They want reform rather than an independent state. In contrast to studies suggesting that ethnic homogeneity or diversity are the ultimate factors in maintaining peace (making it difficult to glean how pluralistic societies such as Nigeria can prosper without literally dividing further), these studies raise the hope that even genocide is not just an act of irrational hatred but a horrific phenomenon that might be averted with better social policies (Shaxson, 2007).

Some scholars have argued that policy makers should look beyond the behaviors of individual actors (whether exploitative oil companies or corrupt rulers) and nebulous collective problems regarding "culture" to address the *systemic* links between social fragmentation, the uneven spoils of resource revenues, and international flows (Shaxson, 2007).

The sorts of policy recommendations recommended for the resource curse overall also apply to contexts plagued by violent conflict. The trick lies in cutting off illegitimate flows of money, such as those of **blood diamonds,** and making it easier for governments and citizens to get the revenues, taxes, services, and jobs they need (Collier, 2000).

BLOOD DIAMONDS ARE NO ONE'S BEST FRIEND

The Kimberley process certification scheme (KPCS) certifies the origin of rough diamonds. KPCS was set up by the United Nations in 2003 to assure consumers that the diamonds they buy are not financing war or human rights abuses, and participating countries include all major diamond importers and exporters. Diamond and jewelry retailers, in turn, sell these diamonds as ethical and conflict-free. Some countries, such as the Republic of Congo, are KPCS members but not allowed to participate because of their inability to prove the origin of their rough diamonds.

Some critics, such as KPCS-cofounding organization Global Witness, argue that the KPCS lacks the power to punish nations, companies, and organizations involved in diamond smuggling, money laundering, and human rights abuses. They also argue that KPCS guidelines are simply too loose. They propose that KPCS adopt stricter guidelines on the diamonds that are allowed to be certified (and the mine conditions that these diamonds come from). They also propose that KPCS receive funding for a permanent secretariat and overall institution building, and that it replace its consensus system with one that enables members to punish those who violate its rules.

Finally, the most controversial policy recommendations are those of military interventions, whether directly by foreign troops attempting to overthrow a dictatorship or indirectly by setting up conditions for a coup.

SUMMARY

Globalization can mean many things, but many think of the freer movement of goods and people across international borders. Free trade and migration can lead to huge leaps in economic growth and well-being. However, it can also lead to a flood of cheaper goods into local markets, hurting business-people, and increasing unemployment. It also raises serious environmental concerns as manufacturers look to less-regulated markets where they are able to manufacture goods without worries about labor conditions or pollution controls. Nations with access to lucrative natural resources that can be traded with other nations may be more likely to be governed by dictators that seek to profit from the sale of such resources.

The prevalence of civil wars and violent conflict, with their devastating effect on health and development, highlights some of the main challenges we currently face in global health. Institutions such as the WHO and the IMF cannot adequately address health and economic policies in low- and middle-income countries on their own. Global trade and the power of the WTO have increased tremendously. Trade is not to be stopped, however, so policy makers must attempt to rewrite trade agreements to better address spillover effects over borders as well as the labor, health, and environmental consequences of economic liberalization. Policy makers must also help to address how the wealth created from commodities such as oil and diamonds gets distributed in a transparent manner in an attempt to use good global governance to avert civil wars.

KEY TERMS

antiglobalization   civil conflict   paradox of
blood diamonds   plenty

DISCUSSION QUESTIONS

1. What do the pathways among natural resources, globalization, and civil conflict look like?

2. What do the pathways between civil conflict and poor population health look like?

3. You are working for a congressional senator or for a large foundation. After a devastating earthquake, your boss would like to give a large aid package to a country with rich oil reserves but, the country has some signs of suffering from the resource curse. Do you still recommend the aid package? What safeguards do you recommend to accompany the aid package?

4. How should large deposits of natural resources be governed? Should intergovernmental organizations play a role? What is the role of consumers in purchasing oil (gasoline), diamonds, and other potentially conflict-ridden commodities?

FURTHER READING

Blattman, C. (2012). Children and war. *Perspectives on Politics*, *10*(2), 403–413.

Paris, R. (2004). *At war's end: Building peace after civil conflict*. New York: Cambridge University Press.

Stearns, J. (2012). *Dancing in the glory of monsters: The collapse of the Congo and the great war of Africa*. New York: PublicAffairs.

REFERENCES

Alden, C. (2007). *China in Africa: Partner, competitor or hegemon?* London: Zed Books.

Blattman, C., & Miguel, E. (2010). Civil war. *Journal of Economic Literature*, *48*(1), 3–57.

Brautigam, D. (2010). *The dragon's gift: The real story of China in Africa*. New York: Oxford University Press.

Burnham, G., Lafta, R., Doocy, S., & Roberts, L. (2006). Mortality after the 2003 invasion of Iraq: A cross-sectional cluster sample survey. *Lancet*, *368*, 1421–1428.

Canavan, A., Vergeer, P., & Bornemisza, O. (2008). *Post-conflict health sectors: The myth and reality of transitional funding gaps*. Amsterdam: Health and Fragile States Network.

Collier, P. (2000). *Economic causes of civil conflict and their implications for policy*. Washington, DC: World Bank.

Collier, P., Elliott, V. L., Hegre, H., Hoeffler, A., Reynal-Querol, M., & Sambanis, N. (2003). *Breaking the conflict trap: Civil war and development policy*. Washington, DC: World Bank and Oxford University Press.

Collier, P., & Hoeffler, A. (1998). On economic causes of Civil War. *Oxford Economic Papers*, *50*(4), 563–573.

Dreze, J., & Sen, A. K. (1989). *Hunger and public action*. New York: Oxford University Press.

Drury, A. C., Krieckhaus, J., & Lusztig, M. (2006). Corruption, democracy, and economic growth. *International Political Science Review*, *27*(2), 121–136.

Dye, C., Scheele, S., Dolin, P., Pathania, V., & Raviglione, M. C. (1999). Global burden of tuberculosis: Estimated incidence, prevalence, and mortality by country. *JAMA*, *282*(7), 677.

Economist. (2003, 22 May). The devil's excrement. Available online at www.economist.com/node/1795921

Economist. (2009, November 12). Hints of a new chapter. Available online at www.economist.com/PrinterFriendly.cfm?story_id=14843563

Farmer, P. (2004). *Pathologies of power: Health, human rights, and the new war on the poor*. Berkeley: University of California Press.

Fearon, J. D., & Laitin, D. D. (2003). Ethnicity, insurgency, and civil war. *American Political Science Review, 7*, 1.

Frieden, T., Sterling, T., Pablos Mendez, A., Kilburn, J. O., Cauthen, G. M., & Dooley, S. W. (1993). The emergence of drug-resistant tuberculosis in New York City. *New England Journal of Medicine, 323*(8), 521–556.

Garrett, L. (2000). *Betrayal of trust: The collapse of global public health.* New York: Hyperion.

Guillermoprieto, A. (2010, October 28). The murderers of Mexico. *New York Review of Books.*

Gylfason, T. (2001). Natural resources, education, and economic development. *European Economic Review, 45*(4–6), 847–859.

Hegre, H., Ellingsen, T., Gates, S., & Gleditsch, N. P. (2001). Toward a democratic civil peace? Democracy, political change, and civil war, 1816–1992. *The American Political Science Review, 95*(1), 33–48.

Hibbert, C. (1980). *The great mutiny: India 1857.* London: Allen Lane.

Humphreys, M., Sachs, J. D., & Stiglitz, J. E. (Eds.). (2007). *Escaping the resource curse.* New York: Columbia University Press.

Iqbal, Z. (2006). Health and human security: The public health impact of violent conflict. *International Studies Quarterly, 60*, 631–649.

Khan, K., Muennig, P., Behta, M., & Zivin, J. G. (2002). Global drug-resistance patterns and the management of latent tuberculosis infection in immigrants to the United States. *New England Journal of Medicine, 347*(23), 1850–1859.

McFerson, H. M. (2009). Governance and hyper-corruption in resource-rich African countries. *Third World Quarterly, 30*(8), 1529–1547.

Midford, P., & de Soysa, I. (2010). *Enter the dragon! An empirical analysis of Chinese versus US arms transfers to autocrats and violators of human rights, 1989–2006.* Trondheim: Norwegian Institute of Science and Technology.

Moss, T. (2011). *Oil to cash: Fighting the resource curse through cash transfers.* Washington, DC: Center for Global Development.

Okonta, I., & Douglas, O. (2001). *Where vultures feast: Shell, human rights, and oil in the Niger Delta.* Seattle: Sierra Club Books.

Ross, M. (2004). How do natural resources influence civil war? Evidence from thirteen cases. *International Organization, 58*(1), 35–67.

Ross, M. (2006). A closer look at oil, diamonds, and civil war. *Political Science, 9*(1), 265.

Ross, M. (2010). *Latin America's missing oil wars.* Washington, DC: World Bank Office of the Chief Economist for Latin America and the Caribbean.

Sandbrook, R., Edelman, M., Heller, P., & Teichman, J. (2007). *Social democracy in the global periphery: Origins, challenges, prospects.* New York: Cambridge University Press.

Shaxson, N. (2007). Oil, corruption and the resource curse. *International Affairs*, *83*(6), 1123–1140.

Shirk, D. A. (2011). *The drug war in Mexico: Confronting a shared threat*. New York: Council on Foreign Relations.

Thoms, O.N.T., & Ron, J. (2007). Public health, conflict and human rights: Toward a collaborative research agenda. *Conflict and Health, 1*(11).

WHO. (2002). *World report on violence and health*. Geneva: WHO.

Zwi, A. B. (2004). How should the health community respond to violent political conflict? *PLoS Medicine, 1*(1), e14.

CHAPTER 13

Frontiers in Global Health

KEY IDEAS

- Health outcomes are shaped by social and physical circumstances on many levels—individual, local, national, and international. Global health solutions must tackle multiple levels at once.

- Health problems interact in dynamic ways.

- Targeted social policy interventions, such as conditional cash transfers and comprehensive neighborhood children's centers, are a promising and growing field in global health.

- Structural approaches work best when they combine environmental changes and increases in public services with individual- and family-based programs such as conditional cash transfers.

In this chapter, we use what you have learned about global health policy up to now as we discuss innovative health policies. We focus on conditional cash transfers, participatory budgeting, and governance and administrative innovations in Brazil, comprehensive early childhood development services in the United Kingdom, and changes to the built environment in New York and San Francisco. We weigh the evidence on the impact of these interventions and the conditions in which they work best, and we conclude with some potential lessons for practice and research.

In just over four decades, Singapore has grown from a tiny backwater city-state with dismal health statistics to become the healthiest nation on earth, when measured in terms of human longevity (Jacobson, 2010). Its visionary but heavy-handed leader, Lee Kuan Yew, achieved this in part by putting strict controls on what people could and could not do. Those who stepped out of line were painfully humiliated with public lashings with a cane for relatively minor infractions, such as graffiti.

Soon, the **rule of law** sets in. By one definition, the rule of law is achieved when relative social order, as measured by low rates of crime or the accurate payment of taxes, becomes the social norm. In Singapore, corruption, overt racial discrimination, and other harmful behaviors are, by and large, rare. In this context, it is quite easy to ensure that exercise, a good diet, and respect for one's neighbor is normative. Also important, a healthy, law-abiding citizenry requires less money spent on policing, health insurance, property insurance, and incarceration.

THE RULE OF LAW AND PUBLIC HEALTH

The rule of law is a legal maxim that no one is immune from or above the law. According to one definition of the rule of law, the laws do not have to be perfect, or even just, but they do have to be consistent, publicly known, transparent, and fairly and equally enforced and implemented for everyone, even the state itself (Raz, 1999; Shklar & Hoffmann, 1998). Some political theorists go beyond such process-oriented, formal principles over how laws are upheld, arguing that the rule of law has normative, substantive implications, such as separation of powers, women's rights, and freedom of assembly and free speech. Others argue that the rule of law should not be confused with justice or human rights (Raz, 1999).

The concept of rule of law has gained attention in international circles since the 1990s. For example, the UN General Assembly has considered the rule of law in different countries an explicit agenda item since 1992.

But the rule of law isn't always a good thing. One must decide which civil liberties are essential to rule of law and which ones can or should be sacrificed in the name of the rule of law. For instance, judicial courts around the world have been weighing whether wiretapping, certain interrogation techniques, campaigns targeted at specific demographic groups, and other violations to rights of privacy and bodily integrity strengthen or undermine national security and the rule of law. In fact, there is a large literature on whether the rule of law is a universal concept because some scholars argue that Asian cultures view good governance as rule by wise and benevolent rulers, not transparent and accountable judicial and legislative systems (Zhu, 2008). Further, the concept or term *rule of law* is primarily known in Anglo-Saxon nations; Sweden and Japan, for example, do not have a formal tradition of rule of law.

Of course, Singapore is an autocratic country that only a select few would choose to live in. One Singaporean was quoted as saying, "We are not North Korea, but we try" (Jacobson, 2010). In the case of Singapore, laws are notoriously clear. There are even indie pop songs about how one cannot chew gum in Singapore, but peppermints melting in your mouth are just fine. However, constitutional amendments also prohibit judicial reviews of the constitutionality of certain laws, and specific laws allow state police forces to make warrantless arrests and to commit suspect drug users without trial. Although electoral processes exist, and the ruling party is slowly losing seats in the parliament, former prime minister Lee Kuan Yew's People's Action Party has dominated Singaporean politics since independence in 1965. Finally, media is largely controlled by the state, so Reporters Without Borders ranked Singapore 146th in media freedom out of 168 countries. To what extent, then, does Singapore abide by rule of law principles? And to what extent were the laws in place essential to economic development and to large strides in life expectancy and health promotion?

The Singapore example suggests that the role of the rule of law in global health is multifaceted. As chapters 6 and 7 argue, democratic accountability appears to make a difference in making sure that policy makers, put bluntly, do not kill their constituents or lead them into conflict and that they help them live better and longer instead. Aside from a set of specific legal and governmental institutions, however, the rule of law is also a lifestyle or a set of shared norms. That broader, more nebulous definition is important in systems theory because it allows researchers to identify patterns in and make predictions about the complex behaviors of interdependent individual agents (governmental agencies, NGOs and civil society groups, different demographic groups of everyday citizens, immigrants and travelers, etc.) in the face of a range of health interventions, natural and unnatural events, and public policies.

Nevertheless, it serves to illustrate approaches to public health policy that are being tried (with much more subtle tactics) in places as different as New York City and Bogotá, Colombia. The idea in these places is to nudge human behaviors so that eventually human behaviors change.

There are different ways of signaling normative behavior that extend beyond crime and into health behaviors. For instance, innovative public health advertising was used in New York City in a way that capitalized on existing trends. Many New Yorkers carry around reusable metal water bottles. This created an opportunity that the department of health could exploit (Chan, 2009). After all, sugary drinks are not only unhealthy to consume, a good deal of pollution is generated (and energy consumed) when the containers are shipped in to the city full and shipped back out again once empty (as garbage). The department of health launched an ad campaign showing fat pouring out of various commercial drinks. This was an effort to create a **tipping point** in which it becomes the norm to drink from a water bottle and purchased beverages are socially shunned.

In epidemiology, one example of the tipping point is **herd immunity** (Anderson & May, 1985; Gladwell, 2001) (see figure 13.1). Herd immunity occurs when enough folks have received a vaccine that the number of people with measles, influenza, or whatever is so low that it no longer commonly spreads from person to person. This can work the other way, too. Once enough people get the flu, it starts to spread like wildfire.

But the tipping point can also apply to social phenomena (Gladwell, 2001). Even the most dyed-in-the-wool anarchist still gets up in the morning and puts clothes on, even if it is an unusually hot day. Why? Because it is what we do in clothes-wearing societies. There are not enough nudists to render nudity a consideration for any but those who make such norms their own community, even where it is legal.

Human behavior, though, is immensely complex. Not only that, but behavior is shaped by a larger and equally complex system of social networks, family dynamics, norms, and laws, to name a few factors, that influence health. Fortunately, public health is a broad discipline that tends to collect an eclectic bunch of political scientists, economists, sociologists, health psychologists, and organizational behavior specialists. The challenge for the future is figuring out how to harness all of this expertise to solve our health problems.

Most fundamentally, we are challenged to think about how the policies and interventions that we create as public health professionals affect our institutions, communities, social support networks, and biological systems. This mode of thinking is called the **multilevel model**. (Not to be confused with multilevel modeling in statistics.)

THE MANY LEVELS OF HEALTH

Going back to the case of Wanda in chapter 2, her mother's premature death was not exactly caused by a DNA mutation. Nor was it caused by an incompetent doctor who might have detected her asthma early enough to prevent it. Some might blame her poor mother for not being as supportive as she could have been or for not getting her daughter out of the neighborhood. A better villain for her asthma, obesity, and elevated risk for heart disease might be the failed social engineering of Robert Moses, the man who conceived the Cross-Bronx Expressway. Or we could attribute it to the government's failure to deliver a quality education that would have gotten her out of her unhealthy living situation. But in reality, the cause is much broader—it is a constellation of health risk factors that arose from a series of policy failures. So, why not blame the campaign finance laws that allow special interest groups to dominate our policy landscape?

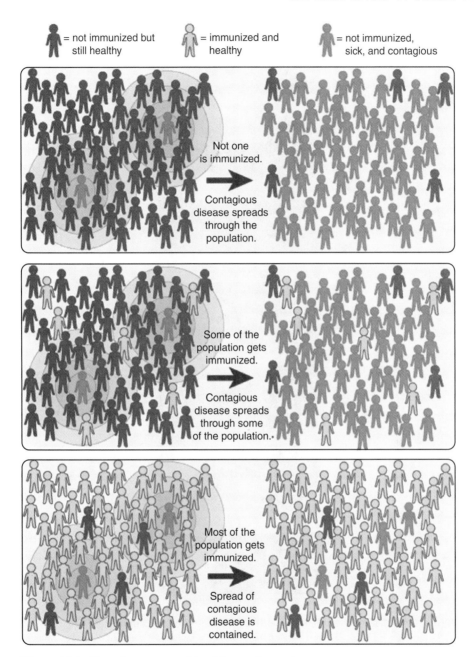

Figure 13.1. How the concept of *herd immunity* works.

Source: Vaccines.gov. (2012). Available online at www.vaccines.gov/basics/protection/index.html.

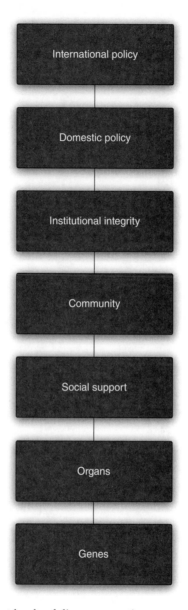

Figure 13.2. The different levels of disease causation or prevention.

The multilevel model (figure 13.2) allows us to think about Wanda's illness through a broader lens (Kaplan, Everson, & Lynch, 2000). In this model, disease is not seen as a failure of biological systems but rather as a complex interplay of genes, organs, social support networks, community factors, and social policies, whether at the international or domestic level.

One team of researchers put this model into play using breast cancer as a test case. They enrolled 230 low-income African American women in Chicago as test subjects. Each of these women had been newly diagnosed with breast cancer. They then developed an animal model, taking a group of rodents and randomly assigning them to conditions similar to those faced by the women or to supportive, nurturing environments. The animals exposed to the high-stress and social isolation environment were much more likely to develop breast cancer over time. This way, the researchers were able to identify the stress hormone receptors in the cell nuclei that were responsible for the higher rate of cancer in the rodents living in the reconstructed high-poverty environment (Gehlert et al., 2008).

This multilevel model has its roots in a brilliant epidemiologic investigation conducted by Rudolf Virchow, a famous pathologist and democracy campaigner in the nineteenth century (Virchow, 1849; Virchow, 2006). When set to investigate a typhus outbreak as a young physician, Virchow not only collected data on who became ill and where, but he also asked detailed questions about the subjects' education, income, housing conditions, and so forth. In fact, the majority of the report focused on the land and its inhabitants rather than the postulated underlying illness. He ultimately concluded from his report that the spread of typhus was the result of overcrowding, which in turn was the result of poverty, which in turn was the result of poor educational opportunities, which, finally arose from a lack of democracy in Otto von Bismarck's Germany. Of course, this did not make him popular with the authorities. Bismarck himself challenged Virchow to a duel. Virchow chose a *Trichinella*-laden sausage as the weapon of choice and Bismarck backed down. Virchow is considered one of the greatest forerunners to the modern public health advocate.

TIDINGS, GOOD OR BAD, COME IN CLUSTERS

In Wanda's case, her health problems were probably not limited to lung cancer. An environment that is high in stress leads to behavioral risks. We have all experienced this around finals week in college. Out come the Snickers bars. (Yes, finals are bad for your health.) In the case of Wanda and her neighbors, their entire lives, not just one week, are filled with stress. And this stress is of the most inevitable and defeating kind. (Although a student can study, Wanda's neighbors are often helpless against crime, malicious landlords, and a job market that demands what they never had the opportunity to achieve.) As a result, they have not exercised or eaten as well as they should have and, as a result of this, developed diabetes, heart disease, and high blood pressure.

Why do these things come together? Well, certainly, the diabetes and high blood pressure are risk factors for heart disease. But the diabetes and high blood pressure shouldn't have any relationship to something as esoteric as a neighborhood. Yet, there they are, again and again, seen in patient after patient in low-income neighborhoods. To top that off, we also see depression popping its head into this mix more often than it should. Though not proven (Berkman et al., 2003), depression may worsen heart disease by adding stress and reducing the body's ability to buffer the damaging effects of stress (Roose & Spatz, 1998). These disease patterns are prevalent at relatively constant but high levels, or **endemic.** They also tend to cluster together in ways that synergize, or magnify, the effect of each factor, such that the total health effect is worse than the sum of the individual health effects. When a number of core health risks that tend to produce predictable sets of health problems, for which the sum of health effects is greater than the parts, you have what is known as a synergistic-endemic condition, called *syndemic* (Milstein, 2008).

Fundamental to most syndemic illnesses is a common set of alternative sociobiological causes (Singer et al., 2006). Again, Wanda's other illnesses are attributable not just to genetic predisposition but also to factors in her family (suboptimal emotional support), community (no access to healthy food), and society (policies that create the family and community risk factors).

There are lots of examples of syndemic patterns. Take HIV and substance abuse, for one. Substance use is a risk factor for HIV, but it also tends to stress the body and is associated with homelessness, poor nutrition, and other infectious diseases (especially when the substance being abused is injected with bloody needles). None of these things is good for you, but they are especially bad in someone with HIV. On top of that, other psychosocial issues often get in the way of taking HIV medications on a regular basis.

Syndemics take very different courses in different development contexts. For instance, in some parts of Africa (but not others), HIV is a disease of affluence rather than poverty, and HIV-related syndemics are less common (Hargreaves et al., 2002; N'Galy & Ryder, 1988). In poorer parts, HIV, TB, and malaria form a syndemic that is complicated by malnutrition. In areas with poor sanitation, hookworm and malaria are common HIV-related syndemics. In wealthy countries, HIV and herpes appear to form a syndemic that leads to rapid progression of HIV into AIDS. As illustrated here, syndemics differ in different development contexts, even when we focus on syndemics related to a single disease, HIV.

The field of syndemic theory focuses on better understanding how different diseases or conditions interact. As we saw in the last section, part of this picture arises from international policies, part from national policies, part from institutions, part from different communities, and part from individual support networks. Syndemic theory not only demands that one account for the multiple levels of disease causation (or cure) but also the dynamic interplay of a large number of variables within each of these levels. Addressing syndemics is therefore best done with the input of experts and computer models that can better help us understand how best to intervene and understand what types of things can go terribly wrong if one is not careful. In other words, it requires a more complex view of the systems that cause disease.

WORKING WITH THE SYSTEM

In the late-1990s, an aid organization set out to eradicate river blindness north of Lake Victoria in sub-Saharan Africa. The idea was simple. If we spray to eradicate the fly and treat people with antiparasitic medication, we can save people from the misery of blindness. So, they sprayed and treated and they eradicated blindness.

There was just one problem. People will live as close to waterways as they possibly can. When a village is next to a river, water does not need to be hauled for hours through the jungle every day. If conditions permit, people will naturally settle on rivers. As it happens, the vector for river blindness, the blackfly *Simulium damnosum,* breeds in fast-moving water, and also generally hangs out near the shoreline. This fly carries a parasite called *Onchocerca volvulus* that causes a disease called *onchocerciasis,* the cause of river blindness (see figure 13.3). Once mostly eradicated, the river was not only a safer place to live, but people also did not have to deal with the damn flies. Thus, as a result of this effort, people moved from inland areas to the shore of the river en masse.

When people live near the water, they also tend to defecate near the water. So, the river quickly became a roaring cesspool. Those living downstream were accustomed to drinking and bathing in the water. Thus, as a result of this humanitarian effort, many people died downstream.

Unintended consequences of noble ideas are commonplace and, as these examples illustrate, some humanitarian aid projects end up doing more harm than good. All of this sounds like grim stuff. But it need not be. A broader, more nuanced view of the systems that make up our society can help stave off these problems.

The field that sets out to help us understand how to avoid such problems is called **systems theory** or **systems dynamics** (Forrester, 1971). Systems dynamics is a concept that has been around for quite a while, but it has only really become possible to fully use as a public health tool with the advent of computers.

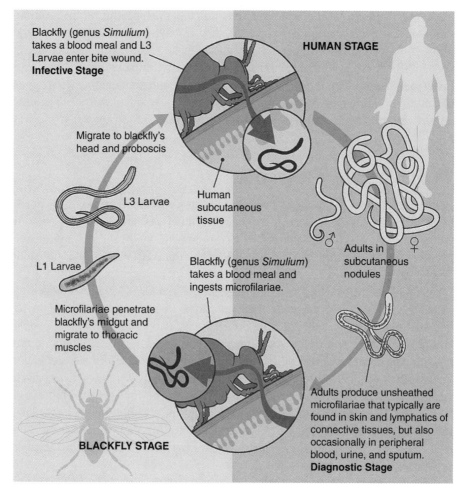

Figure 13.3. The life cycle of the *Onchocerca volvulus*. This is a parasitic worm that is the cause of river blindness.

Source: Wikimedia Commons/Giovanni Maki.

The more that a country develops economically, the more one can afford labor-saving technologies such as dishwashers and washing machines. But work hours tend to increase out of proportion to the savings obtained by automating tasks, thus producing a net decrease in leisure time. These unintended consequences of policies are sometimes called **policy resistance** (Sterman, 2006).

One way of tackling policy resistance is to better understand the complex systems underlying them. If we can imagine all of the potential unintended consequences of any given action, such as treating river blindness, then we can potentially avert some of the problems that might arise (and threaten lives or waste money).

Systems—such as a health system, the economy, or the environment—are complicated, and the elements of systems tend to interact in ways that produce counterintuitive results. This counterintuitive behavior of systems arises from **dynamic complexity.** Dynamic complexity refers to complicated interactions between different elements of a system. Often, these elements push back when you try to fix a problem. For example, as mentioned in chapter 10, penicillin was once used for a huge array of infections. Now, thanks to antibiotic resistance pushing back at us, it is virtually useless against all but a handful of organisms. This process of pushing back is called *negative feedback* (Sterman, 2006).

HEALTHBOUND

Try playing HealthBound (http://forio.com/simulate/cdc/health-bound/run/), and you will see that reality is not always as it seems. This game was developed at the United States Centers for Disease Control and Prevention based on a complex systems model. It is kind of like the old SimCity or SimEarth computer games, but it is based on much more data and much more complex systems, albeit with a relatively poor interface. If you introduce one policy change, you can see how that change will affect different types of health outcomes. Increase funding for health care, and you will see that you do not get much bang for your buck. Increase funding for education, and things look a bit different.

We might not be able to fully overcome it, but if we understand negative feedback, we can at least slow it down. For instance, if we had known that penicillin would soon grow to be ineffective due to its overuse, we might have enacted laws requiring doctors to be more judicious from the start. We might also have moved more quickly to invest in new antibiotics well before the world of microbes began to win its war against us.

Consider another example. If we are planning on reducing congestion on a busy roadway, the intuitive thing to do is to simply widen the road. This is the most common policy approach taken over and over again throughout history and across nations. Surprisingly, though, the more one widens the road, the more congested the road becomes. This is because wider roads reduce barriers to driving. This, in turn, increases the demand for cars. Increased demand for cars tends to increase competition among carmakers and drive down prices, leading to still more cars on the road. Without regulations, carmakers are unlikely to invest in reducing emissions, even if their profits rise and technology advances. Wider roads and cheaper cars also allow people to relocate to cheaper real estate farther from major downtown economic areas. This increases driving time and puts more cars on the road still. People become more and more dependent on the car until it is strange not to own one. So, more infrastructure still is devoted to the car and more cars end up on the road. For instance, a car culture reduces pressure on politicians to build or maintain expensive public transit systems. The end result of this intuitive policy solution? More pollution, worse health outcomes, and, yes, more congestion. Though this cycle has been observed time and time again, policy makers keep widening roads simply because it seems the intuitive thing to do, especially in the short term. With a systems perspective, we can better see how the elements of a system can produce counterintuitive results. Thus, it is always a good idea to hire a systems person before investing millions or billions of dollars in a major change in the way that things are done. This will help avert any unintended consequences.

The "law of unintended consequences" is not really a law, of course. Most of our policies actually work because most are not embedded in systems with a high degree of policy resistance. We have socially evolved from being hunters and gatherers in collections of families to societies with millions of strangers living in relative harmony. Our aviation regulations do a very good job of keeping giant chunks of winged metal from falling out of the air or colliding with one another. But these processes evolved out of trial and error rather than the sudden implementation of a grand policy. For the most part, when something did not work, either it died or we fixed it. Most policies fail not because we did not understand the negative feedback loops, but because policy makers and other actors tend to think in the short term.

It is also true that systems models often warn us of problems that we can do little about. Still, a lot of people lost their lives perfecting the current aviation regulations. The airlines themselves seek to subvert regulations because they hurt their bottom line, and the more governments regulate, the harder industry works to prevent regulation. Legislation was introduced to reinforce cockpit doors a decade prior to September 11, 2001, but the airline industry successfully fought those regulations on the grounds that they would increase costs. It is difficult to see how resistance to such regulations can be overcome in a nation that empowers industry to resist regulations.

Applying Systems Theory Incrementally

Aid agencies may wish to help a nation develop an education system by investing in schools. That nation's department of education may decide that it does not need to invest in schools in a geographic area if there is an aid organization there already. Worse, in the hope of getting more foreign aid for education or at the command of intergovernmental institutions, it may reduce its overall education budget and divert the funding to other priorities. When the aid dries up, there is no department of education, teacher training program, or procurement process that is left behind. The nation therefore languishes. International aid, loans, and trade agreements are often sets of policy interventions that are based on the intuition or focused interests of a few program officers or policy makers, but they are introduced into dynamic systems with complex ripple effects.

Thus, the best intentions can go awry, even when the relationships between different components of a system are relatively straightforward and do not contain negative feedback loops, such as those in the congestion example. But this does not mean that aid should be halted on the grounds that it is destroying national autonomy, fostering corruption, or coaxing governments into diverting funds from critically important programs. After all, many nations are languishing, and if we can understand why, then we can put aid dollars to their best work.

Jay Forrester, a founder of systems dynamics, argues that the human mind must be harnessed for what it does well and computers must be used for what they do well to come up with a better understanding of how systems work (Forrester, 1971). One argument he makes is that we would never send a human into outer space without extensive laboratory experiments and computer models that account for different contingencies. So, why would the United States create a two-trillion-dollar health system without experiments, models, and contingency plans? Why, for that matter, would the WHO decide to make a major investment in scaling up health systems without fully studying, modeling, and testing such an approach? After all, if so many lives and money are in the balance, why would we not?

COST CONTROLS IN THE UNITED STATES HEALTH SYSTEM

One complex problem in the United States is the conflicting goal of providing health care for everyone and improving everyone's health. The way that US democracy works, it turns out, makes it very difficult for everyone to get on board with a centrally controlled health system. As a result, it becomes extremely difficult to control costs overall. Since the 1970s, the United States has moved from one of the top ten nations in terms of life expectancy to somewhere between thirty-fifth and fiftieth place in the world. With this gradual loss in life expectancy, the US health system also went from being among the more expensive in the world to one that costs twice that of the next nearest competitor. Worse, it may well be that all of these additional expenditures are actually partially responsible for the decline in life expectancy.

As it turns out, there is good reason to believe that part of the US decline in life expectancy is attributable to its health system costs (Muennig & Glied, 2010). This is because the provision of health care is a very inefficient way to save lives. You are much better off tackling the causes of poor health, such as a sedentary lifestyle, behavioral risk factors, crime, unsafe conditions in the home or workplace, and so forth. All of these things cost money. For instance, one very good way of improving a nation's health is to install massive public transit systems. This reduces pollution (a major cause of cancer and heart disease), encourages walking, reduces automobile accidents, and improves the quality of life in neighborhoods (e.g., via pedestrian malls, lower noise pollution, etc.). Unfortunately, the United States simply cannot afford these luxuries, which are more common (even in poorer nations) with universal health systems.

This disconnect between how we usually talk about health policy (in terms of medical services for individuals) and what actually affects health (in terms of a whole range of nonmedical policies for a range of overlapping populations rather than individuals) explains part of the puzzle of why the United States spends so much per capita on health care and receives so little in return.

A RISE IN TARGETED SOCIAL POLICY INTERVENTIONS

Another promising field lies in targeted social policy interventions for health and other forms of welfare alike. One idea that has gained traction is to couple welfare payments to classroom attendance and receiving regular medical care, a concept known as *conditional cash transfers* (Adato, Roopnaraine, & Becker, 2011; Cueto, 2009; Fernald, Gertler, & Neufeld, 2008; Paes-Sousa, Santos, & Miazaki, 2011). At first glance, social policies such as payments for primary school attendance may not seem as closely linked to health as clean water, but they may provide the next major boost to life expectancy among many nations tackling chronic diseases.

Such social policies can take very broad forms. Even democracy itself is thought to be life-saving. The Nobel Prize–winning economist Amartya Sen declared that famine is rare in a functioning democracy because mass starvation is not good for anyone's political career (Sen, 1999). Likewise, democracy provides a means for people to demand life-saving programs, such as better schools, roads, and access to medical care.

Innovative social policy reforms have proliferated and gained prominence in public policy debates since the 1990s. Latin American cases have dominated many of these debates. There are several reasons for this. First, many of the largest economies in the region—Brazil, Argentina, and Chile, for example—returned to democratic governance (Shifter, 2009). Second, the structural adjustment crises of the 1980s that ravaged South America highlighted the importance of sustainable social programs to policy makers. Third, some economists had previously conceptualized social programs as arising from economic growth rather than contributing to economic growth, but prevailing opinions began to recognize both pathways as important (Bloom, Canning, & Sevilla, 2004; Sachs, 2002; Waitzkin, 2003). Fourth, there was growing awareness that steep wealth inequalities could lead to civil unrest (Blattman & Miguel, 2010; Collier et al., 2003). Finally, the rise of China led to a demand-driven commodity boom that benefited Latin America economically, opening the door to more expensive, innovative social programs (Nelson, 2011).

Of course, this is not to say that innovative policy interventions are not happening elsewhere. We also look at cases from other low- and middle-income countries, such as India, and from industrialized nations such as the United Kingdom.

Conditional Cash Transfers

Child-centered **conditional cash transfers** (CCTs) attempt to simultaneously promote poverty alleviation and civic responsibility in the short term and investment in human capital in the longer term. In CCT programs, families receive monthly cash payments if they meet certain behavioral criteria, such as sending their primary school–age children to school on more than 85 percent of school days, complying with prenatal visits to clinics, and helping their children receive recommended vaccinations.

For instance, Brazil's Bolsa Família began in rural areas when local governments simultaneously extended after-school programs and paid families with five- to sixteen-year-old children to keep them in school all day rather than have them work in degrading or hazardous conditions. Other components of

Bolsa Família ask that pregnant women attend prenatal medical checkups, complete immunizations for their children, and breast-feed. In Mexico, additional food cash transfers are given after families attend nutrition seminars.

The largest and most well-known programs are Mexico's Oportunidades (formerly known as *Progresa* and the first nationwide program of this kind) and Brazil's Bolsa Família. Bolsa Família alone reached eleven million families, or forty-six million people, in 2006 (Lindert, Linder, Hobbs, & De la Brière, 2006; Soares, Ribas, & Osório, 2010). This constituted 100 percent of the poor and 25 percent of all people in Brazil at the time. Other countries with CCTs include Bolivia, Colombia, Jamaica, and Nicaragua (Lund, Noble, Barnes, & Wright, 2010; Soares, Osório, Veras Soares, Medeiros, & Zepeda, 2009).

Currently, in Bolsa Família, poor families receive monthly benefits of 140 reals (US$88), plus 32 reals per child fifteen or younger (for up to three children). Sixteen- and seventeen-year-olds receive 32 reals (US$21) a month (for up to two children). Families with incomes below the extreme poverty line receive additional cash transfers of 70 reals (US$44). Thus, a very poor family with three children and two teenagers would receive 242 reals (US$153) (Soares, 2011). As a point of comparison, the current minimum wage is 545 reals a month.

These programs have yielded some impressive outcomes. After the implementation of Bolsa Família, Brazil's poverty rate fell from 39 percent in 2001 to 25 percent in 2009 (the lowest rate in decades), and overall income inequalities fell as well (ECLAC, 2010). Secondary school enrollment increased by 13 percent, from 69 percent in 2000 to 82 percent in 2008 (Loyka, 2011). A growing number of Asian, African, and North American governments have followed suit (Schubert & Slater, 2006). The CCT programs' key features appear to be their eligibility rules, coordination with supply-side increases in funding of public services, and administrative structures and transparency.

Eligibility and Conditionalities

The programs' eligibility rules are tied to certain conditions. First, all eligible families must be poor. Brazil's Bolsa Família considers only household income in determining eligibility. This is challenging because many beneficiaries work in the informal sector, so they do not report their income to the government. In Mexico and Chile, social workers use an index to determine eligibility (Soares et al., 2009). Chile's Solidario program is aimed at the indigent, the poorest 225,000 families in the nation.

Solidario builds on the premise that many indigent families do not access public services partly because they face discrimination, lack information, and lack a sense of agency; social workers can help to remedy this by relying more on judgment than workers in Mexico. But requirements include possession of birth certificates, proof of citizenship, marriage certificates and divorce decrees, employment-related requirements, and unemployment affidavits and can increase barriers to access. These barriers to entry often come with high opportunity costs and have been more common in more recent programs, such as one in the Western Cape in South Africa (Lund et al., 2010).

In 2009, Bolsa Família revised its coverage target from 11.1 million to 12.9 million families, despite the fact that poverty rates had fallen. In doing so, it expanded the program's eligibility criteria and working definition of poverty: a family was poor even if its income exceeded thresholds as long as its income was volatile and risked falling below the poverty threshold in a two-year period (Soares, 2011).

Access to Social Services

If families do not meet conditionalities—the criteria they are required to meet in order to receive benefits—they go through five stages of warnings and suspensions before benefits cease. Even then, children under sixteen are not affected, and the warnings trigger a social worker to visit such families. For example, if a sixteen-year-old has partly missed school because she was caring for a younger sibling after their mother got a new job, the social worker helps the family attain alternative child care. The program emphasizes opportunities for greater well-being rather than punitive measures for poor performance.

Mexico's CCTs operate similarly to Brazil's, though they give more generous conditional scholarships to upper secondary school students. As a point of comparison, the CCT ceiling for a very poor family with two teenagers was US$239 in Mexico in 2007, US$91 (PPP) in Brazil in 2003, and just US$33 in 2003 in Chile (Soares et al., 2009).

Chile's Solidario program may seem stingy at first glance. However, it combines CCTs with unconditional family subsidies for the very poor, potable water subsidies (in a country where water provision is privatized in many areas), disability and pension subsidies, and greater access to social services. Chile's Solidario attempts to tackle social exclusion by mandating that social workers work with families to develop action plans for access to employment and to domestic violence programs that may fall outside the parameters of bigger CCT programs. The amount of the CCT is calculated to ensure that the families can afford a certain basket of goods, amenities, and services below which they would be considered socially excluded. The CCT amount decreases and then ceases over a two-year period. Families are then given a graduation bonus and preferential treatment in accessing social services for another three years.

Transparent Administration

Brazil's Bolsa Família was able to achieve notable outcomes because it learned from its mistakes. For instance, its 2003 food subsidy program quickly lost support because it was seen as too bureaucratic; beneficiaries had to provide proof of their purchases to local managers, leading to barriers to access and heavy administrative costs. This led to the recognition that the program was failing. As a result, the Brazilian government unified all welfare programs under Bolsa Família and encouraged civil society to participate (De Janvry, Sadoulet, Solomon, & Vakis, 2006). The government also coordinated the program with the departments of education and health (Lindert et al., 2006).

The central government now bypasses the country's twenty-seven governors and the legislative branch, working with executive branch agencies and municipal agencies instead. Municipal governments must register families and transfer data to individual ministries (such as that of education). A fully updated and accurate registry earns the town a high "decentralized management index" score. Higher scores lead to more funds from the central government, thus reinforcing good behavior. The local government has general guidelines but considerable discretion on how to spend this money. This way, the national government ensures cooperation by simultaneously mandating responsibilities and providing incentives and funding to municipal governments.

In many traditional welfare programs, street-level bureaucrats and social workers perform surveillance over beneficiaries, but there is little bottom-up or peer accountability. In contrast, the money in Bolsa Família is given directly to the households via "citizen cards" mailed to each residence. Families use the citizen card as they would any debit card, withdrawing money at any ATM belonging to Caixa Econômica Federal, a government-owned savings bank. Further, an online portal publishes the names of all people enrolled in the program and their CCT amounts. The federal government also launched a single household database to combine all beneficiary databases for all social programs, including gas and electricity subsidies, Bolsa Família, food subsidies, and youth employment (De la Brière & Lindert, 2003) (see figure 13.4).

Outcomes

The amounts transferred to each family are quite modest, totaling extremely small amounts of the GDP in Chile to roughly 0.5 percent of total GDP in Brazil and Mexico. Nevertheless, these programs have reduced income inequalities in all three countries (Soares et al., 2009). This suggests that when CCT programs achieve good targeting and scale, they can be cost-effective poverty eradication policies.

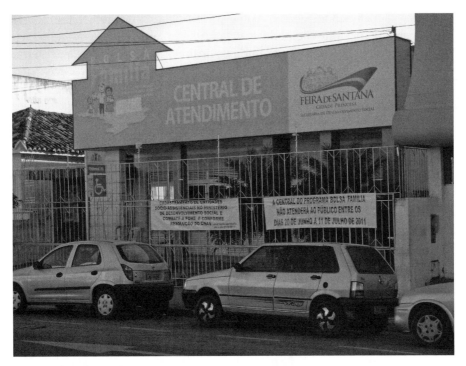

Figure 13.4. A Bolsa Família center in Feira de Santana, Brazil.
Source: Wikimedia Commons/Giovanni Maki.

Although Brazil's Bolsa Família lowered child labor rates, it *raised* adult labor force participation rates, especially among women (Soares et al., 2010). This counters arguments by some critics, including the Brazilian Catholic Church, that the subsidies act as handouts that disincentivize work. The extent to which adults are partly making up for the pay their children no longer earn remains unclear.

As discussed previously, better education translates into greater abilities to earn a living, make choices that yield longer-term benefits, and be an informed citizen. Bolsa Família made the greatest difference for students in northeastern Brazil (the country's poorest region), older students aged between fifteen and seventeen, and girls. Female beneficiary students aged fifteen to seventeen in northeastern Brazil were 28 percent more likely to stay in school (Soares, 2011).

In Mexico, Oportunidades increased school enrollment and lowered dropout rates. However it also lowered academic performance, possibly because low-achieving students became more likely to stay in school (Soares et al., 2010). It is hoped these students still accrue many of the labor market benefits of having a high school degree, but it remains unclear whether the poorer performers are affecting the performance of the other students.

With any luck, these changes improve health outcomes in the longer term, promote greater social cohesion and socioeconomic security, and reduce material deprivation. In terms of more immediate health outcomes, newborns of beneficiary pregnant women were 14 percent more likely to experience longer gestations (fewer premature births), and beneficiary children were 39 percent more likely to avoid malnutrition and achieve normal body mass index scores (Soares, 2011). Nutritional supplements are sometimes shared by everyone in the household, possibly diminishing returns to children under five (Lund et al., 2010). This contrasts with the experiences of Mexico and Colombia, where all beneficiaries under the age of two became significantly less likely to suffer from stunting (Soares et al., 2010). It is unclear exactly what local circumstances—advice on preventing malnutrition, monitoring by health clinicians, governance, culture, and so on—made the difference.

There were also some notable failures. For instance, Bolsa Família's cash payments for vaccinations among children did not seem to improve immunization rates, possibly because vaccination services were not available in some localities. In contrast, immunizations rose dramatically in Colombia and Mexico, where payments were made only within localities that actually offered such services. In Ecuador, the first few years of CCTs were actually unconditional in municipalities where adequate services provision and monitoring had not yet been set up (Soares et al., 2010).

Remaining Problems

These generally promising results hint at several important issues. First, payments work only when quality services are available. For example, payments for school attendance, the cornerstone of Latin American CCT programs, would not make a difference in educational achievement in South Africa, where eight-year-olds achieve an astounding 98 percent average attendance rate (Lund et al., 2010). However, in Kenya, where attendance is low, covering the cost of a school uniform increased attendance by 6.4 percent and reduced dropout rates and teenage pregnancy rates among girls (Glennerster & Kremer, 2011; Kremer, Miguel, & Thornton, 2004).

Opportunity NYC, the New York program that ran from 2007 to 2010, focused on education, health, and work CCTs. In the randomized controlled trial, beneficiary families received an average of US$3,000 a year, and CCTs decreased poverty by 8 percent and extreme poverty by almost half. Programs that linked poor families to existing institutions and provided intensive guidance were quite successful. The most dramatic health outcome, though, was a 10 percent increase in dental visits (to two per year). Other health benefits were similarly small; beneficiaries were 2 percent more likely to hold health insurance (from unusually high baseline rates) and 3 percent more likely to have been treated for a medical condition (Riccio, 2010).

Second, governments recognize that the poverty lines do not accurately differentiate the poor from the nonpoor. This is a problem that led to public scrutiny of Brazil's Bolsa Família. To address this, in 2011, President Dilma Rousseff announced a new "Brazil Without Misery" program aimed at eliminating indigent poverty by 2014. This program will resemble Chile's Solidario program, developing more comprehensive action plans for the poorest. Ideally, this would expand the pool of beneficiaries, to further move Brazil toward a society with a guaranteed basic income.

Third, policy makers are uncertain about the full range of desirable habits that can or should be shaped via conditionalities. Newer proposed conditionalities to tie cash payments to school achievement scores have been controversial. Mandatory "volunteering" in the community has also been tried. (Not only is mandatory volunteering oxymoronic, but it also risks stigmatizing welfare beneficiaries and real volunteers alike.)

Such political questions plagued Opportunity NYC as well, which was criticized by conservatives for "bribing" poor people to do what they should do anyway. Liberals also criticized it for attempting to correct individuals' "poor values" in a "culture of poverty" without adequately addressing larger structural inequalities. Student beneficiaries were 15 percent more likely to have attendance rates of 95 percent or better, but conditionalities tied to outcomes (such as high achievement scores), rather than participation in activities, yielded few results. Few single mothers in the program were able to maintain a job and attend a skills-building course, despite the US$3,000 bonus. Child-care problems, the Great Recession, high unemployment, and the lack of suitable courses were all notable problems. In other cases, full-time workers who met all conditionalities were still unable to raise themselves out of poverty because their jobs did not pay living wages (Goldstein, 2009; Riccio, 2010).

Finally, political and social context also matters. Conditionalities that help adolescents stay in school rather than work full-time in hazardous conditions might be more appropriate in Brazil than in the United States, where students are more likely to drop out for reasons unrelated to the need to work. A program that gave mothers in Rajasthan, India, a kilogram of lentils each time their children received vaccines raised immunization rates from 5 percent to 38 percent (Glennerster & Kremer, 2011), but these conditional lentil transfers would hardly work in other middle-income countries. (For one, in our humble opinion, US lentil soup is much less tasty than Indian dal.)

South African welfare programs have a history of using so-called conditions that are not easily monitored and act as normative injunctions, that is, that the child must be "properly" clothed. At the same time, these welfare benefits are often meager so that parents struggle to meet conditions. Further, past conditionalities demanded that families participated in "livelihood activities" in neighborhoods where such projects did not exist (Lund et al., 2010).

Bolstering Early Childhood Education

Sizable income-related gaps in cognitive development are often present in children even before they attend school (Hart & Risley, 1992). Children from poorer families tend to enter kindergarten far behind their peers with respect to vocabulary and math skills, making it much more difficult to catch up. This gap appears to be primarily attributable to changeable factors, such as maternal health and parenting styles (Waldfogel & Washbrook, 2011). One idea, then, is for governments to enhance these skills for the very poorest children and to help parents (for instance, those with two jobs) cope with the demands of parenting.

There is evidence that such programs not only improve earnings once the children grow up, but that they also reduce criminal behavior, improve health, and reduce the use of social services (Belfield, Nores, Barnett, & Schweinhart, 2006; Muennig et al., 2011; Muennig, Schweinhart, Montie, & Neidell, 2009). In fact, in the United States, one program was shown (in a very small randomized trial) to produce a net benefit of US$1 million dollars over the lifetime of every child in the experimental group.

Sure Start Children's Centres in the United Kingdom attempt to address health disparities by offering services aimed at young children and their families. It has some similarities to Ontario's Early Years Plan in Canada and Head Start in the United States. Sure Start is more comprehensive than Head Start, however. The British government more generally revamped social service programs to (1) make work pay, (2) raise incomes for families with children, and (3) invest in children's services (Waldfogel, 2010).

The first component, making work pay, consisted of establishing a national minimum wage and rendering tax rates more progressive by lowering payroll tax rates for low-income earners. It also established a Working Families Tax Credit. This is similar to the Earned Income Tax Credit in the United States, which provides income supplementation for workers in low-wage jobs. The second component of the antipoverty strategy expands on this strategy by increasing tax credits for families with children, grants to children under ten, and other child benefits. There were also reductions in primary school class sizes, increases in education spending, and a raise of the minimum school-leaving age from age sixteen to eighteen. The most prominent aspect of the campaign probably lay in the Sure Start program's Children's Centres (Waldfogel, 2010).

Between 2002 and 2004, the United Kingdom opened five hundred Children's Centres serving around eight hundred children each. These centers ran independently of local governments and received funds so rapidly that only 9 percent of 1999 moneys were spent that year. In 2005, control was transferred from central to local governments (Melhuish, Belsky, & Barnes, 2010).

Between 1999 and 2008, the United Kingdom experienced a 50 percent drop in children's poverty rates. Health outcomes associated with implementation of the programs included improved mental health and school outcomes among adolescents in single-parent households, a dramatic increase in the consumption of fresh fruits, and decreased spending on tobacco and alcohol by parents (Waldfogel, 2010). The implementation of these social programs was also associated with increased numeracy and literacy among children. Outcomes for parenting behavior (especially in dealing with children's non-compliance, violence, and aggression) were positive and statistically significant in a randomized control trial of similar programs in Wales (Hutchings et al., 2007). Outcomes overall were modest or negligible in 2005 but more pronounced in 2008, suggesting that Sure Start programs improved over time (Mackenbach, 2010; Melhuish et al., 2010). Though they appeared to be largely successful, the British government announced an end to many of these programs and reductions in others due to massive deficits from the Great Recession (Ramesh & Gentleman, 2011).

INNOVATIONS IN ADMINISTRATION AND GOVERNANCE

As the Bolsa Família case suggests, good governance is an integral component of many innovative social policy interventions. Indeed, there has also been a growth in experimental governance structures in the past two decades (de Sousa Santos, 2005; Fung, Wright, & Abers, 2003). Here, we briefly discuss two governance cases: Ceará State in Brazil, where the state government bolstered a preventive care program by bypassing local governments and strengthening civil society instead, and the city of Porto Alegre, Brazil, where city residents decide annual city budgets themselves instead of leaving them up to elected city officials.

In 1987, the Ceará state government launched a new health worker program that managed to lower infant mortality by 36 percent, triple immunization rates, and almost quadruple the number of municipalities with nurse access—all in just five years and all with low-paid, unskilled health workers. It managed to do so by coordinating health worker salaries and the recruitment process via the state capital. This way, local mayors could not distribute these funds or jobs via their patronage networks (a fancy way of saying that they couldn't give them to friends in exchange for favors). It also won over local nurses (the main point of resistance because their jobs were threatened by low-wage workers) by giving them considerable training and supervisory powers over these new health workers. Finally, it launched massive publicity campaigns that encouraged the community, including the many applicants who did not receive the jobs, to respect these new health worker public servants and to hold them accountable via evaluations. All of the public servants felt pressure to perform well and saw the jobs as prestigious, despite their low pay. And they often performed tasks beyond those formally prescribed. This case runs contrary to what decentralization and privatization proponents would have expected. The state government actually increased its involvement in public programs, but it was able to reap some of the typical benefits of decentralization, such as knowledge of local contexts, by empowering local communities to hold civil servants accountable (Tendler, 1997).

Another approach is to include public participation in developing local budgets. Porto Alegre began its first participatory budgeting process in 1989. **Participatory budgeting** is a process in which the people within a community—rather than elite policy makers—help to determine how government funds are spent. In Porto Alegre, a city of roughly 1.5 million people, a disproportionate percentage of government funds historically went to middle- and upper-class neighborhoods. This was true even as slums continued to lack access to potable water and other amenities.

The participatory budgeting process forced elected officials and roughly fifty thousand residents to meet with one another and justify their budget priorities in public, deliberative assemblies. After hearing residents' concerns, delegates translated these concerns into specific program and policy proposals. City officials, in turn, worked with these delegates to make the proposals technically and financially feasible. The resulting budgets from this process are binding. After the process, the proportion of the city budget that went to poor districts and to basic public services rose dramatically (Baiocchi, 2003).

Many of the middle- and upper-class residents who attended neighborhood assemblies voted for projects in slum neighborhoods rather than their own. As a result, sewer and electricity rates rose from 75 percent to 98 percent and the number of schools quadrupled. Health and education budgets increased from 13 percent to almost 40 percent (Bhatnagar, Rathore, Torres, & Kanungo, 2003). An analysis of Brazil's 220 largest cities suggested that participatory budgeting is statistically significantly correlated with lower rates of extreme poverty (Boulding & Wampler, 2010). Participatory budgeting has now spread to over two thousand cities around the world—hundreds in Latin America and dozens in Europe, Africa, Asia, and North America. By building a more equitable distribution of lifesaving resources—such as water, sanitation, education, and public transit—it becomes possible to better tackle the health problems associated with poverty in such nations (Su, 2012; Wampler & Hartz-Karp, 2012).

LESSONS ON SOCIAL POLICY INTERVENTIONS

Social policy interventions are messy. However, tinkering with policies to make them better—as policy makers did with Bolsa Família, the Health Agent Program in Ceará, and Sure Start in the United Kingdom—should not be viewed as a sign of dysfunction. In fact, the governments' responses to the criticisms ultimately rendered the programs successful.

It is also important not to attempt to generalize successful programs from one place across entirely different foreign contexts. Chile, Mexico, and Brazil all launched successful CCT programs but in very different ways: Brazil chose administrative decentralization and income as the sole criteria, Mexico chose centralization and a multidimensional poverty index, and Chile chose social worker empowerment and a multidimensional index (Soares et al., 2009). The real estate brokers' mantra of "location, location, location" matters as much in social policy as it does in housing markets.

Nevertheless, some themes emerge. In all of the successful cases, civil society and the state were mutually reinforcing rather than mutually exclusive. Decentralization only works if central governments have also worked to bypass corrupt networks in local governments, coordinated programs, trained workers, and infused resources into the programs. This increased funding might come about because of newly elected governments or systems of governance (such as participatory budgeting), but it must be institutionalized in a transparent manner.

Structural approaches work best when they combine environmental changes and increases in public services with individual- and family-based programs such as conditional cash transfers. Poor people's risky behaviors might change, but it takes a long time (and many synergistic policies) to shape health outcomes in sustained ways. Still, these cases ultimately demonstrate that thoughtfully designed social policy interventions are worth a shot; when they do work, they tackle the root causes of health disparities in ways medical approaches cannot.

SUMMARY

Population health is shaped by a complex interplay among biology, individual psychology, the social environment, and the physical environment. New frontiers in global public health are being broken as scientists use more complex models for understanding how these factors interact to shape health. Some of these models consider complex feedback loops that can subvert policy makers' intentions. For example, these models have shown that building more roads actually leads to an increase in traffic congestion rather than a reduction.

New policy interventions are being tried that attempt to shape human psychology, relying more on incentives for changing behavior rather than merely providing health information. For example, governments are providing cash welfare benefits on the condition that recipients perform certain tasks, such as seeing a medical provider or enrolling their children in school.

KEY TERMS

conditional cash
   transfers
dynamic complexity
endemic
herd immunity

multilevel model
participatory budgeting
policy resistance
rule of law
syndemic

systems dynamics
systems theory
tipping point

DISCUSSION QUESTIONS

1. You are the new food aid coordinator for a large NGO working to stem a famine in Somalia. How does tackling hunger and malnutrition differ in Botswana, where the rule of law is quite strong, with efforts in Somalia, where the rule of law is quite weak? How does a weak rule of law affect your efforts for the next month? The next year? What might you try to do in response?

2. How can policy makers better address dynamic components of population health, such as building herd immunity or reaching a tipping point in encouraging healthy behaviors? What sorts of multilevel campaigns might be needed to address tobacco use in Indonesia, for instance? What sorts of institutional support would you need in pursuing a successful campaign to dramatically lower tobacco use among youths in Indonesia?

3. At what levels of health do targeted social policy interventions such as conditional cash transfers work best? What other sorts of public policies are needed to ensure that they succeed in improving health outcomes? How should they be governed and monitored?

FURTHER READING

Jones, A. P., Homer, J. B., Murphy, D. L., Essien, J. D., Milstein, B., & Seville, D. A. (2006). Understanding diabetes population dynamics through simulation modeling and experimentation. *American Journal of Public Health, 96*, 488–494.

Singer, M. (2009). *Introducing syndemics: A critical systems approach to public and community health.* San Francisco: Jossey-Bass.

REFERENCES

Adato, M., Roopnaraine, T., & Becker, E. (2011). Understanding use of health services in conditional cash transfer programs: Insights from qualitative research in Latin America and Turkey. *Social Science & Medicine, 72*(12), 1921–1929. doi: 10.1016/j.socscimed.2010.09.032.

Anderson, R. M., & May, R. M. (1985). Vaccination and herd immunity to infectious diseases. *Nature, 318*(6044), 323–329.

Baiocchi, G. (2003). Participation, activism, and politics: The Porto Alegre experiment. In E. O. Wright & A. Fung (Eds.), *Deepening democracy* (pp. 45–76). New York: Verso Books.

Belfield, C. R., Nores, M., Barnett, W. S., & Schweinhart, L. (2006). The HighScope Perry Preschool program. *Journal of Human Resources, 41*(1), 162–190.

Berkman, L. F., Blumenthal, J., Burg, M., Carney, R. M., Catellier, D., Cowan, M. J., et al. (2003). Effects of treating depression and low perceived social support on clinical events after myocardial infarction: The Enhancing Recovery in Coronary Heart Disease Patients (ENRICHD) randomized trial. *JAMA, 289*(23), 3106–3116.

Bhatnagar, D., Rathore, A., Torres, M. M., & Kanungo, P. (2003). *Empowerment case studies: Participatory budgeting in Brazil.* Washington, DC: World Bank.

Blattman, C., & Miguel, E. (2010). Civil war. *Journal of Economic Literature, 48*(1), 3–57.

Bloom, D. E., Canning, D., & Sevilla, J. (2004). The effect of health on economic growth: A production function approach. *World Development, 32*(1), 1–13.

Boulding, C., & Wampler, B. (2010). Voice, votes, and resources: Evaluating the effect of participatory democracy on well-being. *World Development, 38*(1), 125–135.

Chan, S. (2009, September 1). New targets in the fat fight: Soda and juice. *New York Times,* p. A22.

Collier, P., Elliott, V. L., Hegre, H., Hoeffler, A., Reynal-Querol, M., & Sambanis, N. (2003). *Breaking the conflict trap: Civil war and development policy.* Washington, DC: World Bank and Oxford University Press.

Cueto, S. (2009). Conditional cash-transfer programmes in developing countries. *Lancet, 374*(9706), 1952–1953. doi: 10.1016/S0140-6736(09)61640-8.

De Janvry, A., Sadoulet, E., Solomon, P., & Vakis, R. (2006). *Evaluating Brazil's Bolsa Escola program: Impact on schooling and municipal roles.* Berkeley: University of California Press.

De la Brière, B., & Lindert, K. (2003). *Reforming Brazil's cadastro único to improve the targeting of the Bolsa Família program.* Washington, DC: World Bank.

de Sousa Santos, B. (2005). *Democratizing democracy: Beyond the liberal democratic canon*. New York: Verso Books.

ECLAC. (2010). *Social panorama of Latin America*. Santiago de Chile: United Nations Economic Commission on Latin America and the Caribbean.

Fernald, L. C., Gertler, P. J., & Neufeld, L. M. (2008). Role of cash in conditional cash transfer programmes for child health, growth, and development: An analysis of Mexico's Oportunidades. *Lancet, 371*(9615), 828–837. doi: 10.1016/S0140-6736(08)60382-7.

Forrester, J. W. (1971). The counterintuitive behavior of social systems. *Technology Review, 73*(3), 52–68.

Fung, A., Wright, E. O., & Abers, R. (2003). *Deepening democracy: Institutional innovations in empowered participatory governance*. New York: Verso Books.

Gehlert, S., Sohmer, D., Sacks, T., Mininger, C., McClintock, M., & Olopade, O. (2008). Targeting health disparities: A model linking upstream determinants to downstream interventions. *Health Affairs, 27*(2), 339–349. doi: 27/2/339 [pii]10.1377/hlthaff.27.2.339.

Gladwell, M. (2001). *The tipping point*. London: Abacus.

Glennerster, R., & Kremer, M. (2011, March/April). Small changes, big results: Behavioral economics at work in poor countries. *Boston Review, 36*. Available online at www.bostonreview.net/BR36.2/glennerster_kremer_behavioral _economics_global_development.php

Goldstein, D. (2009, August 24). Behavioral theory: Can Mayor Bloomberg pay poor people to do the "right" thing? *American Prospect*. Available online at http:// prospect.org/article/behavioral-theory-0

Hargreaves, J. R., Morison, L. A., Chege, J., Rutenburg, N., Kahindo, M., Weiss, H. A., et al. (2002). Socioeconomic status and risk of HIV infection in an urban population in Kenya. *Tropical Medicine & International Health, 7*(9), 793.

Hart, B., & Risley, T. R. (1992). American parenting of language-learning children: Persisting differences in family-child interactions observed in natural home environments. *Developmental Psychology, 28*(6), 1096–1105.

Hutchings, J., Bywater, T., Daley, D., Gardner, F., Whitaker, C., Jones, K., et al. (2007). Parenting intervention in Sure Start services for children at risk of developing conduct disorder: Pragmatic randomised controlled trial. *BMJ, 334*(7595), 678.

Jacobson, M. (2010). The Singapore solution. *National Geographic*. Available online at http://ngm.nationalgeographic.com/2010/01/singapore/jacobson-text

Kaplan, G. A., Everson, S. A., & Lynch, J. W. (2000). The contribution of social and behavioral research to an understanding of the distribution of disease: A multilevel approach. In B. D. Smedley & S. L. Syme (Eds.), *Promoting health: Intervention strategies from social and behavioral research* (pp. 37–80). Washington, DC: National Academy Press, Institute of Medicine.

Kremer, M., Miguel, E., & Thornton, R. (2004). *Incentives to learn*. Cambridge, MA: National Bureau of Economic Research.

Lindert, K., Linder, A., Hobbs, J., & De la Briëre, B. (2006). *The nuts and bolts of Brazil's Bolsa Família program: Implementing conditional cash transfers in a decentralized context*. Washington, DC: The World Bank.

Loyka, M. (2011). *Inequality and poverty in Latin America: Can the decline continue?* Washington, DC: Council on Hemispheric Affairs.

Lund, F., Noble, M., Barnes, H., & Wright, G. (2010). Is there a rationale for conditional cash transfers for children in South Africa? *Transformation: Critical Perspectives on Southern Africa, 70,* 70–91.

Mackenbach, J. P. (2010). The English strategy to reduce health inequalities. *Lancet, 377*(9782), 1986–1988.

Melhuish, E., Belsky, J., & Barnes, J. (2010). Evaluation and value of Sure Start. *Archives of Disease in Childhood, 95*(3), 159–161.

Milstein, B. (2008). *Hygeia's constellation: Navigating health futures in a dynamic and democratic world*. Atlanta: Centers for Disease Control and Prevention.

Muennig, P., & Glied, S. A. (2010). What changes in survival rates tell us about US health care. *Health Affairs*. doi: hlthaff.2010.0073 [pii]10.1377/hlthaff.2010.0073.

Muennig, P., Robertson, D., Johnson, G., Campbell, F., Pungello, E. P., & Neidell, M. (2011). The effect of an early education program on adult health: The Carolina Abecedarian Project randomized controlled trial. *American Journal of Public Health, 101*(3), 512–516. doi: 10.2105/AJPH.2010.200063.

Muennig, P., Schweinhart, L., Montie, J., & Neidell, M. (2009). Effects of a prekindergarten educational intervention on adult health: 37-year follow-up results of a randomized controlled trial. *American Journal of Public Health, 99*(8), 1431–1437. doi: AJPH.2008.148353 [pii]10.2105/AJPH.2008.148353.

Nelson, J. M. (2011). Social policy reforms in Latin America: Urgent but frustrating. *Latin American Research Review, 46*(1), 226–239.

N'Galy, B., & Ryder, R. W. (1988). Epidemiology of HIV infection in Africa. *Journal of Acquired Immune Deficiency Syndrome, 1*(6), 551–558.

Paes-Sousa, R., Santos, L. M., & Miazaki, E. S. (2011). Effects of a conditional cash transfer programme on child nutrition in Brazil. *Bulletin of the World Health Organization, 89*(7), 496–503. doi: 10.2471/BLT.10.084202.

Ramesh, R., & Gentleman, A. (2011, 28 January). Cuts will force 250 Sure Start centres to close, say charities: 60,000 families could lose local centre despite "family-friendly" coalition agenda. *The Guardian*.

Raz, J. (1999). *Practical reason and norms*. New York: Oxford University Press.

Riccio, J. (2010). *Sharing lessons from the first conditional cash transfer program in the United States*. Ann Arbor, MI: National Poverty Center.

Roose, S. P., & Spatz, E. (1998). Depression and heart disease. *Depression and Anxiety, 7*(4), 158–165.

Sachs, J. D. (2002). Macroeconomics and health: Investing in health for economic development. *Revista Panamericana de Salud Pública, 12*(2), 143–144.

Schubert, B., & Slater, R. (2006). Social cash transfers in low-income African countries: Conditional or unconditional? *Development Policy Review, 24*(5), 571–578.

Sen, A. (1999). *Development as freedom*. New York: Knopf.

Shifter, M. (2009). Managing disarray: The search for a new consensus. In A. F. Cooper & J. Heine (Eds.), *Which way Latin America? Hemispheric politics meets globalization*. Tokyo: United Nations University Press.

Shklar, J. N., & Hoffmann, S. (1998). *Political thought and political thinkers*. Chicago: University of Chicago Press.

Singer, M. C., Erickson, P. I., Badiane, L., Diaz, R., Ortiz, D., Abraham, T., & Nicolaysen, A. M. (2006). Syndemics, sex and the city: Understanding sexually transmitted diseases in social and cultural context. *Social Science & Medicine, 63*(8), 2010–2021.

Soares, F. V. (2011). Brazil's Bolsa Família: A Review. *Economic & Political Weekly, 46*(21), 55–60.

Soares, F. V., Ribas, R. P., & Osório, R. G. (2010). Evaluating the impact of Brazil's Bolsa Família: Cash transfer programs in comparative perspective. *Latin American Research Review, 45*(2), 173–190.

Soares, S., Osório, R. G., Veras Soares, F., Medeiros, M., & Zepeda, E. (2009). Conditional cash transfers in Brazil, Chile and Mexico: Impacts upon inequality. *Estudios Economicos, 1*, 207–224.

Sterman, J. D. (2006). Learning from evidence in a complex world. *American Journal of Public Health, 96*(3), 505–514. doi: AJPH.2005.066043 [pii]10.2105/AJPH.2005.066043.

Su, C. (2012). Whose budget? Our budget? Broadening political stakeholdership via participatory budgeting. *Journal of Public Deliberation, 8*(2), Art. 1. Available online at www.publicdeliberation.net/jpd/vol8/iss2/art1

Tendler, J. (1997). *Good government in the tropics*. Baltimore: Johns Hopkins University Press.

Virchow, R. (1849). Notes on the typhoid epidemic prevailing in Upper Silesia. *Archiv für pathologische Anatomie und Physiologie und für klinische Medizin, 2*, 143–322.

Virchow, R. C. (2006). Report on the typhus epidemic in upper Silesia. *American Journal of Public Health, 96*(12), 2102.

Waitzkin, H. (2003). Report of the WHO Commission on Macroeconomics and Health: A summary and critique. *Lancet, 361*(9356), 523–526.

Waldfogel, J. (2010). *Britain's war on poverty*. New York: Russell Sage Foundation.

Waldfogel, J., & Washbrook, E. (2011). Early years policy. *Child Development Research, 343016,* 1–12.

Wampler, B., & Hartz-Karp, J. (2012). Participatory budgeting: Diffusion and outcomes across the world. *Journal of Public Deliberation, 8*(2), Art. 13. Available online at www.publicdeliberation.net/jpd/vol8/iss2/art13

Zhu, Y. (2008). *How east Asians view democracy.* New York: Columbia University Press.

Index